Family and Community Health

A Developmental Approach

Bassim Hamadeh, CEO and Publisher
John Remington, Acquisitions Editor
Sean Adams, Project Editor
Miguel Macias, Senior Graphic Designer
Alisa Munoz, Licensing Associate
Natalie Piccotti, Senior Marketing Manager
Kassie Graves, Vice President of Editorial
Jamie Giganti, Director of Academic Publishing

ISBN: 978-1-63487-917-0 (pbk) / 978-1-63487-918-7 (br)

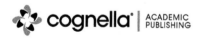

Family and Community Health

A Developmental Approach

First Edition

Sue K. Adams, Ph.D.

University of Rhode Island

Sarah W. Feldstein Ewing, Ph.D.

Oregon Health & Science University

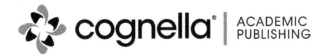

Acknowledgments

This book would not be possible without the assistance of some very intelligent women with whom we have had the privilege of mentoring and working aside:

Genevieve Dash, M.S., Rachel Feragne, B.S., Lindsey Hylek, B.A., Rosemary Reilly-Chammat, Ed. D., Meredith Rose, L.S.W., M.L., Caroline Segal, Ph.D., and Vanessa Somohano, M.A.—Thank you for your contributions in helping to make this book a reality.

And to our children: Benjamin, Nathaniel and Alexander; Ber, Amy and Elliott—May you always know that although we are proud of our accomplishments in the workplace, our greatest masterpieces are our children.

Contents

CHAPTER ONE

Health in the United States

Coauthors:
Sue K. Adams, Ph.D., Rosemary Reilly-Chammat, Ed.D.

@CDCgov

What Is Health?

If you were to ask someone what it means to be healthy, the most common response would be "to not be sick." Although this answer has merit, it is simplistic. Being healthy is much more than merely the absence of disease. Would a person who is physically fit but suffers from severe depression with suicidal thoughts be considered healthy or unhealthy? Would a person who has well managed diabetes and who is genuinely happy be considered healthy or unhealthy? Viewing health as a dichotomous construct where you can only check one box—healthy or unhealthy—is very limiting. In addition, how we define health has many implications for how we understand illness and intervene to help maximize quality of life. Although there are many definitions of health, the most widely accepted definition used throughout the world incorporates these larger concepts. According to the World Health Organization (WHO), the definition of health is "a state of complete physical, mental and social well-being and not merely the absence of disease or infirmity."[1]

The Importance of Community Health

Health can be conceptualized as affecting the individual, family, or community. In the United States, federal and state laws and regulations often guide the health of people within their communities, and many health issues occur at the community level. In general, community health efforts work on a broad level, supporting healthful practices where people live, learn, work, and play by using the community's assets to support and sustain healthful practices. According to the Centers for

1

Disease Control's (CDC) Division of Community Health, four principles guide the work in community health: 1) maximizing public health impact, 2) advancing health equity, 3) using and expanding the evidence base, and 4) engaging the community. Community health is provided and led by members of the community who have established relationships with the community and have insights into the needs of individuals living within the community. Community health leaders use their established relationships to support individual and collective behavior change. Community engagement is at the heart of community health, and it is only when people work together collectively that optimal health can be achieved. Partnerships create pride and ownership of community-level efforts.

International, National, and Local Health Agencies

Many community health efforts are organized using a top-down approach. That means that the federal or state governments fund particular community agencies, which then fund community-health programs. Once the funding has been allocated on a large scale, community-level efforts help to ensure that federal and state mandates are implemented to the betterment of the community to maximize public health impact. Each community is distinct in its assets and challenges, and some communities face greater barriers than others due to socioeconomic status of its members, housing, job opportunities, healthy foods, places to be active, and the like. Targeted community health efforts ensure that support is aligned to each specific community's needs. Some communities need more support than others to adequately ensure optimal health for all.

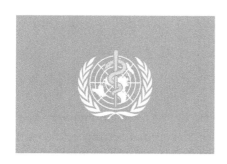

FIGURE 1.1 **The emblem of the World Health Organization**

At the international level, the World Health Organization (WHO) is the largest international health organization, and its mission is to help all people attain the highest possible level of health. While the WHO focuses on the health of people around the world, the United States has its own national health agencies that promote the health and welfare of American citizens. The primary agency is the Department of Human Health and Services (HHS), and within HHS are 11 operating divisions that focus on different populations and topic areas. One particularly important division that focuses on health promotion is the Centers for Disease Control and Prevention (CDC). The CDC's mission is "to keep Americans safe and healthy where they work, live and play." The CDC has expanded its global perspective so that it can "track diseases, research outbreaks, respond to emergencies of all kinds, and use what they learn from this work to develop and advocate public health policies that strengthen America's health and resilience."[2]

At the state level, each state has its own department of health dedicated to promoting, protecting, and maintaining the health and welfare of its residents. States work diligently to collect information about the health of their communities, create policies to address the

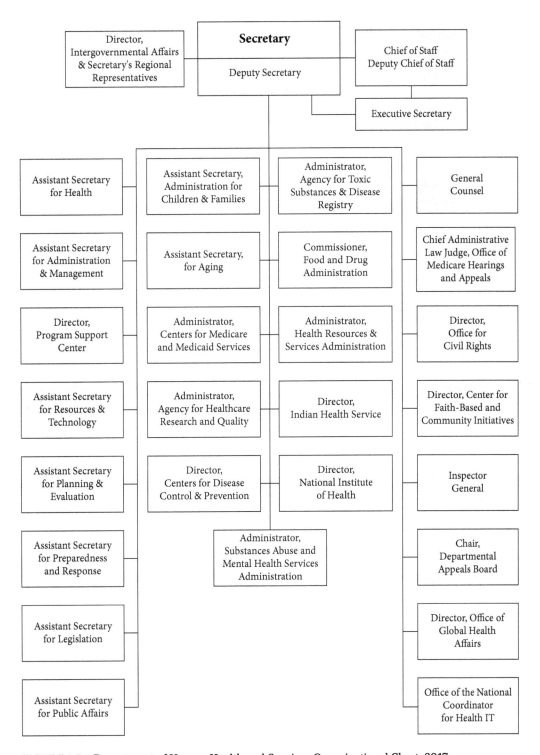

FIGURE 1.2   Department of Human Health and Services Organizational Chart, 2017

health needs of their citizens, and implement public health services in their communities. This information is often funneled down to local-level health departments who implement local health programs and clinical services. Local health departments are also responsible for overseeing public infrastructure, detecting and reporting diseases, collecting birth and death rates, and overseeing public health campaigns such as immunization clinics, safety belt checks, and car seat checks.

School-based Health Centers

School-based health centers (SBHCs) are another example of local, community-based efforts to improve health. SBHCs provide health services to students (pre K-12) and may be offered on-site (i.e., school-based centers) or off-site (i.e., school-linked centers). SBHCs are often established in schools that serve predominantly low-income communities and have the following characteristics: 1) SBHCs **must** provide primary health care and **may** also include mental health care, social services, dentistry, and health education, 2) primary care services may be provided by a single clinician, or comprehensive services may be provided by multi-disciplinary teams, 3) services may be available only during some school days or hours and may also be available during non-school hours, 4) student participation requires parental consent, and services provided for individual students may be limited for specific types of care, such as reproductive or mental health, 5) services may be provided to school staff, student family members, and others within the surrounding community, and 6) services are often provided by a medical center or provider independent of the school system.

Since school-based health centers generally serve schools that have a higher percentage of children from low-income families, they strategically attempt to promote health equity. The National Alliance for School Based Health Care's 2013–14 Census of SBHCs reported that there are currently 2,315 SBHCs that serve students and communities in 49 of 50 states and the District of Columbia. The number of SBHCs nationally grew 20% since the 2010–11 Census of SBHCs, with 385 new centers. SBHCs are supported through a combination of federal, state, and local funds, school district funds, private foundations, and reimbursement for services through health insurance.[3]

Neighborhood Health Stations

Another type of promising, evidence-based community health effort is called the Neighborhood Health Station (NHS). Dr. Michael Fine from the state of Rhode Island developed the Neighborhood Health Station, with the first groundbreaking in 2014 in the small urban town of Central Falls, RI, and the second ground-breaking in 2016 in the small rural town of Scituate, RI. The NHS builds upon the services provided within a Federally Qualified Community Health Center, which by definition is a health center that provides a comprehensive array of services to a population identified as high need. The NHS is different from a traditional health center as it is built around the needs of the community, rather than the needs of the provider or health entity. In Rhode Island, the Neighborhood Health Stations offer comprehensive and integrated wrap-around services including primary care, walk-in primary care, dental care, a pharmacy, physical therapy, pediatric care, occupational therapy, mental health services, OB/GYN services, radiology and more. Rhode Island's two Neighborhood Health Stations serve over 14,000 patients and provide 50,000 health care visits per year. It is expected that when the NHSs are running at full capacity in 2018, they will serve more than 90% of the population of these two towns. With a focus on primary care but also functioning as a hub of sorts for health care services in the community, the stations should reduce expensive health care costs for individuals and the community at large.[4]

Health Prevention and Intervention Models in the U.S. Health Care System

Today's health care system is largely driven by an intervention model in which people receive health care after they become sick. However, prevention and/or the delay of illness are becoming increasingly necessary to control health care costs. Community-level efforts can focus on each level of prevention: primary, secondary, and tertiary. The three tiers enable health practitioners to consider improving outcomes in spite of challenging health conditions.

Primary Prevention

The aim of primary prevention is to prevent disease before it occurs. Practicing healthy behaviors is a primary prevention strategy. Tobacco use, physical inactivity, and poor diet are among the three leading causes of death, contributing to many chronic diseases and premature death. Therefore, primary prevention efforts would include avoiding tobacco use, engaging in physical activity, and eating a nutritious diet. Similarly, primary prevention efforts also include wearing seat belts in a car to prevent injury or death in a motor vehicle accident, practicing safe sex to prevent sexually transmitted infections including HIV, and immunizations to protect against infectious diseases.

Secondary Prevention

Secondary prevention aims to reduce the impact of a disease or injury that has already occurred. Many preexisting chronic illnesses are just that—chronic and long-lasting—and secondary prevention aims to halt the progression of the disease as soon as a person has been diagnosed. For example, a person who had a heart attack may be advised to take daily aspirin and eat a more nutritious diet to reduce the likelihood of future heart attacks. Many secondary prevention efforts, such as healthy eating, exercise, and regular cancer screenings, are also primary prevention strategies.

Tertiary Prevention

Tertiary prevention aims to soften the impact of an ongoing illness, injury, or complex health problem. These efforts improve a person's ability to function, their quality of life, and their life expectancy, and decrease the risk of re-injury. For example, a person diagnosed with severe depression may engage in regular group and individual therapy as a way to help reduce the severity of future debilitating episodes by providing the tools to be able to better cope with depression. Determining whether a behavior is a primary, secondary, or tertiary prevention strategy depends on the context and often how close the prevention effort is to the onset of the disease.

	Primary Prevention	Secondary Prevention	Tertiary Prevention
Definition	An intervention that is implemented before there is evidence of a disease or injury	An intervention that is implemented after a disease has begun, but before there are symptoms	An intervention that is implemented after a disease or injury is established
Purpose	Reduce or eliminate causative risk factors	Early identification through screening and treatment	Prevent the disease or injury from getting worse
Example	Encourage exercise and healthy eating to prevent individuals from becoming overweight	Check body mass index (BMI) at every well visit to identify individuals who are overweight or obese	Enroll overweight or obese individuals in a weight loss program to prevent long term negative consequences

FIGURE 1.3   Primary, secondary and tertiary prevention model

The concept of preventative care is certainly not a new construct, although it is one that is gaining momentum in the current day. A poem written by Joseph Malins in 1895 entitled *The Ambulance Down in the Valley*,[5] defines the conceptual and practical importance of efforts to prevent health calamities before they occur:

'Twas a dangerous cliff, as they freely confessed,
Though to walk near its crest was so pleasant;
But over its terrible edge there had slipped
A duke and full many a peasant.
So the people said something would have to be done,
But their projects did not at all tally;
Some said, "Put a fence 'round the edge of the cliff,"
Some, "An ambulance down in the valley."

But the cry for the ambulance carried the day,
For it spread through the neighboring city;
A fence may be useful or not, it is true,
But each heart became full of pity

For those who slipped over the dangerous cliff;
And the dwellers in highway and alley
Gave pounds and gave pence, not to put up a fence,
But an ambulance down in the valley.

"For the cliff is all right, if you're careful," they said,
"And, if folks even slip and are dropping,
It isn't the slipping that hurts them so much
As the shock down below when they're stopping."
So day after day, as these mishaps occurred,
Quick forth would those rescuers sally
To pick up the victims who fell off the cliff
With their ambulance down in the valley.

Then an old sage remarked: "It's a marvel to me
That people give far more attention
To repairing results than to stopping the cause,
When they'd much better aim at prevention.
Let us stop at its source all this mischief," cried he,
"Come, neighbors and friends, let us rally;
If the cliff we will fence, we might almost dispense
With the ambulance down in the valley."

"Oh he's a fanatic," the others rejoined,
"Dispense with the ambulance? Never!
He'd dispense with all charities, too, if he could;
No! No! We'll support them forever.
Aren't we picking up folks just as fast as they fall?
And shall this man dictate to us? Shall he?
Why should people of sense stop to put up a fence,
While the ambulance works in the valley?"

But the sensible few, who are practical too,
Will not bear with such nonsense much longer;
They believe that prevention is better than cure,
And their party will soon be the stronger.
Encourage them then, with your purse, voice, and pen,
And while other philanthropists dally,
They will scorn all pretense, and put up a stout fence
On the cliff that hangs over the valley.

Better guide well the young than reclaim them when old,
For the voice of true wisdom is calling.

> *"To rescue the fallen is good,*
> *But 'tis best to prevent other people from falling."*
> *Better close up the source of temptation and crime*
> *Than deliver from dungeon or galley;*
> *Better put a strong fence 'round the top of the cliff*
> *Than an ambulance down in the valley.*

Source: Joseph Malins, "The Ambulance Down in the Valley." Copyright in the Public Domain.

Health Impact Pyramid

As suggested in Malins' poem, it is possible to prevent people from falling or help them after they fall. The reality of the U.S. health care system is that it largely focuses on intervention efforts, treating a disease after it occurs. Thomas Frieden proposed a conceptual framework, The Health Impact Pyramid, which outlines a five-tiered public health action plan to treat disease[6]. It promotes health by focusing on different levels or tiers of interventions, rather than solely relying on the individual to make behavior change efforts.

At the base tier of the pyramid are socioeconomic factors, such as poverty and education. Frieden proposes that interventions aimed at this layer of change will have the widest impact on population health. For instance, creating communities that have access to good

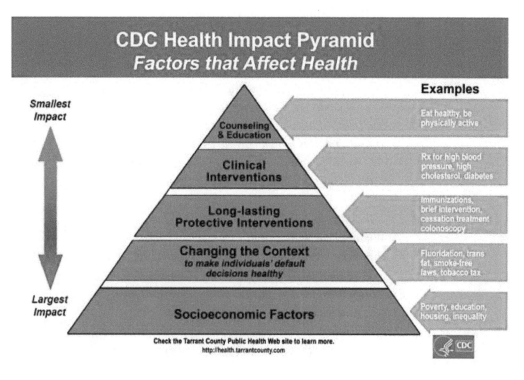

FIGURE 1.4   The Health Impact Pyramid

paying jobs will increase socioeconomic status and afford people the resources to live in healthy communities and make healthier choices for their families. There are many ways that communities can adopt programs and policies that promote health across the lifespan.

The second tier of the pyramid addresses interventions that change the environmental context to encourage healthier choices. By making healthy options the default choice regardless of education, income, or other societal factors, all people living in the community have access to the intervention. For instance, providing fluoride in the public water supply reduces tooth decay and direct and indirect health-related costs, while not putting the burden on individuals to change their behavior in a significant way.

The third tier of the pyramid involves a one-time or infrequent intervention that does not require ongoing maintenance or clinical care. Examples include childhood immunizations or cancer screenings, which can help prevent or detect illness. These, however, are less globally effective than tier 1 or 2 interventions because they require health care providers to reach people individually.

This leads us to the fourth tier, which represents ongoing clinical interventions, typically for chronic illnesses that require constant medical intervention. For instance, a person with diabetes requires regular clinical intervention of insulin to control his or her blood sugar. Issues related to adherence to medications and access to health care services impact the effectiveness of these interventions and make it less likely to efficiently reach large groups of people.

Finally, the fifth tier includes counseling and educational interventions. When people in a community do not have access to global interventions, they have to rely on individual behavior change to improve health. For instance, not having fluoride in the water means that individuals must get and fill prescriptions and take a fluoride pill daily, which is much more difficult to accomplish than drinking water.

Frieden proposes that working with individuals will have the least public health impact because fewer people receive the intervention, and targeting socioeconomic factors will be the most effective. This model underscores the interconnectedness of the preventative health care system. Each level of the pyramid could play a role in improving health within communities. Counseling and educational interventions are, however, widely available and are effective when consistently and repeatedly delivered. Are there certain health issues that would be more effectively treated by Tier 1 interventions versus Tier 5 interventions? How would you systemically address a health issue with each tier of the pyramid? And how could the Health Equity Pyramid be used to address disparities in community health?

Epidemiological Definitions

Epidemiology is "the study of the distribution and determinants of health-related states or events in specific populations, and the application of this study to the control of health problems."[7] Basic knowledge of epidemiology is important for any professional who works with community members to promote health and wellness. Within epidemiology, definitions give professionals consistent language and tools for measuring the presence of disease across time. *Morbidity* refers to the unhealthy state of an individual or is another term for the presence of illness. A person can have multiple morbidities, also known as co-morbidities, at the same time. For example, a person with asthma may have symptoms of asthma (i.e., asthma morbidity), obesity, and anxiety. This is in contrast to *mortality*, which is another term for death. Specifically, a mortality rate is the number of deaths due to a disease relative to the entire population. *Prevalence* of disease symptoms is often used to measure how many people in a population have a disease. For instance, the prevalence rate of people with diabetes is calculated by taking all old and new cases of diabetes and dividing that number by the total population. Prevalence rates are helpful when trying to understand how many people have experienced a certain illness for a period of time and are often used to inform public health programs. *Incidence* is the number of newly diagnosed cases of a disease. For example, we could calculate the number of new cases of influenza in the past week, and that would be the incidence rate. Incidence rates are helpful when trying to identify cases of acute diseases, which peak and then resolve themselves over a few days or week.

Healthy People 2020

Many national, state and local agencies and individuals are working to promote health across the United States. With so many agencies involved in health-promotion efforts across the United States, there was a need for planning, coordination, and consistency in health promotion efforts across the country. As a result, in 1979 the U.S. Surgeon General's Report, *Healthy People: The Surgeon General's Report on Health Promotion and Disease Prevention*, recommended that agencies develop a national health-promotion and disease-prevention initiative to help improve the health of all Americans.[8] To achieve this, experts developed

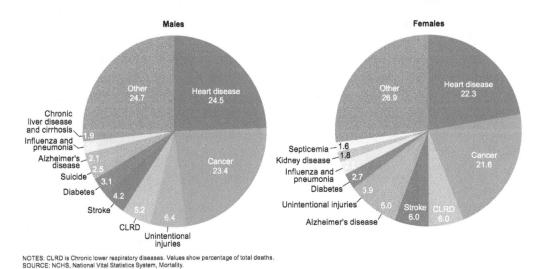

NOTES: CLRD is Chronic lower respiratory diseases. Values show percentage of total deaths.
SOURCE: NCHS, National Vital Statistics System, Mortality.

FIGURE 1.5   Percent distribution of the 10 leading causes of death, by sex: US, 2014

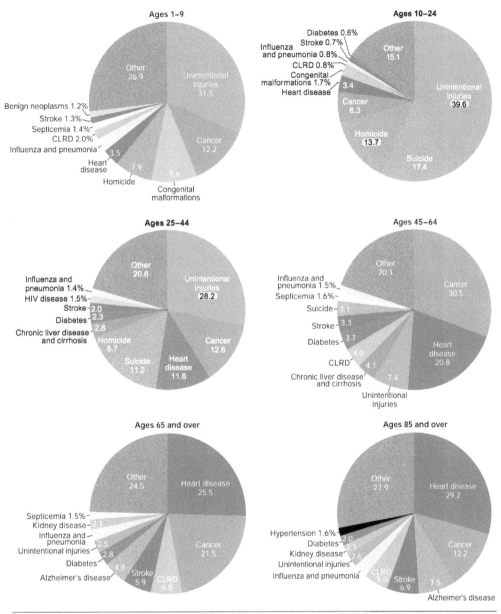

Ages 1–9

- Other 26.9
- Unintentional injuries 31.5
- Benign neoplasms 1.2%
- Stroke 1.3%
- Septicemia 1.4%
- CLRD 2.0%
- Influenza and pneumonia
- Heart disease 3.5
- Homicide 7.9
- Congenital malformations 9.6
- Cancer 12.2

Ages 10–24

- Diabetes 0.6%
- Stroke 0.7%
- Influenza and pneumonia 0.8%
- CLRD 0.8%
- Congenital malformations 1.7%
- Heart disease 3.4
- Other 15.1
- Unintentional injuries 39.6
- Cancer 6.3
- Homicide 13.7
- Suicide 17.4

Ages 25–44

- Other 20.6
- Unintentional injuries 28.2
- Influenza and pneumonia 1.4%
- HIV disease 1.5%
- Stroke 2.0
- Diabetes 2.3
- Chronic liver disease and cirrhosis 2.8
- Homicide 5.7
- Suicide 11.2
- Heart disease 11.6
- Cancer 12.6

Ages 45–64

- Other 20.1
- Cancer 30.5
- Influenza and pneumonia 1.5%
- Septicemia 1.6%
- Suicide 3.1
- Stroke 3.3
- Diabetes 3.7
- CLRD 4.0
- Chronic liver disease and cirrhosis 4.1
- Unintentional injuries 7.4
- Heart disease 20.8

Ages 65 and over

- Other 24.5
- Heart disease 25.5
- Septicemia 1.5%
- Kidney disease 2.1
- Influenza and pneumonia 2.5
- Unintentional injuries 2.8
- Diabetes 4.8
- Alzheimer's disease 5.9
- Stroke
- CLRD 6.5
- Cancer 21.5

Ages 85 and over

- Other 27.9
- Heart disease 29.2
- Hypertension 1.6%
- Diabetes 2.0
- Kidney disease 2.1
- Unintentional injuries 2.6
- Influenza and pneumonia
- CLRD 5.0
- Stroke 6.9
- Alzheimer's disease 7.5
- Cancer 12.2

NOTES: CLRD is Chronic lower respiratory diseases; HIV is Human immunodeficiency virus. Values show percentage of total deaths.
SOURCE: NCHS, National Vital Statistics System, Mortality.

FIGURE 1.6   Percent distribution of the 10 leading causes of death, by age: US, 2014

"management by objectives" guidelines, which refer to setting clear, objective, and measurable goals for each illness-specific priority area. Agencies work together to identify the top health issues impacting Americans, to identify effective interventions to reduce the rate of illness, and to identify assessment techniques to measure progress toward the goal.

Many states also use the Healthy People report to create tailored goals for specific health issues in their states.

Every 10 years, a report is produced that aggregates, or combines, the data collected from various agencies and identifies if progress has been made toward reducing health issues. Based on that data, Healthy People sets new national goals and objectives for improving the health of Americans. Over the past four decades, *Healthy People 1990*, *Healthy People 2000*, *Healthy People 2010*, and *Healthy People 2020* have been published. As health goals are achieved, Healthy People typically increases the goal for that objective. If the goals are not met, Healthy People evaluates the reasons why they have not been met and continues to work toward progress.

The most current version, *Healthy People 2020*, is the latest iteration developed under the leadership of the Federal Interagency Workgroup, which consists of the U.S. Department of Health and Human Services and 15 other lead agencies, such as the Centers for Disease Control and the U.S. Department of Education.[9] According to *Healthy People 2020* the vision is simple—to promote a society in which all people live long, healthy lives. The mission of *Healthy People 2020* strives to:

- Identify nationwide health-improvement priorities
- Increase public awareness and understanding of the determinants of health, disease, and disability and the opportunities for progress
- Provide measurable objectives and goals that are applicable at the national, state, and local levels
- Engage multiple sectors to take actions to strengthen policies and improve practices that are driven by the best available evidence and knowledge
- Identify critical research, evaluation, and data-collection needs.

Healthy People 2020 also has overarching goals, including to:

- Attain high-quality, longer lives free of preventable disease, disability, injury, and premature death
- Achieve health equity, eliminate disparities, and improve the health of all groups
- Create social and physical environments that promote good health for all
- Promote quality of life, healthy development, and healthy behaviors across all life stages.

Healthy People 2020 contains 42 topic areas with more than 1,200 objectives. Leading Health Indicators (LHI) have also been identified, which are high-priority health issues that affect the most Americans. They include mental health, reproductive and sexual health, nutrition, physical activity and obesity, among others. The good news is that between 2000 and 2010 there was significant progress toward the goals in the areas of health communication, heart disease and stroke, immunization and infectious diseases, occupational safety and health, and tobacco use. Two areas have made little progress toward goals: 1) physical activity, nutrition, and obesity and 2) arthritis, osteoporosis, and chronic back conditions.

National Health Data

Researchers, practitioners and policy makers use many types of nationally collected health data to inform their work. Below are descriptions of the most widely used and recognized datasets.

Community Preventive Services Guide

Similar to Healthy People 2020, the Community Preventive Services Guide is a collection of evidence-based findings of the Community Preventive Services Task Force.[10] This resource enables community health practitioners to select interventions that improve health and prevent disease in their state, community, community organization, business, health care organization, or school. Community Guide reviews are designed to answer three questions: 1) what has worked for others and how well? 2) what will the intervention approach cost, and what is likely to be achieved through the investment? and 3) what are the gaps in evidence? For example, one community-level health effort that the Community Preventive Services Task Force recommends is the implementation and maintenance of school-based health centers in low-income communities. This recommendation is based on a systematic review of all available studies that were conducted—with oversight from the Task Force—by scientists and subject matter experts from the CDC in collaboration with a wide range of government, academic, policy, and practice-based partners.

National Health and Nutrition Examination Survey (NHANES)

The National Health and Nutrition Examination Survey (NHANES)[11] began in 1960 and was designed to assess the health and nutritional status of adults and children in the United States. NHANES interviewers go to the homes of a nationally representative sample of approximately 5,000 families per year across the United States. Using a combination of interviews and physical examinations, they collect demographic and health information for each member of that household. Results are used to inform and guide national public health policy on a range of health topics such as infant mortality, heart disease, stroke, and drug overdose.

Behavioral Risk Factor Surveillance System (BRFSS)

The Behavioral Risk Factor Surveillance System (BRFSS)[12] is a telephone survey that collects data on United States residents pertaining to health-related risk behaviors, chronic health conditions, and the use of preventive services. BRFSS also collects data on health issues that may be emerging in communities, such as vaccine shortages and communicable illnesses. BRFSS is used to inform health promotion programs at both the municipal and state levels. Sponsored by multiple federal agencies, the BRFSS is the nation's premier surveillance system and the largest continuously conducted health survey system in the world.

Youth Risk Behavior Surveillance System (YRBSS)

The Youth Risk Behavior Surveillance System (YRBSS)[13] was developed in 1990 to monitors six types of health-risk behaviors that contribute to the leading causes of death and disability among youth and adults, including

- Monitor behaviors that contribute to unintentional injuries and violence
- Sexual behaviors related to unintended pregnancy and sexually transmitted infections, including HIV infection
- Alcohol and other drug use
- Tobacco use
- Unhealthy dietary behaviors
- Inadequate physical activity

YRBSS is a biennial survey conducted in odd-numbered years and is conducted at both the national and state levels. The most common version of the YRBSS is administered to high school students, and versions also exist for middle school and college students (e.g., The National College Health Risk Behavior Survey).

U.S. Census Bureau National Health Interview Survey

The U.S. Census Bureau's mission is "to serve as the leading source of quality data about the nation's people and economy." Every ten years, the Census Bureau counts every resident of the United States. Among its many purposes, the Census informs the reallocation of resources within the state and local governments, such as funding for neighborhood improvements, public health, education, transportation and other essential community services. In addition, the Census conducts the National Health Interview Survey (NHIS) which is an extensive survey used to track health status, health care access, and progress toward achieving national health objectives. Key health topics include medical conditions, health insurance, doctor's office visits, physical activity and other health-related behaviors. The NHIS also helps monitor progress toward national health objectives such as Healthy People 2020. It is used to evaluate the effects of health policies and programs at a national and state level. It also helps to track changes in health risk behaviors and health care utilization.

Health Disparities

One of the overarching goals of Healthy People 2020 and the Community Preventive Services Task Force is to achieve health equity, eliminate disparities, and improve the health of all groups of people living in the U.S. At the core of this goal is the topic of health disparities. A *health disparity* is defined as "a particular type of health difference that is closely linked with social, economic, and/or environmental disadvantage. Health disparities adversely affect groups of people who have systematically experienced greater obstacles to health based on their racial or ethnic group; religion; socioeconomic status; gender; age; mental health; cognitive, sensory, or physical disability; sexual orientation or gender identity; geographic location; or other characteristics historically linked to discrimination or exclusion."[14] In other words, a health disparity exists when certain groups of people get sick more often than others. As you saw in the definition, there are many different types of health disparities, and they should be labeled accordingly. More women than men diagnosed with

Alzheimer's is a *gender* health disparity. Black Americans having higher rates of obesity than white Americans is a *racial* health disparity. Families living in urban neighborhoods having higher rates of asthma than families living in suburban neighborhoods is a *geographic* and/or *socioeconomic* health disparity. It is also important to note that many health disparities overlap in type; that is, they may be both racial and geographic, as the causes of health disparities are often driven be a complexity of factors. Healthy People 2020 aims to not only eliminate health disparities but also achieve health equity, which is defined as attaining the highest level of health for all people.

Determinants of Health

The underlying premise for why health disparities exist is due to a confluence of powerful factors that interact to influence health. These factors are known as *determinants of health*. Determinants of individual and population health include biology, genetics, individual behavior, access to health services, socioeconomic status, physical environment, discrimination, racism, cultural beliefs, religion, literacy levels and legislative policies, social supports, employment and poverty, among others.[15] Historically, the medical approach to health care has focused on the biological and genetic factors that predispose individuals to illness. In the past few decades, however, there has been increased emphasis on the impact that

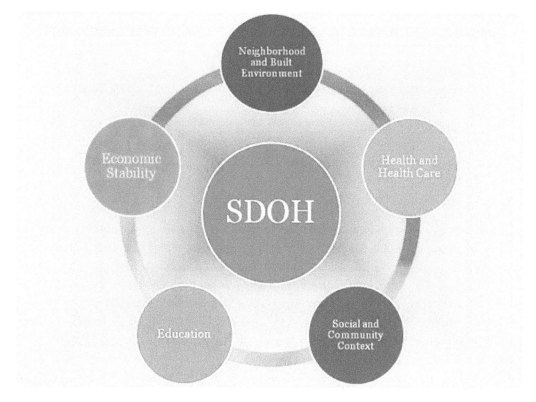

FIGURE 1.7   Social Determinants of Health

social environments have on health. As a result, Healthy People 2020 added a new topic area—*social determinants of health*.

Social Determinants of Health

The social determinants of health topics were added to Healthy People 2020 as a way to bring attention to the impact of social and physical environments on health and wellness in all Americans. Social determinants of health are "the conditions in which people are born, grow, live, work and age and the wide set of forces and systems shaping the conditions of daily life."[16] Researchers have estimated that social factors such as education, poverty, racial segregation, and lack of social supports account for approximately 1/3 of total deaths in the U.S. each year.[17] According to Healthy People 2020, social determinants of health include

- Availability of resources to meet daily needs (e.g., safe housing and local food markets)
- Access to educational, economic, and job opportunities
- Access to health care services
- Quality of education and job training
- Availability of community-based resources in support of community living and opportunities for recreational and leisure-time activities
- Transportation options
- Public safety
- Social support
- Social norms and attitudes (e.g., discrimination, racism, and distrust of government)
- Exposure to crime, violence, and social disorder (e.g., presence of trash and lack of cooperation in a community)
- Socioeconomic conditions (e.g., concentrated poverty and the stressful conditions that accompany it)
- Residential segregation
- Language/Literacy
- Access to mass media and emerging technologies (e.g., cell phones, the Internet, and social media)
- Culture.

Additionally, it is widely accepted that the conditions and environments in which people live and spend their days affect their short- and long-term health outcomes. These "place" determinants include home, school, work, neighborhoods, and churches, and how individuals socially interact with others in these places can influence health. Physical environments that have more economic resources dedicated to development and maintenance of infrastructure, public safety, health services, healthy food, and toxin-free environments will promote better public health outcomes. According to Healthy People 2020, physical determinants of health include

- Natural environment, such as green space (e.g., trees and grass) or weather (e.g., climate change)

- Built environments such as buildings, sidewalks, bike lanes, and roads
- Worksites, schools, and recreational settings
- Housing and community design
- Exposure to toxic substances and other physical hazards
- Physical barriers, especially for people with disabilities
- Aesthetic elements (e.g., good lighting, trees, and benches).

Eliminating health disparities and achieving health equity will require addressing these social and environmental determinants on a population-based level and working toward communities that have access to fair and equitable resources to promote wellness for all Americans.[18]

Understanding Access to Health Services

Although the work of communities, states, and local and federal governments is to make health care services available to all Americans, equitable access to health care continues be a challenge to many. As a result, access to health care is a leading health indicator in Healthy People 2020. Access to health care has been linked to many important outcomes, including physical, social and mental health, quality of life, life expectancy, prevention of disease and disability, and the detection and treatment of disease. Below, we will discuss some of the factors that impact access to health care, as well as continuity of care across time.

Health Insurance Coverage

Recent state and federal efforts have focused on universal or near universal insurance coverage as key to accessing health care. Medical insurance is one of the most essential factors to accessing health care. People who lack medical insurance coverage are less likely to receive medical care due to the inability to pay large medical bills. They are also more likely to wait to seek care until their health is so compromised that they require emergency services. A direct correlate of not having health insurance is poorer overall health status and earlier age of death compared to insured counterparts.

Primary Care Services

Another focus of recent efforts related to accessing health care includes ensuring that every person has access to a primary care provider. Primary care providers include pediatricians, family practice doctors, general practitioners, and internal medicine doctors. Primary care providers are in high demands and short supply in our current medical system, as the number of medical students who choose primary care fields has declined. Nurse practitioners and physician assistants also play important roles and often fill the need when medical doctors are not available. Having a regular primary care provider is an important gateway to the medical system, as a primary care provider is the person who knows the patient's medical history and has developed a trusting relationship with the patient. Primary care providers who are trusted and respected have a higher likelihood of being able to guide their patients through challenges to their health, such as motivating patients for behavior change or encouraging them to follow through with referrals.[19]

Let's spend some time reviewing some of the national data pertaining to the topics discussed above. The National Health Interview Survey reported that 83.2% of Americans had health insurance in 2008. The data target for the year 2020 is 100% of people with coverage. Furthermore, the Medical Expenditure Panel Survey reported that 76.3% of persons had a regular primary care provider in 2007. The Healthy People 2020 target is 83.9%. Question for the reader: Why do you think that the Healthy People 2020 target for medical insurance is 100% and the target for every person to have a primary care provider is 83.9%?

Timeliness of Care

Timeliness of care includes the responsiveness of the health care system to meet the needs of the population it is designed to serve. Timeliness includes wait times in physician offices, lag times between identified needs and specific tests and/or treatments, and the physical distance and length of time to access health care services. Treatment lag times and patient dissatisfaction result in clinically significant delays in care. These factors can drive up health costs and lead to mistrust and frustration with the health care system.

Responsiveness to the Community

One could argue that it is an ethical and professional duty of health care providers to provide services to the community in ways that the community can understand. For instance, health care and health education information needs to be communicated in languages that are represented within the patient populations. An even higher ideal would be for health care providers to reflect the culture and diversity of the community in which they are located. Providers who understand cultural norms and more are better able to establish relationships with the patients whom they serve, resulting in better health outcomes. Racial and ethnic minorities, older adults, and people who identify as lesbian, gay, bisexual, or transgender would benefit from seeing health care providers who are sensitive to their concerns and can communicate in ways that resonate with their varied needs. The reality, however, is that health care providers themselves often lack diversity, making it ever more important that their training reflects culturally sensitive practice.

Theories and Models for Understanding Health and Human Behavior

The Biopsychosocial Model

Prior to the 1980s the accepted model for understanding the health of individuals was reductionist and purely biomedical; that is, diseases were the result of changes at the cellular and physiological level. In 1977, Dr. George Engel argued that people were more than their biology and that psychological and social factors were important indicators of health outcomes. Engel pioneered the idea that understanding health and illness must be done within the full context of the person's life.

Dr. Engel used the example of a 60-year-old overweight man who rarely exercises. The man's younger and physically fit brother visits for the week. After a snow storm, the man's wife complains that he never shovels the snow and knowingly glances over at the brother to do the shoveling. With his masculinity threatened, the man picks up a shovel, begins shoveling the driveway, and 15 minutes later suffers a heart attack and dies. Engel argues that focusing on the purely biological reasons for the heart attack (e.g., blood clots) disregards the social (e.g., competition with the brother) and psychological (e.g., threat to his masculinity) factors that impacted the man's health.

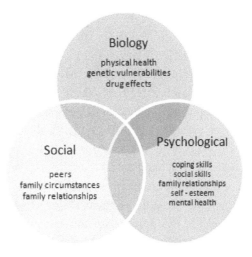

FIGURE 1.8   The Biopsychosocial Model of Health

Although many now take this way of thinking for granted, Dr. Engel paved the way for understanding the role of social, psychological, and contextual factors in disease and illness. Although there are some critics of this model, it has become the norm for how medical students are trained and has informed the development of fields of study which integrate psychological and social factors into understanding physical health (e.g., health psychology, public health, etc.).

Ecological Model of Health Behavior

Ecological models of health behavior focus on how people interact with their environments and how these interactions affect health and well-being. These environments include multiple levels or determinants, including intrapersonal (biological, psychological, family situation), interpersonal (social interactions with family and friends, culture), organizational (school and workplace), community (neighborhood, physical environment), and policy (government, agencies, laws).[20] The central tenet of the ecological model of health behavior is that the combination of individual-level, environmental, and policy-level interventions will lead to the most significant health behavior change.

The ecological model of health behavior has four core principles:

1. *Multiple levels of factors influence health behaviors*: Each level or determinant plays a role in shaping health behavior. There are some factors, such as the physical environment or sociocultural context, which cut across multiple levels.

2. *Influences interact across levels*: Factors in each level work together or interact to affect health. For example, a child who is genetically predisposed to anxiety may also have anxious parents. If their community recently experienced a threatening event, such as child abduction, and the community perceives that the police did not act as proactively as needed, this may interact to increase anxiety in the child and the family.

3. *Multi-level interventions are the most effective in changing behavior:* The best way to change behavior is to address the behavior at each level. For instance, the most effective intervention for healthy eating in urban settings includes putting healthy fruits and vegetables in schools and convenience stores, having physicians assess and educate people about eating habits, creating motivational television campaigns promoting healthy eating, working with individuals to change beliefs about healthy eating, and implementing policies that make healthy food choices more affordable. Simply doing only one of these strategies would decrease the likelihood of changing eating habits.

4. *Interventions must target specific behaviors:* Although some lessons may apply to other health behaviors, interventions generally need to target a specific behavior. For example, campaigns encouraging flu shots to promote health would not necessarily translate into checking one's body for cancerous moles, and providing free condoms at a college health center would not necessarily lead to decreased rates of binge drinking. Each intervention must be tailored at multiple levels.

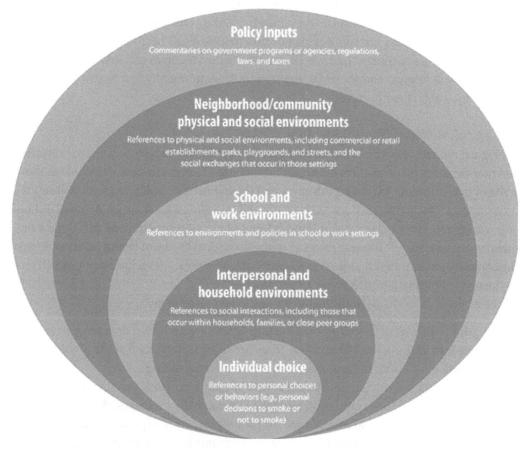

Policy inputs
Commentaries on government programs or agencies, regulations, laws, and taxes

Neighborhood/community physical and social environments
References to physical and social environments, including commercial or retail establishments, parks, playgrounds, and streets, and the social exchanges that occur in those settings

School and work environments
References to environments and policies in school or work settings

Interpersonal and household environments
References to social interactions, including those that occur within households, families, or close peer groups

Individual choice
References to personal choices or behaviors (e.g., personal decisions to smoke or not to smoke)

FIGURE 1.9   The Ecological Model of Health Behavior

The biggest challenge with the ecological model of health behavior is that determining which factor or factors caused the changes can be difficult, as they all interact. However, when health care providers and researchers create intervention approaches that focus on multiple levels of change, it becomes more likely that health behaviors will improve.

Risk and Resilience

Risk and resilience are broad concepts used to describe factors that either put people at risk for harm or protect them from harm. By definition, risk is "a condition of being open to something undesirable or harmful." Risk factors and threatening events often combine and accumulate over time. For example, the amount of stress experienced after moving to a new school may put a child at risk for anxiety, but moving to a new school due to parental divorce could have a significantly worse outcome. Risk factors are also multidimensional and can include physical, psychological, social, and economic factors that impact health. Risk factors are also classified as modifiable and unmodifiable. *Modifiable risk factors* include environmental and behavioral factors over which a person has some degree of control, such as smoking cigarettes or lack of exercise. *Unmodifiable risk factors* include factors that cannot be changed, such as genetics, race, personality type, and age. By contrast, resilience is defined as "the ability to avoid negative outcomes by doing well in the face of adversity."[21] To illustrate this point, think about a person you know who has experienced significant adversity but remains happy, optimistic, and goal oriented. This person may be considered "a fighter" or "an inspiration" and epitomizes what it means to be resilient. If a person does not experience adversity in life, he or she cannot be considered resilient. As we move through the book, we will identify risk and resiliency factors that impact a variety of health conditions, although many common risk factors impact multiple health conditions.

Conclusion

This chapter represents an overview of community health care, how it is delivered and funded in the United States, factors that contribute to health inequity, and theories and models that help to explain health and behavior change. The information described in this chapter is the foundation for the rest of the book. As you continue to read, you will be asked to apply these concepts to a range of topics that affect millions of Americans. As residents of the United States, we should all have a basic understanding of how individual behaviors, families, communities, and government policies affect health so that we can promote health and wellness throughout our lives.

In concluding this chapter, we would like to end with a few more statistics and thoughts to ponder. The United States spends more on health care than any other developed nation, yet outcomes and life expectancy are not better. Why is that? One difference between the United States and other developed countries is that the U.S. spends more money on health care services than on social services such as transportation, housing, education, employment opportunities, food availability, mental health, and safe neighborhood environments.[22]

If health were strictly a result of biology this concept would not be an issue. However, a person's environment, psychological well-being, social environment, and governmental policies all influence health. It is challenging to focus on health and wellness if one's basic needs are not being met.

Case Study

APPLYING DETERMINANTS OF HEALTH TO 21ST CENTURY EVENTS: FLINT, MICHIGAN WATER CRISIS

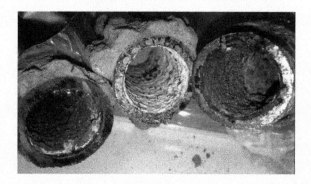

FIGURE 1.10   Corrosion in Flint Water Pipes

Perhaps you have heard about the Flint, Michigan Water Crisis which began in April of 2014 and led to the mass lead poisoning of hundreds of children and families between April of 2014 and December of 2015. To provide a bit of context, Flint, Michigan was economically devastated when General Motors (GM) moved its manufacturing plant to Mexico. GM employed approximately 80,000 Flint residents. Much of Flint's population lost their jobs, and the remaining low-income and largely minority population has been living in extreme poverty ever since. Flint is suffering from a devastating economic loss which affects every area of life.

In 2014, Flint officials decided to switch the water supply from Lake Huron to the Flint River. The water in the Flint River was known to be very corrosive—so corrosive, in fact, that the water was not used by the automotive industry because it was corroding metal parts. The corrosive water should have been treated with an anti-corrosion chemical that would have prevented it from absorbing lead from leaching into the water system, but it was not. This was in direct noncompliance with the Environmental Protection Agency's Lead and Copper Rule, which requires corrosive water to be treated. When untreated, corrosive water entered the pipes, lead from the interior of soldered water pipes leached into the water system. Residents already lived in environments at risk for elevated lead levels, including living in older homes painted with lead paint manufactured before 1979, living in urban areas with elevated levels of lead in the soil, and poor nutrition which increases the rates of lead absorption into the body. The decision to switch Flint's water supply appeared to be financially driven. Government officials sought to save money with little regard for community health.

Lead poisoning has both short- and long-term effects on the body, but the symptoms generally develop slowly. In the short-term, chronic lead exposure leads to loss of appetite, a metallic taste in the mouth, stomach cramps, pale skin, fatigue, headache, joint pain, dizziness, numbness, seizures and anxiety, among others. Longer-term symptoms include anemia, nervous system damage, kidney disease, reproductive issues, birth defects, behavioral disorders such as poor attention and hyperactivity, developmental disabilities, decreased IQ, and death. These symptoms are irreversible, which makes lead exposure so costly to individuals, families, and society as a whole. Additionally, because lead mimics the chemical structure of calcium and is absorbed very quickly in children who are chronically hungry and deprived of nutrients, one might expect that children living in Flint would be at increased risk for lead absorption. It is state law that children be tested annually for lead exposure. Dr. Mona Hanna-Attisha, a local Flint pediatrician, examined blood lead levels (BLL) from children living in Flint before the water change to after the water change. Although the Centers for Disease Control recommends that BLL should be under 5 µg/dL, Dr. Hanna-Attisha found that the children living in the affected area has BLL three-times higher than before the water diversion.[23] If parents brought their children to the doctor with these symptoms, it is likely that their physical and behavioral issues would have been linked to issues related to poverty, rather than lead poisoning.

Ultimately, the Flint Water Advisory Task Force reported that the Flint water crisis was "a story of government failure, intransigence, unpreparedness, delay, inaction, and environmental injustice," with multiple agencies failing to enforce drinking water regulations and protect the public health.[24]

The Flint community has developed a multi-pronged approach to helping affected families, as well as preventing future situations like this. First, the Flint Water Advisory Task Force recommended the creation of a Flint Toxic Exposure Registry, which will allow exposed children and adults to receive follow-up care such as routine lead screenings in their homes, as well as screenings for school readiness. They also recommended a fund dedicated to providing health-related services to Flint residents, who will undoubtedly require some level of ongoing care. Dr. Hanna-Attisha established the Flint Child Health and Development Fund with the purpose of supporting optimal health and development of children and families. Lastly, this public health tragedy shed light on the fact that federal, state, and local agencies must improve their efforts to ensure environmental justice. The American Academy of Pediatrics has set forth clear recommendations that the U.S. Environmental Protection Agency and Department of Housing and Urban Development should reassess their protocols for "identifying and mitigating residential lead hazards (e.g., lead-based paint, dust, and soil) and lead-contaminated water from lead service lines or lead solder and revise downward the allowable levels of lead in house dust, soil, paint, and water to conform with the recognition that there are no safe levels of lead."[25] However, recommendations must be turned into policy and action, and law and policy makers must put public health ahead of personal interests in order to effectively promote change and well-being.

Flint and Healthy People 2020

The disaster in Flint serves as a reminder of some important points regarding our environment. First, water is the world's most essential and vulnerable resource. Some scientists believe that with no alternative for water, the wars of the future will be over water. In other words, water equals power. Once water is polluted or wasted, we have less access to this precious resource. As such, Healthy People 2020 aims to 1) increase the proportion of Americans who receive clean drinking water that meet the standard of the Safe Drinking Water Act, 2) reduce waterborne disease outbreaks, 3) conserve water, and 4) increase the number of beaches that are open and safe for swimming. Second, more research is needed to understand how exposure to toxic substances and hazardous waste impacts health. With regard to lead exposure, Healthy People 2020 aims to reduce blood lead levels in children ages 1–5 years old. Reducing exposure to toxins, protecting water sources, and minimizing exposure to contaminated water sources are fundamental aspects of environmental health.

Notes

1 WHO Definition of Health. (2003). Retrieved January 30, 2017, from http://www.who.int/about/definition/en/print.html

2 CDC's Work Saves Lives Everywhere, Every Day. (2014, March 19). Retrieved January 30, 2017, from https://www.cdc.gov/about/24-7/savinglives/

3 2013–14 Census of SBHCs Report. (2014). Retrieved January 30, 2017, from http://censusreport.sbh4all.org/

4 Alquist, S. (2013–2014) First neighborhood health station breaks ground in Central Falls. *School Based Health Alliance.* Retrieved from: http://www.rifuture.org/1st-neighborhood-health-station/

5 Australian Nursing Federation (2009) *Primary health care in Australia: A nursing and midwifery consensus view.* Retrieved from: http://anmf.org.au/documents/reports/PHC_Australia.pdf

6 Frieden, T. R. (2010). A framework for public health action: the health impact pyramid. *American Journal of Public Health, 100*(4), 590–595.

7 Epidemiology. (n.d.). Retrieved January 30, 2017, from http://www.who.int/topics/epidemiology/en/

8 Healthy People 2020 [Internet]. Washington, DC: U.S. Department of Health and Human Services, Office of Disease Prevention and Health Promotion. Retrieved from: https://www.healthypeople.gov/2020.

9 U.S. Department of Health and Human Services. The Secretary's Advisory Committee on National Health Promotion and Disease Prevention Objectives for 2020. Phase I report: Recommendations for the framework and format of Healthy People 2020 [Internet]. Section IV: Advisory committee findings and recommendations [cited 2010 January 6]. Retrieved from: http://www.healthypeople.gov/sites/default/files/PhaseI_0.pdf.

10 Your online guide of what works to promote healthy communities. (n.d.). Retrieved January 30, 2017, from https://www.thecommunityguide.org/

11 National Health and Nutrition Examination Survey. (2017, January 25). Retrieved January 30, 2017, from https://www.cdc.gov/nchs/nhanes/index.htm

12 Behavioral Risk Factor Surveillance System. (2016, August 26). Retrieved January 30, 2017, from https://www.cdc.gov/brfss/index.html

13 Youth Risk Behavior Surveillance System (YRBSS). (2016, August 11). Retrieved January 30, 2017, from https://www.cdc.gov/healthyyouth/data/yrbs/index.htm

14 Disparities. (2010). Retrieved January 30, 2017, from https://www.healthypeople.gov/2020/about/foundation-health-measures/Disparities

15 Determinants of Health. (n.d.). Retrieved January 30, 2017, from https://www.healthypeople.gov/2020/about/foundation-health-measures/Determinants-of-Health

16 Determinants of Health. (n.d.). Retrieved January 30, 2017, from https://www.healthypeople.gov/2020/about/foundation-health-measures/Determinants-of-Health

17 Galea, S. et al., (August 2011) Estimated deaths attributable to social factors in the United States. *American Journal of Public Health, 101*(8):1456–1465, doi:10.2105/AJPH.2010.300086.

18 Marmot, M. et al., (8, November, 2008) Closing the gap in a generation: Health equity through action on the social determinants of health, *The Lancet, 372*(9650),1661–1669.

19 Martin, L., Williams, S., Haskard, K., DiMatteo, M. (2005) The challenge of patient adherence. *Therapuetics and Clinical Risk Management.* Retrieved from: https://www.ncbi.nlm.nih.gov/pmc/articles/PMC1661624/

20 Sallis, J. F., Owen, N., & Fisher, E. B. (2008). Ecological models of health behavior. *Health Behavior and Health Education: Theory, Research, and Practice, 4*, 465–486.

21 Masten, A. S. & Coatsworth, J. D., (1998). The development of competence in favorable and unfavorable environments: Lessons from research on successful children. *American Psychologist, 53*(2), 205–220.

22 The Commonwealth Fund. (2015) U.S. Health Care from a Global Perspective. Retrieved From: http://www.commonwealthfund.org/publications/issue-briefs/2015/oct/us-health-care-from-a-global-perspective

23 Campbell, C., Greenberg, R., Mankikar, D., & Ross, R. D. (2016). A case study of environmental injustice: The failure in Flint. *International Journal of Environmental Research and Public Health, 13*(10), 951.

24 Flint Water Advisory Task Force. (2016). *Flint Water Task Force final report.* Lansing, MI: Office of Governor Rick Snyder.

25 Lanphear, B. P., Lowry, J. A., Ahdoot, S., Baum, C. R., Bernstein, A. S., Bole, A., & Trasande, L. (2016). Prevention of childhood lead toxicity. *Pediatrics*, e20161493.

Figure Sources

1 Figure 1.1: Source: https://commons.wikimedia.org/wiki/World_Health_Organisation#/media/File:Flag_of_WHO.svg.

2 Figure 1.2: Source: http://www.hhs.gov/about/agencies/orgchart/.

3 Joseph Malins, "The Ambulance Down in the Valley." Copyright in the Public Domain.

4 Figure 1.4: Source: https://www.cdc.gov/nchs/data/nvsr/nvsr65/nvsr65_05.pdf.

5 Figure 1.5: Source: https://www.cdc.gov/nchs/data/nvsr/nvsr65/nvsr65_05.pdf.

6 Figure 1.6: Source: https://www.mapc.org/our-work/expertise/public-health/
health-impact-assessments/.

7 Figure 1.7: Source: https://www.healthypeople.gov/sites/default/files/SDOH.png.

8 Figure 1.8: Copyright © MrAnnoying (CC BY-SA 4.0) at https://commons.wikimedia.org/wiki/
File:Biopsychosocial_Model_of_Health_1.png.

9 Figure 1.9: Source: https://www.cdc.gov/pcd/issues/2013/images/12_0204_01.gif.

10 Figure 1.10: Source: www.flickr.com, Copyright © 2017 by VCU CNS.

CHAPTER TWO

Asthma

Author:
Sue K. Adams, Ph.D.

@LungAssociation

Imagine this: On a frigid winter day you are supposed to board a train to visit some friends, but you are running late. As you get to the station, you see the train pulling into the station. You start running toward the train so that you do not miss it. As you breathe in the cold, dry air, you start to feel your airways burn. Every time you inhale, your throat makes a whistling noise, and you are thinking, "I'm having an asthma attack, but I don't have my medications. This is not good." Your heart is racing, and you start to panic. You board the train, and as you sit down you realize that your chest feels tight, like someone with large hands is squeezing your lungs. You begin to cough—sometimes you cough up mucus, and sometimes it is a dry, hacking cough. You start to panic because you do not have your inhaler, and you do not know when you will get your next breath, and you are stuck on a moving train with strangers. Your thoughts are racing. Will someone help you if you need it? What if you need to go to the hospital? Luckily, after about 7–10 minutes of these physical feelings and thoughts, you notice that it is easier to breath, although your breathing will not go back to normal for a day or two after this asthma attack. For some, this is what it feels like to have asthma.

What Is Asthma?

Asthma is one of the most prevalent chronic illnesses in the United States, and the number of new cases continues to grow each year. According the Centers for Disease Control and the American Academy of Allergy, Asthma, and Immunology, 17.7 million adults, or 7.4% of the population, has asthma. Of that, 6.3 million children (8.3% of children) have asthma, with teenagers between 12 and 14 representing the most cases during childhood.[1] Asthma is also a very costly disease. With 10.5 million people visiting doctor's offices every year due to asthma attacks, 1.8 million people visiting an emergency room, and over 3,600 people dying of asthma each year, asthma costs the U.S. about $3,300 per person with asthma each year. These costs are related to a number of factors, including medical expenses, missed school, missed workdays, and early death. Overall, asthma cost the US approximately $56 billion in 2007, and that number increases every year.[2]

By definition, asthma is a chronic respiratory disease in which the airways become inflamed and enlarged.[3] In normal lungs, air is inhaled through the nose and mouth and passes through the trachea, or windpipe. The air then moves into the bronchi, which is the large airway. The bronchi branches into smaller and smaller tubes, eventually leading the air into small sacs called the alveoli. The alveoli pass oxygen to the blood and remove carbon dioxide. When a person has an asthma attack, three processes occur in the lungs and airways that impair oxygen exchange. Each of these processes interact to cause an asthma attack:

1. Inflammation: People with asthma experience inflamed, or swollen, airways. As the airways swell, they become narrow, making it harder to breath in oxygen.

2. Bronchoconstriction: The airways are surrounded by smooth muscles. During an asthma attack, the muscles around the airways get tight, squeezing the airways from the outside and restricting airflow.

3. Mucus: During an asthma attack, cells in the airway make more mucus than normal. The mucus is a thick and sticky substance (similar to nasal mucus) and can further narrow the airways.

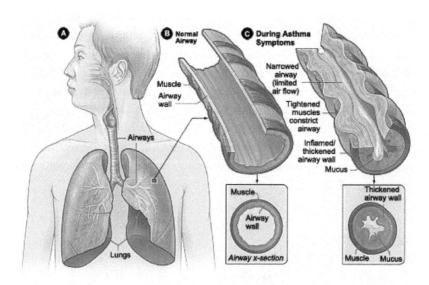

FIGURE 2.1   Normal airways vs. airways of someone with asthma

Health Disparities in Asthma

Many racial, ethnic, and gender health disparities exist in asthma. As you continue reading this section, begin to think about what factors may contribute to these health disparities. Although asthma disproportionately affects individuals from ethnic minority backgrounds, non-Hispanic blacks of all ages have the highest rates of asthma. According to the U.S. Department of Health and Human Services Office of Minority Health, in 2014 almost 2.4 million non-Hispanic blacks reported that they have been diagnosed with asthma, which is approximately 15% of black Americans. Black children are four times more likely to be admitted to the hospital for asthma than white children, and African Americans are three times more likely to die from asthma-related causes than whites. Alarmingly, Hispanic children, particularly Puerto Ricans, have the highest rates of asthma, ranging between 18% and 35% of Puerto Rican children living in Connecticut and New York.[4]

Gender health disparities also exist, with women more likely to develop asthma than men (11.5% versus 5.3%), and boys are more likely to have asthma than girls. More specifically, African American women are 20% more likely to have an asthma attack than non-Hispanic white women.[5] These are only some of the health disparity statistics, and they often vary depending on the source of data. However, the bottom line is clear—black and Puerto Rican men, women, boys, and girls living in the United States are disproportionately affected by asthma. This is an alarming trend, and we must continue to consider how social, environmental, socioeconomic, cultural, and behavioral factors contribute to these patterns.

Healthy People 2020

In an effort to decrease respiratory diseases in Americans, Healthy People 2020 has set forth multiple objectives to decrease Asthma and Chronic Obstructive Pulmonary Disease (CPOD), which is defined as nonreversible airflow limitation. For asthma, objectives include reducing asthma deaths, hospitalizations, emergency room visits, activity limitation, and missed days of school and work while increasing the number of Americans who receive appropriate asthma care consistent with national guidelines and formal patient education. A final objective is increasing the number of states with comprehensive asthma surveillance systems to track cases of asthma. Since 2007, the national statistics have remained below the desired goals, and, therefore, Healthy People 2020 will continue to support efforts to work toward goal attainment by the year 2020.

Biological and Environmental Factors that Contribute to Asthma

Asthma is a complicated condition, and one that is caused by a number of factors. Many people are genetically susceptible to asthma and their environments "pull the trigger" to cause the disease. Genetically, asthma clearly runs in families. Approximately ten genes have been identified that have a significant effect on a person's susceptibility to asthma.[6] These genes make the bronchial tubes oversensitive or can cause inflammation resulting from exposure to specific allergens. It also appears that genetics makes certain groups of people, such as blacks and Puerto Ricans, more likely to develop asthma and not respond to traditional asthma medication as well as whites do.[7] Genetics can also contribute to allergies or increased sensitivity to certain substances. When allergies affect the nose, it is referred to as "hay fever," but when they affect the bronchial tubes, it is referred to as asthma.

Asthma Triggers

Asthma is often triggered, which means that a person's asthma is likely to flare when he or she comes in contact with certain allergens, irritants, or changes in the environment. For people who have allergies, contact with their allergens (e.g., pollen, cats or dogs) may trigger an asthma attack. For others, however, strong emotions can cause asthma attacks. Identifying asthma triggers and staying away from triggers is an important part of asthma management. Below is a list of the most common triggers.

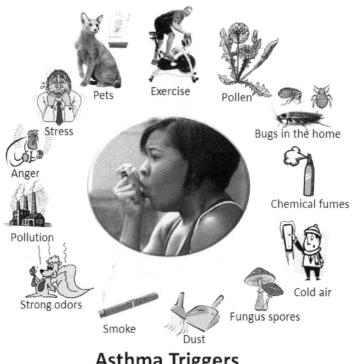

Asthma Triggers

FIGURE 2.2   **The most common asthma triggers**

Cockroaches

Did you know that cockroaches have been around since the time of the dinosaurs, and that they can live for up to a month without food and a week without water? Cockroaches tend to live in warm, dark areas (often in cities or rural areas) and will eat most anything, with the most delicious treats being human food. These critters scurry into people's homes, eat food crumbs, and then defecate (or poop). The cockroach droppings then turn into dust, people breathe the dust, and the dust is what triggers asthma. To avoid this scenario, be sure to wipe up your spills and clean up after you eat.

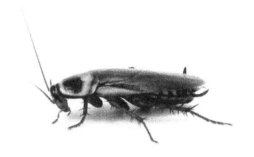

FIGURE 2.3   Asthma trigger: Cockroach

Dust Mites

Dust mites are microscopic organisms found everywhere that humans inhabit. Dust mites feed on dust, but where does dust come from you? Most dust (75–90%) is made up of dead skin cells. The average human sheds between 30,000 and 40,000 skin cells per minute, and dust mites savor this tasty meal. That also means that dust mites are present in places where people spend a lot of time, such as bedrooms. Therefore, we would expect mattresses, carpets, and even stuffed animals to have large concentrations of dust mites.

Pollen

From spring through fall, many people succumb to seasonal allergies. Allergies are often triggered by a variety of pollens, such as grass, tree, and weed pollens. Many people with asthma will also experience

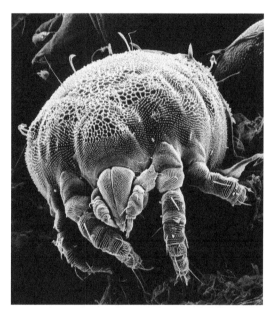

FIGURE 2.4   Asthma trigger: Dust mite

asthmatic episodes during this time. Additionally, pollen is wind-borne and can easily come into homes and schools through open windows. Be sure to keep your home clean, close the windows on high pollen days, and take prescribed allergy and asthma medications during susceptible times of year.

Mold

Fungi release mold spores into the air and are typically found in damp areas of the home, such as bathrooms, basements, air conditioners, humidifiers, and compost piles. Mold spores can be released at any time of the year but usually get worse during the hot and humid months. If a person is allergic to mold, these tiny spores can induce both allergies and asthma. In an effort to minimize a person's allergic response, thoroughly dry out damp places in the home.

Emotions

People who have asthma may feel that they have more symptoms when they are stressed. This is not "all in their heads," as stress-induced asthma is a documented condition. People who experience stressful events or strong emotions such as anger, excitement, or intense happiness are more likely to experience physiological changes that can trigger an asthma attack, specifically causing a narrowing of the airway. They may also cry, which increases mucus secretions in the sinuses and lungs. People who are really stressed may also forget to take their medications or be more likely to get sick, all of which can make asthma worse. For these people, stress reduction strategies such as deep breathing, relaxation, exercise, and/or psychotherapy can be particularly helpful in managing symptoms.

Exercise

Exercise-induced asthma (EIA) symptoms can start soon after a person begins vigorous exercise. Exercises that involve breathing cold, dry air such as skiing or running outdoors will make asthma flare more than exercise in warmer, humid air. EIA symptoms will usually peak in severity five to 10 minutes after a person stops exercising and can resolve within 30 minutes, even if the person does not take medication.[8] Interestingly, professional athletes who have asthma are at particular risk for asthmatic episodes when they are competing, as they are more likely to be breathing through their mouths. However, the mouth does not do as good of a job as the nose at filtering environmental irritants, which allows the irritants to get into the lungs and trigger a more severe reaction. Therefore, all athletes should strictly use their asthma medications, should wear scarves or masks over their mouths in cold air, and always ease into and out of exercise with warm-ups and cool-downs.

Smoking

Cigarette smoke is the number-one indoor air pollutant and plays a serious role in exacerbating a person's asthma. A person who has asthma should seriously consider quitting smoking as the smoke may directly cause inflammation (first-hand smoke). Furthermore, small children who are exposed to cigarette smoke are at an increased risk for developing asthma at some point in their childhood. It is also important to remember that smoking in front of a child or a person with asthma is only one form of transmission (second-hand smoke). Parents who smoke outside still have cigarette smoke in their clothing, hair, and on their person (this is third-hand smoke—think of how you smell after you leave a nightclub). Children breathe in these irritants when they cuddle with their parents, though I am sure that their parents do not mean them harm.

Signs and Symptoms of Asthma

The signs and symptoms of an asthma attack are what can be seen on the outside of the person or felt within the person. Remember that many processes have already been happening internally that have already affected the person's lung function. Signs and symptoms vary across individuals, but below is a description of the most common.

Coughing

Why do people cough? Coughing helps expel mucus and other irritants from the lungs. The person's body is trying to expel all of the extra mucus out of the body, helping to clear the airway and lungs for the exchange of oxygen. Coughing is often worse at night or early in the morning.

Wheezing

This is a whistling sound that happens when a person breathes. This is a very raspy sound usually heard when the person is inhaling due to narrowing of the airways.

Chest Tightness

As a person's airways become more inflamed, filled with mucus, and constricted, a person's chest might start to feel tight. Typically, people feel like they are unable to move air in and out of their lungs.

Shortness of Breath

People who experience shortness of breath usually describe this as trying to take a deep breath but not being able to fill their lungs or get enough air into their lungs.

Fatigue

Asthma can trigger fatigue mainly due to decreased oxygen levels. When asthma narrows the airways, the lungs will not be able to exchange air into the blood stream properly. When oxygen levels are too low, a person's body will not have the energy to function properly, and the person will feel very tired.

Asthma Across Development

Childhood

As a first step to answer why certain groups of people are more likely to develop asthma, we must also discuss issues related to poverty. In states across the U.S., cities with the highest proportion of families living in poverty have the highest proportions of people diagnosed with asthma. Historically, one of the major reasons for this disparity was lack of health coverage. Even with universal access to health care, a lack of quality health care providers in minority communities to provide continuous care impacts asthma outcomes. Minority children often are under-prescribed medications, and their families may not have the money to fill prescriptions. Research also shows that children from minority backgrounds are less able to adhere to medications.[9] Why would this be? Parental beliefs about the role and usefulness of medications play a critical role. Why would a parent give a child a medication that he or she does not believe works or will harm the child? Parents may also have concerns about negative side effects of the inhaled corticosteroids. Even if health care providers explain that side effects are limited, parents may not trust health care providers due to historical untruths told by doctors (e.g., The Tuskegee Project). Combined with the fact that as much as 40% of asthma in minority populations is due to living unhealthy environments full of environmental triggers, children and adults living in poverty are at considerable risk for asthma health disparities.

School Considerations

For many, nighttime asthma attacks are common. More than 59% of children with asthma have missed school, with these children missing an average of four days of school per month.[10] Given the sheer number of days of missed learning, it is important to consider how nighttime asthma attacks may impact a child's ability to function in school. First, disrupted sleep may make it harder for the child, particularly an adolescent, to awaken in the morning for school. Many parents will allow their children to stay home due to missed sleep. Second, if children do attend school, sleep deprivation may make it harder to pay attention. Teachers may notice that children have trouble focusing their attention on learning. Adolescents may appear visibly tired—they may be struggling to keep their eyes open! When children are sleep deprived, however, their bodies counter fatigue by becoming hyperactive.

Teachers should know the students in their classes who have asthma, as teachers play an important role in aiding asthma management at school. For instance, teachers should note any trends in absences and school performance due to sleep deprivation. Conversations with parents about the reasons for absences can potentially open the door for the school nurse to consult with parents about improved asthma management. Similar to school management of other diseases, parents should consult with the school about their child's asthma and provide the school with an Asthma Action Plan. If children are able to self-administer quick relief medication, they should have it handy at all times during the day. However, for children who cannot self-administer their medications or who may not want to due to embarrassment of drawing attention to themselves, teachers should remain vigilant of the signs and symptoms of asthma. Sending children to the school nurse for their medications at the first signs of asthma will help to better control symptoms. Also consider sending children to run "special errands" if they do not want their peers knowing about their condition. Finally, teachers should consider the set-up of their classrooms to be asthma friendly. Children with asthma probably should not sit near open windows in the spring or near the dusty chalkboard. Findings ways to minimize exposure to asthma triggers can go a long way in controlling asthma.

Physical Education

For all children, exercise is an essential component of long-term physical and psychological health, and all children with asthma should be supported to participate in physical education activities. If a child's asthma is well controlled, he or she should have little problem engaging in exercise. As we know, though, often asthma is not well controlled, and physical education teachers need to be aware of the signs and symptoms of asthma.

A child should never be forced to "tough it out," but rather, make sure the child follows the action plan and is administered medication as needed. Therefore, it behooves physical education teachers to understand how to properly administer asthma medication. Teachers should also encourage the child to breath through the nose rather than the mouth and engage in indoor activities. Long-distance running and outdoor adventure sports can be among the most triggering activities, so children with asthma generally do well with activities such as swimming or any team games that provide bursts of activity with time to recover. As my six-year-old boy tells me on a regular basis, Physical Education is his favorite subject of the day, so be creative and have fun!

Adults and Older Adults

Work-related Asthma or Occupational Asthma

Some adults have what is called "Monday Morning Asthma." This is asthma that is caused or made worse as a result of exposure to substances in their workplaces, and the symptoms typically get worse on Monday morning when the person returns to work. It is estimated that 1.9 million cases of adult asthma are workplace related, which accounts for 16% of adult asthma. This type of asthma is highest among people 45–64 years old.[11] The types of workplace asthma are surprising, and occupations include bakers, beauticians, farmers, pharmaceutical workers, grocery workers, veterinarians, postal workers, and hospital workers, to name a few. However, the most severe workplace asthma symptoms are related to latex. As more people develop latex allergies, asthmatic episodes also increase.

Asthma and the Flu

Influenza, otherwise known as the flu, can be particularly dangerous for people with asthma. Of the 830 children who died of the flu between 2004 and 2014, 16% were diagnosed with asthma.[12] Children who have asthma are hospitalized for the flu at higher rates than those without asthma. We also see similar, disproportionate trends in the elderly, with older adults more likely than those without asthma to develop pneumonia after they have the flu. The good news is that the flu vaccine can be a powerful tool in reducing influenza-related complications in all people, especially people with asthma. All young children, older adults, and those with serious medical conditions including asthma should seriously consider getting a flu vaccine. However, they should receive the inactivated vaccine in the form of a shot (not the nasal spray). Finally, some common medications such as those for hypertension, heart disease, arthritis, and glaucoma, as well as aspirin, can trigger asthma. Older adults should provide their doctors with a list of medications at each visit.

How Asthma Affects the Family

Families must work together to manage asthma symptoms. Like most things in parenting, a fine balance needs to be maintained between being too controlling and not being controlling enough. With asthma, parents may already be concerned about their children's health and fear that a child will have a severe episode that results in hospitalization or death. Some parents respond by being very structured in managing their children's asthma. For some families, this works well, particularly if the child is young, and we see good asthma control. As children get older, however, they often prefer to take responsibility for their asthma management. Once again, for some families this works well, and for others it does not. When parents *overestimate* the level of responsibility that their adolescent can handle, we see increased nonadherence to medications and more asthma symptoms. Asthma can also affect the family's functioning and increase stress in the family. For instance, the family may have to manage the demands of asthma management by avoiding certain situations and allergy proofing the home (for example, getting a dog may never be an option). Some researchers have found that parents who have children with very severe asthma report poorer quality of life.[13] Across all parts of the lifespan, families and couples who have good communication patterns and work together to manage asthma tend to experience better asthma management and fewer symptoms.

Psychological and Social Effects of Asthma

Not knowing when you will be able to take your next breath can be a frightening experience. It comes as no surprise that people with asthma are twice as likely to develop anxiety and depressive disorders.[14] Asthmatics, especially children, may live with anticipatory anxiety about when the next asthma attack will occur. People with asthma are also more likely to be diagnosed with panic attacks,[15] and panic attacks can sometimes be confused with asthma attacks since they feel very similar in the body. Furthermore, if a person with asthma does not have well-controlled asthma, he or she may change behavior in an attempt to prevent an asthma attack. The person may experience activity restriction—for example, a child may not be able to attend sleepovers because his or her friend has a cat. An adult may not be able to go out with friends because her friends smoke or may go hiking in the woods. Social isolation can have a profound effect on one's mental health, which in turn could make asthma worse. People with asthma may also be chronically exposed to fearful or catastrophic thoughts, leading to increased anxiety over time.[16] Family exposure to asthma may also produce environments that overwhelm family members with medical care and financial demands, or lead to feelings of learned helplessness, all of which could contribute to depression.

The Role of Individuals, Families and Communities in Promoting Asthma Management

You may have heard that "you can outgrow asthma." That is not exactly true. Asthma cannot be cured. Although a person's symptoms may change over time, lung physiology is permanently altered after someone develops asthma. Therefore, the goal for asthma management is asthma control, which is the degree to which asthma symptoms are minimized by 1) detecting symptoms, 2) avoiding asthma triggers, and 3) adhering to medication.

Medical Management of Asthma

Asthma medications are an essential component of asthma management. Medical management of asthma is very similar in children, adults, and the elderly. In general, there are two types of medications—long-term controller medications and quick-relief medications. These medications come in different forms, including mist inhalers, dry-powder inhalers, pills, shots, and nebulizers.

Long-term controller medications need to be taken daily to help prevent symptoms. These medications reduce airway inflammation and mucus production, which help to prevent asthma symptoms from starting. Pediatric asthma patients are only adherent to approximately 50% of their prescribed medications.[17] Elderly patients also exhibit low adherence rates. Nonadherence is caused by a number of factors, including concerns about the side effects of long-term corticosteroid medications, misunderstanding the treatment regimen, and/or forgetfulness.

As a result, it is important to educate patients about the fact that these medications are generally safe when taken as prescribed. Inhaled corticosteroids are different from illegal anabolic steroids and are not addictive. They can have mild side effects such as mouth infections called thrush, cataracts (i.e., clouding of the lens of the eye), and osteoporosis (i.e., weakening of the bones). Research also shows that inhaled corticosteroids may possibly slow children's growth, but only temporarily.[18]

Quick-relief medications are taken as needed at the first sign of an asthma attack. These medications act very quickly and help to relax the tight muscles around the airway, otherwise known as bronchoconstriction, to help a person breath again. These medications should never be used in instead of long-term controller medications because they do not reduce inflammation or swelling. If a person has exercise-induced asthma, his or her physician may recommend taking quick-relief medication before exercise. Common side effects include tremor, shakiness, nervousness, headache, restlessness, irritability, muscle aches and throat/nasal irritation.[19]

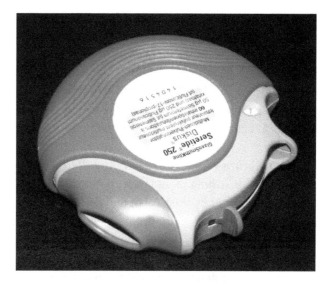

FIGURE 2.5   Asthma diskus device and inhaler used for treatment

Spacers

All children who use inhalers should use spacers, or an extension tube. Spacers are attachments that fit over the mouthpiece of an inhaler. The medication enters the chamber of the spacer and becomes trapped in the chamber for several seconds, creating a fine mist of medication. This allows the person to breathe in the medicine ensuring that it travels to the lungs. If a child does not use a spacer, it is likely that the medication will land on his or her tongue and not make it to the lungs where it is needed. Adults who have difficulty taking medications should also use spacers.

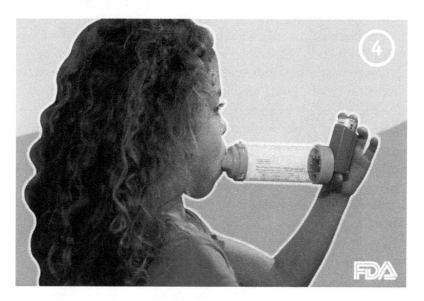

FIGURE 2.6 **An example of the proper use of a spacer**

Peak Flow Meter

Peak flow meters are an important component of asthma management, especially if a person has moderate to severe asthma. A peak flow meter is a device that a person exhales into to determine lung function. When determining a person's optimal lung function, he or she will use this device for a two- to three-week period to determine his or her personal "zones." This will be used to determine the zones of the Asthma Action Plan, helping a person to identify if her breathing is good, just OK, or really bad and in need of medical attention.

Asthma Action Plan: Green, Yellow, Red Zones

All people with asthma should have an Asthma Action Plan. An action plan is a written plan developed together by the patient and doctor. It describes the steps to be taken to manage and control asthma symptoms. Since asthma management is unique for every individual, each asthma management plan must be tailored to the person.

The Asthma Action Plan is typically broken up into three color-coded sections or zones. A person determines which zone he or she is in based on symptoms and peak flow meter results. The Green Zone means that a person is doing well, having an easy time breathing, is not coughing or wheezing, and can go to school or work. The Yellow

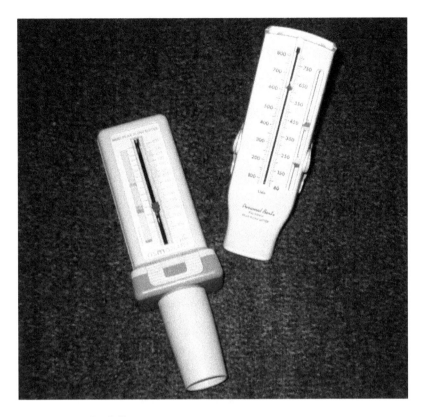

FIGURE 2.7   **Peak flow meters**

Zone means that the person should use caution—he or she may have the first signs of a cold or mild coughing or wheezing. The Red Zone indicates danger—the person needs medical help because his or her breathing is fast and hard, he or she cannot breathe, and medications are not helping. People who fall in the Green and Yellow Zones should take their medications as prescribed. People in the Red Zone should take their medications as prescribed and call their health care provider or go to the emergency room immediately.[20]

Community Interventions

Asthma educators use a number of methods to teach children and adults about asthma, as well as to ensure that communities provide safe spaces for breathing. Examples of community outreach efforts include traditional asthma education programs, efforts to make workplaces tobacco-free, 5K runs that raise money for asthma research, and the systematic monitoring of air quality and air quality alert systems, to name a few. The most effective community prevention and intervention programs are multidisciplinary, as you will see in the three programs described in more detail below.

My Asthma Action Plan
Age ≥5 years

Patient Name: _____

Medical Record #: _____

Physician's Name: _____   DOB: _____

Physician's Phone #: _____   Completed by: _____   Date: _____

Long-Term-Control Medicines	How Much To Take	How Often	Other Instructions
		_____ times per day EVERY DAY!	
		_____ times per day EVERY DAY!	
		_____ times per day EVERY DAY!	
		_____ times per day EVERY DAY!	

Quick-Relief Medicines	How Much To Take	How Often	Other Instructions
		Take ONLY as needed	NOTE: If this medicine is needed frequently, call physician to consider increasing long-term-control medications.

Special instructions when I feel ● good, ○ not good, and ● awful.

GREEN ZONE

I feel *good*.

{My peak flow is in the GREEN zone.}

My Personal Best Peak Flow

PREVENT asthma symptoms everyday:

☐ Take my long-term-control medicines (above) every day.

☐ Before exercise, take _____ puffs of _____

☐ Avoid things that make my asthma worse like: _____

YELLOW ZONE

I do *not* feel *good*.

{My peak flow is in the YELLOW zone.}

My symptoms may include one or more of the following:

- Wheeze
- Tight chest
- Cough
- Shortness of breath
- Waking up at night with asthma symptoms
- Decreased ability to do usual activities
- _____

80% Personal Best

CAUTION. I should continue taking my long-term-control asthma medicines every day AND:

☐ Take _____

If I still do not feel good, or my peak flow is not back in the Green Zone within 1 hour, then I should:

☐ Increase _____

☐ Add _____

☐ Call _____

RED ZONE

I feel *awful*. {My peak flow is in the RED zone.}

Warning signs may include one or more of the following:

- It's getting harder and harder to breathe
- Unable to sleep or do usual activities because of trouble breathing

50% Personal Best

Unable Peak Flow Meter

MEDICAL ALERT! Get help!

☐ Take _____ until I get help immediately.

☐ Take _____

☐ Call _____

Danger! Get help immediately! Call 9-1-1 if you have trouble walking or talking due to shortness of breath or lips or fingernails are gray or blue.

FIGURE 2.8   Sample Asthma Action Plan

Asthma Camp

A number of states in the U.S. offer free, overnight asthma camps for children and adolescents who have asthma. Due to the severity of their asthma, many of these young people have not been able to attend overnight camps. Barriers to attendance at traditional camps include exposure to asthma triggers (e.g., lots of trees), lack of trained staff to oversee the medical management of the disease, and parental concerns about sending medically fragile children to camp. Asthma camps, however, are unique as they are staffed by trained pulmonologists, counselors, nurses, respiratory therapists, psychologists, and volunteers. During the camp, children engage in developmentally appropriate lessons that teach them that they can be in control of their asthma. They learn about what happens in the lungs during an asthma attack, about medication management, how to identify warning signs and symptoms of asthma, and how to put all of these tools together to promote asthma control. Often, a pediatric pulmonologist will also review their medications and adjust them as needed, and researchers collect data about the effectiveness of the information provided to help support that the camp is effectively teaching children about asthma. If you are interested in volunteering for an asthma camp, you can visit www.asthmacamp.org.

Asthma Video Games

The city of Lungtropolis is under attack by a mob of mucus, and it is your job to save the city! During the game, children learn how to become "asthma change agents" and control the mucus mob by identifying signs, symptoms, and triggers of asthma. This is an example of a fun, interactive way for children to learn about asthma management, all while in the comfort of their own homes. In one randomized control study, researchers found that children who played Lungtropolis had higher Asthma Control Test scores, asthma knowledge scores, and self-efficacy. Lungtropolis is funded by the American Lung Association and can be downloaded for free at www.lungtropolis.com.

The Controlling Asthma in American Cities Project (CAACP)

The Controlling Asthma in American Cities Project was designed to extend traditional medical services to communities and households in underserved communities with high asthma morbidity.[21] This program is an example of taking evidence-based asthma interventions, adapting them in culturally appropriate ways, and integrating them into the communities. Seven U.S. cities took part in the project, and in each city doctor's offices, schools, daycares, pest control companies and pharmacies joined forces to offer asthma education to children and families. This project is an example of a multi-disciplinary approach to help solve a complex problem!

Clean Air Act

At a national and global level, lawmakers enacted the Clean Air Act that sets air quality standards regulated by the Environmental Protection Agency (EPA). The overarching goal of the Clean Air Act is to regulate smog, soot, and other air toxins released by industry and automobiles into the air. These regulations must be enacted at a national level, as air pollution crosses state borders. Although progress has been made to clean up the air, large industry has challenged the courts to weaken regulations for dirty power plants, oil refineries, and other polluting facilities. At the writing of this book (2016), the future of the EPA is also questionable. Regardless of our political structure, change-makers must continue to fight to protect the air, which will undoubtedly affect the quality of lung functioning.

Conclusion

Asthma is a complex disease influenced by a number of factors, most broadly including genetics and the environment. Asthma is a chronic condition that never goes away. Thus, the goal is to control asthma symptoms by knowing the symptoms, staying away from triggers, and adhering to medications. However, a number of socioeconomic and environmental factors may interfere with the ability to achieve asthma control. To help promote healthy lung functioning, it is important to have a comprehensive understanding of how one's biology, environment, and beliefs about medications interact to influence the presence of asthma symptoms. Health care providers, community agencies and families must all collaborate to promote optimal asthma management.

Case Study

Amy is a 65-year-old, white, retired woman. As a child, Amy was diagnosed with breathing problems but did not receive a formal asthma diagnosis. As a child, she would experience bouts of wheezing, coughing, and difficulty breathing, especially when she was sick. As Amy entered into her late teens, she "outgrew" her asthma and did not experience any asthma-type symptoms for many years. However, Amy continues to recognize the symptoms of asthma, as her six-year-old grandson was diagnosed with the disease two years ago. At the age of 64, Amy became very alarmed when she began having difficulty breathing and began wheezing. She thought it was due to a respiratory illness that she caught from one of her grandchildren. It could not possibly be that her asthma was returning after 50 years? No way—she was always told that people outgrow asthma!

Her physician confirmed that she was experiencing asthma. Her childhood symptoms had reappeared. She worked with her physician to figure out what medications worked for her and what lifestyle changes would help keep her symptoms from flaring. This was an isolating time for Amy. Her husband passed away two years ago, and all of her children lived outside the home. Her main sources of company were her cat and dog, but unfortunately, allergy testing showed that Amy had allergies to both, and she was advised to give them up for adoption. She could not bring herself to do that, though.

Amy was prescribed a Ventolin inhaler and a long-term controller medication in pill form. Amy finds the pill much easier to take, although she reported that she forgets to take it a few times per week. Amy reported that it is difficult to take the "puffer" with her arthritic hands. Amy gets wheezy only a few times per week and thinks that is "good enough," even though on those days she is unable to leave the house and see her grandchildren.

Notes

1 Asthma Statistics. Retrieved January 16, 2017, from http://www.aaaai.org/about-aaaai/newsroom/asthma-statistics

2 Barnett, S.B. & Nurmagambetov, T.A. (2011). Costs of asthma in the United States: 2002–2007. *Journal of Allergy and Clinical Immunology, 127*(1): 145–152. doi: 10.1016/j.jaci.2010.10.020

3 What is asthma? (2014, August 4). Retrieved January 16, 2017, from https://www.nhlbi.nih.gov/health/health-topics/topics/asthma

4 The Asthma and Allergy Foundation of America, (2005, January). *Ethnic disparities in the burden and treatment of asthma* (Rep.). Retrieved January 16, 2017, from http://www.aafa.org/media/Ethnic-Disparities-Burden-Treatment-Asthma-Report.pdf

5 Ledogar, R. J., Penchaszadeh, A., Garden, C. C., & Garden, I. (2000). Asthma and Latino cultures: different prevalence reported among groups sharing the same environment. *American Journal of Public Health, 90*(6), 929.

6 Ober, C., & Hoffjan, S. (2006). Asthma genetics 2006: The long and winding road to gene discovery. *Genes and Immunity, 7*(2), 95–100.

7 Lara, M., Akinbami, L., Flores, G., & Morgenstern, H. (2006). Heterogeneity of childhood asthma among Hispanic children: Puerto Rican children bear a disproportionate burden. *Pediatrics, 117*(1), 43–53.

8 Molis, M. A., & Molis, W. E. (2010). Exercise-induced bronchospasm. *Sports Health, 2*(4), 311–317. http://doi.org/10.1177/1941738110373735

9 McQuaid, E. L., Kopel, S. J., Klein, R. B., & Fritz, G. K. (2003). Medication adherence in pediatric asthma: reasoning, responsibility, and behavior. *Journal of Pediatric Psychology, 28*(5), 323–333.

10 Taras, H., & Potts-Datema, W. (2005). Childhood asthma and student performance at school. *Journal of School Health, 75*(8), 296–312.

11 Asthma Statistics. Retrieved January 16, 2017, from http://www.aaaai.org/about-aaaai/newsroom/asthma-statistics

12 Greenhawt, M. J. (2014). Influenza vaccination in asthmatic patients. *Journal of Allergy and Clinical Immunology, 133*(4), 1233.

13 McQuaid, E. L., Walders, N., Kopel, S. J., Fritz, G. K., & Klinnert, M. D. (2005). Pediatric asthma management in the family context: The family asthma management system scale. *Journal of Pediatric Psychology, 30*(6), 492–502.

14 Kuehn, B. (2008). Asthma linked to psychiatric disorders. *JAMA, 299*,158–160.

15 Scott, K.M., Von Korff, M., Ormel, J., Zhang, M., Bruffaerts, R., Alonso, J., Kessler, R. C., Tachimori, H., Karam, E., Levinson, D., Bromet, E. J., Posada-Villa, J., Gasquet, I., Angermeyer, M. C., Borges, G., de Girolamo, G., Herman, A., Haro, J.M. (2007). Mental disorders among adults with asthma: Results from the World Mental Health Survey. *General Hospital and Psychiatry, 29*, 129–133.

16 Katon, W.J., Richardson, L., Lozano, P., & McCauley, E. (2004). The relationship of asthma and anxiety disorders. *Psychosomatic Medicine, 66*, 349–355.

17 McQuaid, E. L., Kopel, S. J., Klein, R. B., & Fritz, G. K. (2003). Medication adherence in pediatric asthma: Reasoning, responsibility, and behavior. *Journal of Pediatric Psychology, 28*(5), 323–333.

18 Brand, P. L. P. (2001). Inhaled corticosteroids reduce growth. Or do they? *European Respiratory Journal, 17*(2), 287–294.

19 Albuterol Oral Inhalation. (2016, February 15). Retrieved January 16, 2017, from https://med-lineplus.gov/druginfo/meds/a682145.html

20 Well, D. (2010). Asthma Action Plan. *Nursing Standard, 28*(36).

21 Herman, E. J. (2011). Conceptual framework of the controlling asthma in American cities project. *Journal of Urban Health: Bulletin of the New York Academy of Medicine, 88*(Suppl 1), 7–15. http://doi.org/10.1007/s11524-010-9473-1

Figure Sources

1 Figure 2.1: Source: https://upload.wikimedia.org/wikipedia/commons/4/4a/Asthma_attack-illustration_NIH.jpg.

2 Figure 2.2: Copyright © 7mike5000 (CC BY-SA 3.0) at https://commons.wikimedia.org/wiki/File:Asthma_triggers_2.PNG.

3 Figure 2.3: Source: https://commons.wikimedia.org/wiki/File:Blatella_germanica_(German_cockroach).jpg.

4 Figure 2.4: Source: https://pixabay.com/p-989500/?no_redirect.

5 Figure 2.5: Source: https://commons.wikimedia.org/wiki/File:Seretide250.jpg.

6 Figure 2.6: Source: https://commons.wikimedia.org/wiki/File:Treating_Kids_with_Asthma.jpg.

7 Figure 2.7: Source: https://commons.wikimedia.org/wiki/File:Two_Peak_Flow_Meters.jpg.

8 Figure 2.8: Copyright © HealDove (CC BY-SA 2.5) at https://commons.wikimedia.org/wiki/File:Asthma_action_plan.jpg.

CHAPTER THREE

Obesity

Coauthors:
Lindsay Hylek, B.A., Sue K. Adams, Ph.D., Sarah W. Feldstein Ewing, Ph.D.

@ObesitySociety

Although some argue that the obesity epidemic stems from a lack of individual self-control, research demonstrates that obesity is far more complex than any one factor. Biological, psychological, social, cultural, and community-specific factors drive the obesity epidemic. In this chapter, we will explore how these factors interact and contribute to the obesity epidemic in the United States.

What Is Obesity?

Defining Overweight and Obesity—Body Mass Index (BMI)

The WHO defines overweight and obesity as "abnormal or excessive fat accumulation that presents a risk to health."[1] Body mass index (BMI), a person's weight in kilograms (kg) divided by his or her height in meters squared (m^2), is a commonly used screening tool for unhealthy levels of body fat. Adults fall within the overweight range if their BMI is between 25.0 and 29.9 and obesity range if their BMI is above 30. Unlike adults, child and adolescent BMIs are calculated using an age- and sex-specific percentile for both weight and height–for example, a girl's weight would be compared to other girls her age, and she would be assigned a percentile score. Children and adolescents are considered overweight if their BMI is between the 85th and 95th percentile for youths of the same age and sex. They are considered obese if their BMI is at or above the 95th percentile.[2]

Although BMI is a useful and simplistic measure, it is not a formal measure of body fatness, which may vary depending on individual factors such as bone or muscle mass. For example, at their peak fitness level, Tom Cruise (BMI=26) and

Obesity and Body Mass Index (BMI)

$$BMI = \frac{weight\ (kg)}{height\ (m^2)}$$

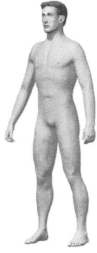 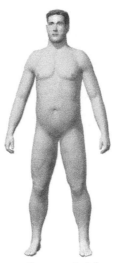 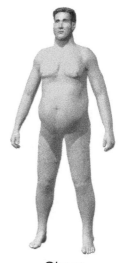

Normal
<25 kg/m²

Overweight
25 – 29 kg/m²

Obese
≥ 30 kg/m²

FIGURE 3.1   Illustrations of BMI Categories

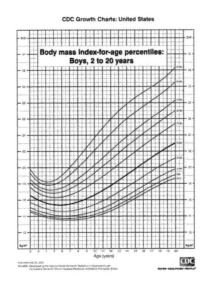

FIGURE 3.2   BMI percentiles for boys

George Clooney (BMI=29) were considered overweight and Arnold Schwarzenegger (BMI=33) and Dwayne "The Rock" Johnson (BMI=33) were considered obese.[3] Thus, some people argue that body fat percentage, as well as other markers like waist circumference, should be used to categorize weight status. However, BMI data is easy to collect and allows for population comparisons, which is why large organizations like the National Institute of Health (NIH) have adopted it as a standard measure. More accurate measures of body fat exist, although they require more training and have higher costs associated with their use. Examples include skin fold calipers (which uses calipers to pinch and measure body fat), hydrostatic weighing (which uses water displacement to measure body fat), and machines such as the BOD POD® (which uses air displacement to determine body fat versus lean muscle).

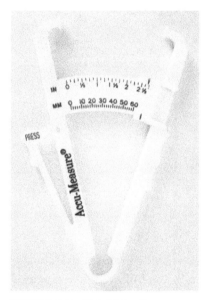

FIGURE 3.3   **Skinfold calipers**

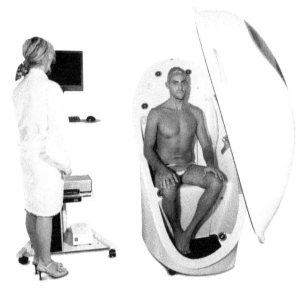

FIGURE 3.4   **BOD POD (Air Displacement)**

The Obesity Epidemic: Worldwide and U.S. Obesity Trends

Obesity is largely preventable, yet millions of people suffer from it worldwide. According to the WHO, about 1.9 billion adults, or 39% of the world's adult population, were overweight in 2014. Of these, about 600 million adults, or 13% of the world's adult population, were obese.[4] Overall, the global prevalence of adult obesity doubled between 1980 and 2014. In the United States alone, roughly 155 million adults, or 69% of the U.S. adult population, were overweight as of 2012. Of these, roughly 79 million adults, or 35% of the U.S. adult population, were obese. Approximately 24 million children and adolescents, or 32% of the U.S. pediatric population, were overweight. Of these, approximately 13 million children and adolescents, or 17% of the U.S. pediatric population, were obese.[5] Alarmingly, between 1990 and 2010, the number of overweight and obese preschool children increased by 60%.[6] Such dramatic increases within a relatively short period of time prompted a swift response to what has been termed the "obesity epidemic" in the United States and beyond.

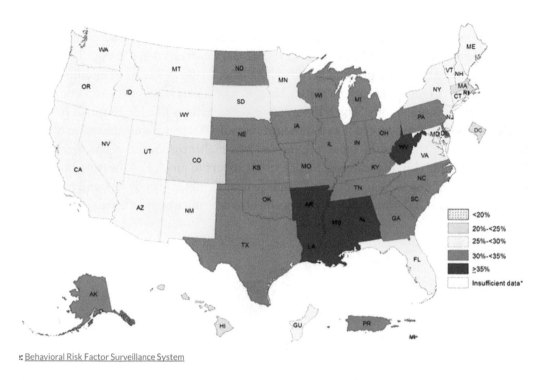

FIGURE 3.5   Prevalence of self-reported obesity among U.S. adults by state (BRFSS, 2014–2016)

Health Disparities in Obesity

Adult obesity is more prevalent among certain racial and ethnic groups; non-Hispanic blacks have the highest age-adjusted rates of obesity at 47.8%, followed by Hispanics at 42.5%, non-Hispanic whites at 32.6%, and non-Hispanic Asians at 10.8%. Childhood and adolescent obesity is most common among Hispanics at 22.4%, followed by non-Hispanic blacks at 20.2%, non-Hispanic whites at 14.1%, and non-Hispanic Asians at 8.6%.[7] According to the 2013 Youth Risk Behavior Surveillance System, 11.3% of black youth and 9.3% of Latino youth did not eat vegetables during the week compared to 4.5% of white youth. African Americans were also 70% less likely to engage in physical activity than Caucasians.[8] Thus, it becomes much more difficult for African Americans and Hispanics to achieve a healthy energy balance between calories consumed and energy expended.

Healthy People 2020: Goals for Decreasing Obesity Rates

Healthy People 2020 set forth 30 specific objectives which aim to "promote health and reduce chronic disease risk through the consumption of healthful diets and achievement and maintenance of healthy body weights [and] improve health, fitness, and quality of life through daily physical activity."[9] The overarching goal is simple: If Americans

Prevalence of Self-Reported Obesity Among Non-Hispanic White Adults by State and Territory, BRFSS, 2014-2016

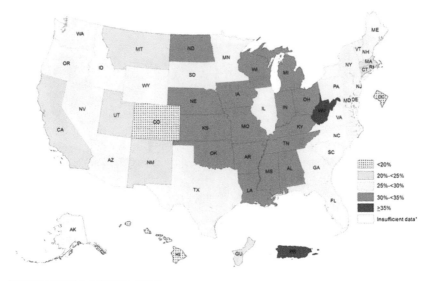

Source: Behavioral Risk Factor Surveillance System

FIGURE 3.6 **Prevalence of self-reported obesity among non-Hispanic White adults by state (BRFSS, 2014–2016)**

Prevalence of Self-Reported Obesity Among Non-Hispanic Black Adults by State and Territory, BRFSS, 2014-2016

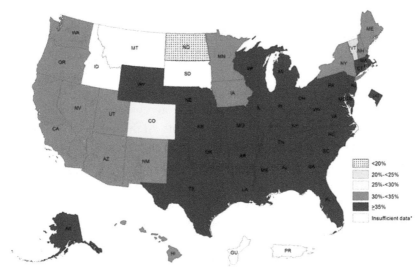

Source: Behavioral Risk Factor Surveillance System

FIGURE 3.7 **Prevalence of self-reported obesity among non-Hispanic Black adults by state (BRFSS, 2014–2016)**

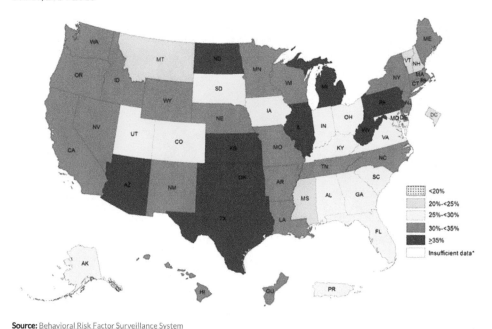

Prevalence of Self-Reported Obesity Among Hispanic Adults by State and Territory, BRFSS, 2014-2016

	<20%
	20%-<25%
	25%-<30%
	30%-<35%
	≥35%
	Insufficient data*

Source: Behavioral Risk Factor Surveillance System

FIGURE 3.8   **Prevalence of self-reported obesity among Hispanic adults by state (BRFSS, 2014–2016)**

are more active and eat nutrient-rich foods, there will be less disease morbidity and mortality across multiple diseases including heart disease and cancer, among others. This is why increasing physical activity and nutrition are among Healthy People 2020's top goals.

As of 2014, a progress review revealed a significant decrease in the consumption of added sugars, that more adults were engaged in leisure-time aerobic activity, and that recreational computer use had declined among high school students. At the same time, weight status data for children, adolescents, and adults showed little or no change; total vegetable consumption showed little to no change; disparities persisted in weight status by age, race, and income as well as food and nutrient consumption by age, sex, race, and income; and obesity prevalence was higher among non-Hispanic black, Hispanic, and lower-income populations.[10] Although there is some reason to be optimistic, the reality is that since Healthy People first began, obesity has steadily increased. Despite large-scale efforts, obesity remains a major national public health issue in the United States.

Obesity Classified as a Disease
In 2013, the American Medical Association voted in favor of classifying obesity as a disease. At the time, a lot of controversy surrounded whether or not obesity should be classified as

a medical condition that needs treatment. Specifically, experts in the field took issue with the implication that the body is malfunctioning. In the article "Is Obesity a Disease?" David L. Katz, MD, MPH made the analogy of drowning to illustrate this argument:

> We don't, for instance, label drowning a disease. It is, clearly, a legitimate medical condition worthy of treatment and insurance coverage. But the fault lies with the situation, not with ourselves—in the sense that human bodies are simply not adapted to spend too much time under water.
>
> Obesity is the same. It is rampant in the modern world not because of changes in our bodies, but because of changes in the modern world. The causes are all around us; we are drowning in them! We are drowning in excess calories and labor-saving technologies.
>
> My preference would be to catalog obesity as a form of drowning—in calories rather than water—because that would combine medical legitimacy with an appropriate focus on the environmental causes. To appreciate the danger of calling it a disease: consider an effort to develop drugs to treat drowning, rather than focusing on fences, lifeguards, and swimming lessons.[11]

Many professionals agreed with Dr. Katz, asserting that adopting a healthy lifestyle can reverse obesity. Individuals in this camp argued that obesity is not a disease but a precondition for diseases.

Those in favor of classifying obesity as a disease believed that the pros outweighed the cons. They believed that classifying obesity as a disease would be a way of increasing its legitimacy and, thus, lead to a number of positive outcomes. Insurance coverage is one benefit; not only would the classification help obese people defer costs associated with obesity, but it would also help health care providers get reimbursed for preventative measures, such as counseling patients on making lifestyle changes, as well as treatment. Furthermore, the vote would encourage public policymakers, as well as public and private funders, to expand access to resources. The hope was that the classification would decrease stereotyped perceptions and reduce stigmatization of obesity.

Causes of Overweight and Obesity

Two-thirds of adults and one-third of children and adolescents are overweight in the United States, which raises the question, how did the obesity epidemic happen? What factors contribute to weight gain? Obesity is fundamentally caused by an energy imbalance between calories consumed and expended.[12] However, there are other biopsychosocial factors that contribute to its cause.

Biological Factors

Family history is a major determinant of weight. Studies have shown that children of overweight parents have an 80% chance of being overweight as well.[13] Although the nature versus nurture debate applies, the research is clear that genetic factors play an important role in obesity. Research on identical twins who were raised apart has shown that overweight and obesity tend to run in families. One reason is that genes predispose individuals to gain weight, even when they consume an appropriate number of calories. Genes can also affect the amount of fat stored and where extra fat is carried on the body.[14] Endocrine abnormalities, such a thyroid malfunction or hyperfunctioning of the adrenal gland, can lead to obesity as well. An underactive thyroid is a condition in which the thyroid gland does not make enough thyroid hormone. This lack of thyroid hormones slows down the metabolism and

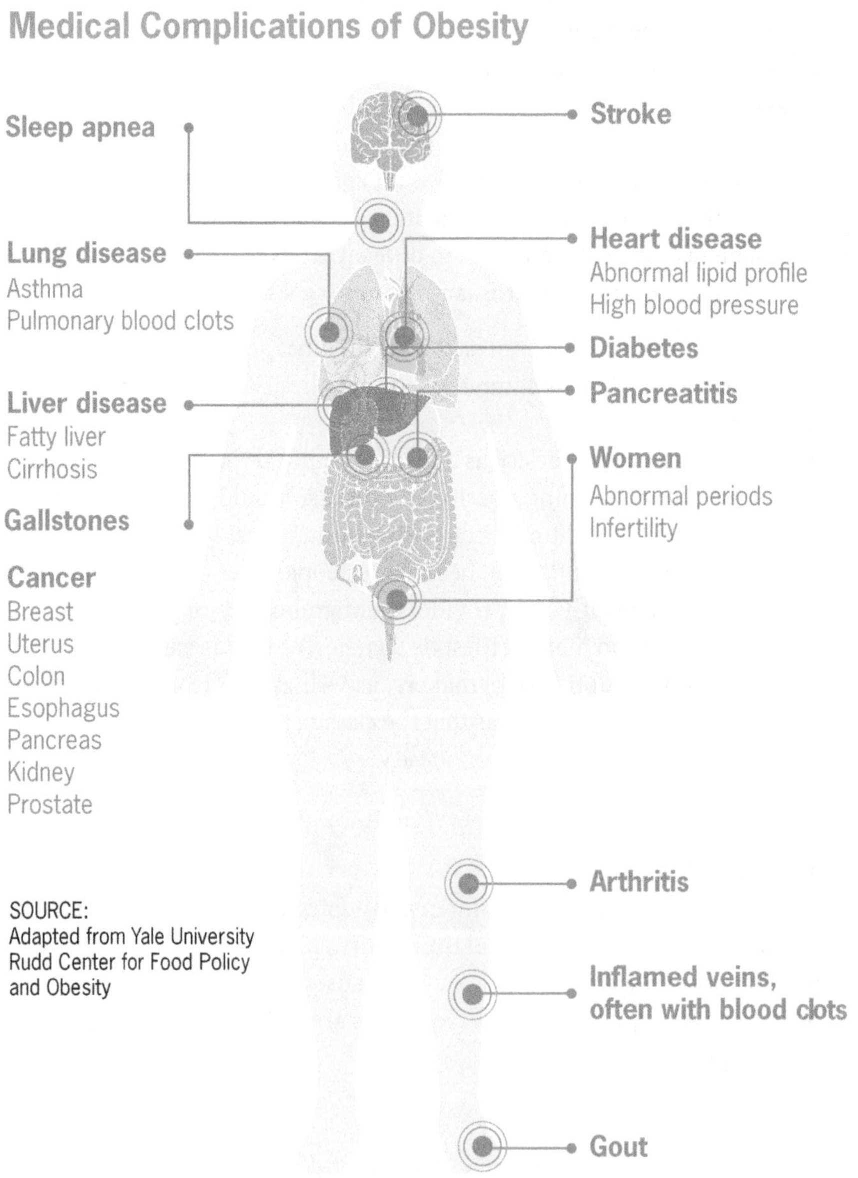

Medical Complications of Obesity

Sleep apnea

Stroke

Lung disease
Asthma
Pulmonary blood clots

Heart disease
Abnormal lipid profile
High blood pressure

Diabetes

Liver disease
Fatty liver
Cirrhosis

Pancreatitis

Gallstones

Women
Abnormal periods
Infertility

Cancer
Breast
Uterus
Colon
Esophagus
Pancreas
Kidney
Prostate

SOURCE:
Adapted from Yale University
Rudd Center for Food Policy
and Obesity

Arthritis

Inflamed veins,
often with blood clots

Gout

FIGURE 3.9   Medical complications associated with Obesity

increases fatigue, which causes weight gain. Cushing's syndrome is a condition in which the body's adrenal glands make too much of the hormone cortisol. Excess cortisol leads to weight gain, resulting in excess upper-body fat with thinner arms and legs. Polycystic Ovary Syndrome (PCOS) is another health condition that has been linked with overweight and obesity and affects 5 to 10% of women of childbearing age. With PCOS, high levels of androgen hormones (e.g., estrogen and testosterone) lead to weight gain, excess hair growth, and reproductive issues.[15] Apart from the medical causes of obesity, prescription medication can also contribute to weight gain by increasing appetite. These drugs include corticosteroids, female hormone treatments, antidepressants and anti-psychotic drugs, and insulin and insulin-stimulating drugs. Overall, biological factors may play a part in 70 to 80% of obesity cases.[16]

Psychological Factors

If an individual has a family history of mental illness, he or she may be genetically predisposed to develop one as well. Mental disorders, such as depression and anxiety, often make it more difficult to maintain an exercise routine and control food consumption. For instance, people with Major Depression Disorder generally find it difficult to get out of bed in the morning, let alone motivate themselves to exercise. Moreover, overeating has an emotional component, which is where the expression "eat your feelings" originates. When negative emotions—such as sadness, loneliness, stress, anger, fear, or boredom—arise, some individuals cope with these feelings with food. Whether the process is conscious or subconscious, it can become an ingrained compulsion. For example, emotions may be so closely tied to eating habits that people automatically reach for comforting sweet or savory food without thinking about it. This habit can lead to an unhealthy cycle where negative emotions trigger overeating, overeating causes feelings of guilt and shame, and these new negative emotions trigger overeating once again.

Mental illness may promote excessive weight gain, and/or obesity may induce psychopathology. The stigmatization of obesity in our society perpetuates this phenomenon. Overweight individuals often internalize stereotypes, such as "fat people are lazy," and suffer from low self-esteem, putting themselves at risk for mood disorders or substance abuse.[17] Fortunately, support systems, like supportive families, serve as protective mechanisms against psychological stressors. Family has been shown to alleviate stress, increase self-confidence and feelings of value, and decrease feelings of loneliness and isolation among individuals. Building a strong support system can foster positive mental health to protect individuals against weight gain and vice versa.

Societal Factors

Although genetics play an important role in the development of obesity, family *environment* is said to have a stronger influence on weight in most cases.[18] Why? Children adopt their parent's behavior from the day they are born, and eating patterns are usually engrained in children by the time they are preschool aged. If parents model proper nutrition and fitness practices, then their children are more likely to overcome their genetic predisposition for weight gain. According to weight-loss specialists, small changes in the household go a long way. For example, experts claim that removing high-fat and high-sugar foods from the kitchen and replacing them with fruits, vegetables, and other healthy snack food leads to better food choices. In addition, simply sitting down to eat meals as a family at home is said to facilitate mindful eating and help prevent weight gain. In terms of healthy exercise habits, parents are encouraged to plan activities like family nature walks and limit sedentary activity like watching television. However, creating a supportive home environment is not easy, especially for parents who struggle to eat right and exercise. Breaking bad habits and adopting new lifestyle changes, no matter how small, is difficult but so important.

Overweight and Obesity Across Development
Children and Adolescents
While some children experience physical consequences of obesity, the most widespread consequences are psychosocial. At an early age, obese children become targets of discrimination. Cultural stereotypes are a driving force of this phenomenon. Studies show that children as young as six have already internalized negative stereotypes associated with overweight and obesity, such as laziness and sloppiness.[19] Another driving force of this bullying is society's preoccupation with thinness, which is predominant in preteens on the verge of adolescence. One study revealed that 10-to-11-year-old girls and boys ranked overweight peers the lowest when asked who they would prefer to be friends with. In fact, they preferred peers with a variety of disabilities over "fat peers."[20] Despite the negative connotations of obesity, overweight children do not usually develop low self-esteem until adolescence.[21] Acquiring negative self-image at such an impressionable time in the lifespan has lingering effects.[22] Obese adolescents are far more likely to become obese adults and continue to be at risk, both psychologically and socially.

Children and adolescents with BMIs at the overweight and obese level are at risk for mental health disorders and other psychological, as well as social, complications. These include, but are not limited to depression; anxiety; substance use disorders; low quality of life; low self-esteem; feelings of worthlessness or inferiority; body dissatisfaction; disordered eating and unhealthy weight-control behaviors; peer victimization; negative stereotyping, stigmatization, and teasing; fewer friends; behavior problems; poor concentration levels; poor academic performance; and school absenteeism.[23] Children also suffer from obesity-related health conditions such as type 2 diabetes, atherosclerosis (plaque buildup in the arteries), dyslipidemia (high blood triglycerides and high cholesterol), high blood pressure, metabolic syndrome, gallbladder disease, liver disease, asthma, allergies, sleep apnea, sleep disordered breathing, orthopedic complications such as knee and joint pain, iron deficiency, early onset puberty, and poor health-related quality of life.[24]

Adults
For adults under the age of 70, obesity is second only to tobacco in the number of deaths caused per year in the United States.[25] BMIs at the overweight and obese level are a major

risk factor for a number of health conditions and other health complications at this stage in life. Obese adults are at risk for all of the medical conditions previously listed for children. In addition, they are at risk for heart disease, stroke, kidney disease, arthritis, chronic back pain, mobility limitations (e.g., pressure joints and limbs), up to 11 types of cancer (e.g., endometrial, breast, and colon cancers), reproductive complications (e.g., irregular periods and infertility), pregnancy-related complications (e.g., birth defects, gestational diabetes, and preeclampsia), increased risk of hospitalization, increased all-cause mortality, and premature death by up to nine years.[26] Consequently, the medical costs of obesity have exceeded $147 billion dollars per year, which is an additional $1,429 per year for obese versus average-weight individuals.[27] Although adults also experience many of the same psychosocial consequences as children and adolescents, obese adults also experience lower employment rates, lower salary, employer discrimination, work impairment, time away from work, lower chances of marriage, high chances of divorce, and disruption from work, family, and social life.[28]

Pregnancy

Obesity puts both women and babies at risk for several complications during pregnancy, childbirth, and post childbirth. During pregnancy, obesity increases the likelihood of the mother developing gestational diabetes, preeclampsia (high blood pressure that can lead to kidney or liver failure or stroke), blood clots, and sleep apnea. The developing fetus is also at increased risk for short- and long-term complications, such as heart and neural tube defects, preterm birth before 39 weeks of gestation, stillbirth (a heart wrenching situation in which a full-term baby dies in utero), and being born at a very large weight. Macrosomia increases the chances that the baby will get stuck in the birth canal or break collarbones at delivery. Although most pregnant women receive adequate monitoring during pregnancy, even diagnostic tests such as ultrasounds or monitoring the baby's heart rate can be harder to achieve when there is too much body fat on the abdomen. Women who are obese also tend to experience longer labors than women who are average weight and are at increased risk for needing a cesarean section. Because it may be harder to determine the proper place for the cesarean incision, complications from the surgery, such as severe infections and blood loss, are more likely, including severe infections and blood loss. These potential complications increase the cost of health care utilization and require mothers-to-be to exhibit higher levels of diligence in eating healthy, gaining less weight during pregnancy, and engaging in regular exercise.[29]

Older Adults

As human beings age, their metabolism slows down, and it becomes more difficult for individuals to lose weight. Older adults need to consume fewer calories and exercise more frequently than when they were younger to lose weight.[30] For people 65 and older, hormonal changes that occur during aging may cause fat accumulation. For example, aging is associated with decreases in hormone secretions, reduced responsiveness to thyroid hormones, declines in testosterone, and resistance to leptin (the hormone that makes you feel full).

Other physical consequences of aging, such as impaired vision or hearing, may make it more difficult for older adults to participate in weight-loss programs. In these cases, it is essential for family members and/or caregivers to participate in these programs as well. Furthermore, older adults may suffer psychologically from widowhood, loneliness, isolation, or depression, which can set back weight loss goals.[31] All things considered, if individuals are overweight or obese by the time they enter older adulthood, they are much more likely to maintain this status. At this stage, the life-threatening health problems associated with obesity begin to outweigh the nonfatal ones.

Family Functioning

Aspects of poor family functioning may include poor communication, poor behavior control, and high levels of family conflict. Poor family functioning is associated with increased risk of overweight and obesity in children and adolescents. In addition, children and adolescents who are already overweight or obese are more likely to come from poorly functioning families.[32] Family health is very important in establishing proper nutrition and exercise habits. However, some parents do not recognize when their children are overweight or even obese. A recent study revealed that 95% of parents of overweight boys and 93% of parents of overweight girls said that their kids were "about the right weight."[33] This misperception was most common among African-American and low-income parents. The issue here is that parents compare their children to peers, as opposed to medical standards, and draw the conclusion that they fall into a healthy weight range. Due to lack of awareness of childhood overweight and obesity, parents may not intervene when appropriate. It is particularly important that the obesity epidemic is approached through a family systems lens. It will be difficult for future generations to achieve and maintain a healthy weight if their primary role models are overweight or obese._

The Role of American Culture

A major obstacle for families looking to attain an ideal weight is that American culture as a whole does not support healthy lifestyle habits. In part, U.S. standards actually work against its citizens. Below we will discuss some cultural factors that impact the health of Americans.

Bigger Portions, More Calories

Some individuals point to increases in standard portion sizes as a leading cause of obesity. Food portions at American restaurants, fast food places, gas stations, movie theaters, and supermarkets have doubled or tripled since the 1970s.[34] At the same time, Americans are dining out more frequently; about 50% of meals are consumed outside of the home in the United States.[35] As a result, Americans consume more calories than they did in the past. To illustrate this point, suppose someone ate a bagel and a medium coffee with sugar and milk for breakfast, two pieces of pepperoni pizza and a large soda for lunch, and a chicken Caesar salad and a large soda for dinner. With today's portions, they would be consuming

1,595 more calories that day than if they ate the same meals 20 years ago. Over the course of one year, these larger portions could amount to more than 500,000 extra calories (which, by the way, is the equivalent of 2,400 donuts!).[36] Other examples of food-portion-size increases include hamburgers (by 23%), a plate of Mexican food (by 27%), soft drinks (by 52%), and snacks like potato chips, pretzels, and crackers (by 60%).[37] Researchers believe that food portions have been gradually getting larger due to "value sizing"; consumers want to get more food per dollar. Unfortunately, when people are served food to eat, they have a hard time listening to their bodies and stopping when they are no longer hungry. People are more likely to finish what they have in front of them than take part of their meal to-go. Thus, consumers get more for their dollar at the cost of their waistline.

Even for individuals who eat mostly home-cooked meals, restaurants become a problem when they distort consumers' perception of what is "normal." Consequently, parents may perpetuate childhood obesity through poor food choices and inaccurate conceptions of typical portion sizes. These misconceptions are especially problematic when considering the "clean-plate club." The idea behind the clean plate was invented during the Hoover era to discourage children from wasting food after World War I. Today, some parents still instruct their children to eat everything on their plate before leaving the table. However, this practice prevents children from noticing when they are full and listening to their bodies telling them to stop eating. As a result, children normalize overeating by consuming the entirety of the large portions in front of them.

Processed Foods: Fast, Cheap, and Unhealthy

In conjunction with larger quantities of food, the United States has also seen an increase in the consumption of processed foods over the past 20-plus years. Eating a whole-foods, plant-based diet is optimum for good health. However, Americans eat less than the recommended amount of whole grains, fruits, and vegetables. At the same time, they consume more than the recommended amount of meat, oils, added sweeteners, and refined grains.[38] Part of the problem is that the federal government provides large subsidies to crops like corn, soy, and wheat, which are used to feed factory-farmed animals or manufacture processed foods. This practice, in combination with the efficiency of the packaged food industry, keeps unhealthy, processed food cheap and limits the supply of affordable fruits and vegetables.

In addition to lower prices, processed foods have the added benefit of labor and time; they are easier and faster for the consumer to make. For instance, it is much more convenient for parents to purchase Kraft "Easy" Mac & Cheese and pop it in the microwave than buy ingredients for homemade whole-grain pasta with light cream sauce to cook at home. For busy parents, juggling the demands of work and home can make fast food an appealing choice.[39] Schools also struggle to feed students healthy food. Tight budgets force cafeteria workers to serve a great deal of food in a short period of time. Thus, processed food becomes an efficient, low-cost solution.

Another part of the problem lies in how processed food is marketed by the food industry. The food industry spends over $36 billion a year marketing food that is primarily unhealthy.

Children are often the targets of advertising for high-calorie, high-fat snacks and sugary drinks.[40] Ultimately, parents control the supply lines in that they decide which foods to buy and serve their children. However, it is difficult for parents to make the right food choices when their children pressure them to buy the nutrient-poor food advertised on television, or when those foods are strategically placed at "eye level" at the supermarket.[41] In order to teach children how to maintain a healthy weight, parents must hold the line when it comes to processed food.

A major issue here is that processed foods, like macaroni and cheese, are not only nutrient-scarce, but also contain a number of harmful ingredients. Instead of pasta, cheese, butter, and milk—all you need to make macaroni and cheese—Kraft "Easy" Mac & Cheese contains 22 ingredients including MSG, palm oil, artificial colors, and preservatives. Some say that these additives make processed food addicting, have adverse effects on activity and attention in children, increase the risk of kidney disorders, and more.[42] Unlike Europe, which requires companies to put warning signs on products with ingredients such as food dye, the U.S. Food and Drug Administration (FDA) is less strict on food labeling. Part of the issue is that the FDA is under-funded and does not have the resources to test questionable ingredients.[43] Another part of the problem is that government organizations, like the U.S. Department of Agriculture (USDA), have conflicts of interest because they are tied to American food and drug industries.[44]

Inactive Lifestyle

Many Americans are not very physically active. Why? With the invention of electronic devices like televisions, computers, and video games, as well as convenience devices like remote controls, washing machines, and dishwashers, Americans started leading much more sedentary lifestyles than their parents and grandparents. Leisure activities like binge-watching shows have taken the place of activities like playing basketball with friends. As a result, people are not burning enough calories to maintain or lose weight. In fact, more than two hours a day of regular television viewing has been linked to overweight and obesity.[45] Moreover, certain luxuries have become so normalized that people forget that they have alternative options. For example, some people have become so dependent on cars that they drive even if their destination is less than a half-mile away. Once again, children look to their parents as role models and adopt their behavior. If parents drive to and from their desk job to come home and watch television, then their children will probably end up doing the same.

Not only are people less active at home but also at work and school. With modern technology, many American adults have fewer physical demands at work. To make matters worse, people often say that they do not have time for physical activity because of long work hours and time spent commuting. As for American children, no federal law requires physical education in schools. Lack of funding led to cuts in physical education classes and recess, limiting the amount of energy children expend during the school day.[46] Indeed, motivating children, adolescents, and adults alike is an uphill battle in today's society.

Lower Incomes and Food Insecurity

Of the ten states with the highest obesity rates, nine rank among the nation's poorest.[47] Wealth inequality contributes to the prevalence of obesity in black and Latino communities where a disproportionate number of families live below the poverty line. For every two dollars that Caucasians make, African-Americans and Hispanics make one dollar. With such limited monetary resources, low-income populations often face food insecurity resulting in a lack of resources to secure access to adequate food. Indeed, one in four African-American and Hispanic families are food insecure.[48] While food insecurity and obesity are strongly correlated in some studies, they are not necessarily causally linked with one another. Nevertheless, food insecurity can make it even more difficult to secure access to affordable, healthy food. Thus, the impoverished are not only subject to the same cultural changes as other American families (e.g., increased portion sizes and sedentary lifestyles) but also face unique challenges that come with poverty.[49]

"Soul Food" and the Legacy of Slavery in America

Slavery plays a historical role in eating patterns for African Americans, which explains, in part, why non-Hispanic blacks have the highest rates of obesity. Enslaved Africans worked from dawn until dusk, burning as many as 3,000 calories per day, and yet they received inadequate food from slave owners. For example, some slaves were only provided a pack of corn meal and a half pound of salted pork weekly. As a result, slaves retaliated by supplementing their diets with food they hunted or grew themselves, such as crab meat or okra. Through cooking, African Americans were able to reclaim some of their unique culture. Even after slavery was abolished, African Americans took pride in turning survival food into delicacies by seasoning it, battering it, frying it, etc. Examples include BBQ ribs, grits and eggs, collard greens, ham hocks, corn bread, mac and cheese, black-eyed peas, and sweet potato pie. Overtime, this food began to hold significant weight in the black community as a unifying force. During the Black Power movement, the term "soul food" emerged to describe what had become traditional African-American cuisine. Since then, soul food has also been described as "comfort food" because it is said to make people feel good (emotionally, not physically). Many individuals used this comfort food as a coping mechanism throughout the history of nlack marginalization in American society.

Fewer Supermarkets

As previously mentioned, food insecurity makes it difficult for poor families to consume an adequate amount of nutritious food. However, other factors contribute to this phenomenon as well. There are fewer supermarkets, farmers' markets and healthy food options in predominately minority, low-income neighborhoods. By definition, these areas are called "food deserts" because they systemically lack healthy options. At the same time, these areas have a greater availability of fast food restaurants, especially near schools.[50] In fact, only 8% of black families live in communities with one or more supermarkets compared to 31% of white families.[51] Latino families have one-third the number of supermarkets as non-Latino neighborhoods.[52] As a result, it is more difficult for residents to buy high-quality fruits, vegetables, whole grains, and low-fat dairy products.

Unreliable Transportation

Another reason that families with lower incomes struggle to eat a balanced diet is lack of reliable transportation. According to the USDA, "vehicle access is perhaps the most important determinant of whether or not a family can access affordable and nutritious food."[53] Poverty-stricken families are less likely to have their own vehicle to use for regular food shopping. Regular purchases become restricted to whatever someone can carry on foot or public transit, or parents are confined to one large, monthly shopping trip with a friend or family member who owns a car. Subsequently, food choices are limited to nonperishable items because transportation is too costly with regards to both time and money for these individuals.

Expensive Perishables

Lastly, when healthy food is available, low-income families can rarely afford it. Perishable items like fresh produce are much more expensive due to the potential for going bad quickly. Families need to maximize their calories per dollar, so instead they buy cheap, energy-dense food that will last for a long time but with less nutritional value. Calories per dollar is particularly important for families with more mouths to feed, and low-income families usually have more children than high-income families.[54] The result is overconsumption of foods with refined grains, added sugars, and high fat content. Often, parents will eat less or skip meals to stretch their budget, so they end up overeating when food does become available. These chronic ups and downs in food intake contribute to weight gain. Moreover, they can lead to disordered eating behaviors, an unhealthy preoccupation with food, and metabolic changes that promote fat storage.[55]

Media and Advertising

African-Americans and Hispanics are disproportionately exposed to more marketing for obesity-promoting products.[56] Specifically, these advertisements encourage the consumption of unhealthy foods (e.g., fast food and sugary beverages) and promote sedentary activity (e.g., television shows and video games). Disturbingly, children are often the target of these marketing efforts and highly susceptible to their ploys. According to one study, 71% of youth-targeted brands, like Pop Tarts, Doritos, and Skittles, focused on African-American and Latino communities.[57] Studies have shown that black children end up seeing twice as many calories advertised in food commercials as white children as a result[58] and are less likely to see ads for healthier foods like fruits, vegetables, yogurt, juice, and water than the general population.[59] Taken together, according to Jennifer Harris of the Rudd Center for Food Policy and Obesity at the University of Connecticut, "Black and Latino kids have higher rates of obesity. … If the [food] companies are purchasing more advertising in [ethnically] targeted media, then they could actually be contributing to the health disparities in these communities with their marketing practices."[60]

Less Green Space, More Danger

Neighborhoods with fewer public parks and recreation centers are largely occupied by African-American and Hispanic families, which becomes problematic when children without access to green space are at 20% to 45% greater risk of becoming overweight.[61] Parks that are available in lower-income neighborhoods often have fewer natural resources like grassy areas as well as more disrepair, trash, and noise. Limited access to resources makes it difficult to lead a physically active lifestyle. Furthermore, these communities often encounter safety concerns like heavy traffic or higher rates of criminal activity. The threat of violence decreases the amount of outdoor activity that African-American and Hispanic families engage in, and they are more likely to stay indoors and engage in sedentary activities like watching television or playing video games.[62]

The School Environment

Other factors that contribute to disparities in physical activity include lack of physical education classes and recess, as well as fewer organized sports. Children in lower-income communities spend even less time in physical education classes and recess than the general population. In addition, participating in organized sports is expensive with regards to both time and money and can be difficult to logistically coordinate. For parents who do not have reliable transportation, after-school activities become troublesome. Additionally, about 90% of students eat lunch at school, and 89.9% of parents believe that cafeteria food at their child's school is either very or somewhat healthy according to a recent USDA survey. However, 99% of American public schools participate in the National School Lunch program, and 94% of those schools failed to meet the USDA standard for healthy school meals. With children consuming 40 to 50% of their daily calorie intake at school, it is not surprising that increases in "junk" food availability in school correlated with the rise in pediatric obesity.[63]

The Role of Communities in Promoting Health and Wellness

Addressing Gaps in Obesity Prevention and Treatment

Obesity can be treated in many ways, including medical strategies such as gastric bypass and gastric-banding surgeries, and intensive behavioral health promotion strategies that promote weight loss and exercise. The State of Obesity released policy recommendations in its 2014 Special Report on Racial and Ethnic Disparities in obesity. The organization advocated for increased support at the federal, state, and local levels; partnering with black and Latino residents to determine priorities and develop culturally sensitive and sustainable solutions; financing to attract additional grocery stores with healthy food; limiting the amount of advertising of foods and beverages with low nutritional value; and more.[64] Below, we will discuss some of the federal, state, and local initiatives that are helping to put these recommendations into action.

Let's Move!

The Let's Move! initiative is an example of an intervention for elementary and middle school students to help parents and childcare providers meet weight-related guidelines. It started two years into Barack Obama's presidency, when Michelle Obama declared that decreasing the number of overweight children nationwide was her primary objective as First Lady. At the time, she asserted that "the physical and emotional health of an entire generation and the economic health and security of our nation is at stake."[65] In 2010, she launched the Let's Move! initiative, which targeted children as young as two years of age. The aims of Let's Move! included educating parents on modeling healthy lifestyle choices, providing healthier food in schools, increasing access to healthy, affordable food, and encouraging children to be physically active.

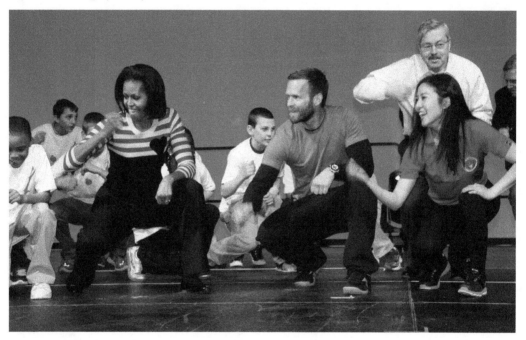

FIGURE 3.10   Michelle Obama and the "Let's Move!" initiative

Nationwide: SNAP and WIC

The Supplemental Nutrition Assistant Program (SNAP) was originally implemented by the Food and Nutrition Service branch of the USDA to address food insecurity back in the late 1930s.[66] It continues today, offering nutritional assistance to help low-income families gain access to more affordable, healthy food nationwide. In conjunction with SNAP-Ed, it also provides economic benefits to aid state agencies, nutrition educators, and community organizations in helping families make informed decisions about food choices. Similar to SNAP, the Women, Infants, and Children (WIC) program was executed by the USDA in the early 1970s to provide supplemental foods, health care referrals, and nutrition education to low-income mothers and their offspring who are at nutritional risk.[67] In 2012, 35%

of SNAP recipients were Caucasian, 23% were African-American, 15% were Hispanic, and 21% were classified as unknown.[68] In 2012, 41.5% of WIC recipients were Hispanic, regardless of race, and 19.8% were African-American.[69] As a result of these programs, the consumption of nutritious food increased among participants.

City-wide Initiatives

Individual cities and states have taken action against health discrepancies in obesity as well. For instance, the city of Philadelphia created strategies to increase access to healthy foods and physical activity by establishing a comprehensive, district-wide wellness policy, removing soda and sugar-sweetened drinks from public school vending machines, banning deep fryers and whole milk in school kitchens, enforcing calorie transparency on restaurant menus, and more. Their efforts lead to a 5% reduction in obesity rates among children in grades K through 12 with a 7.6% drop in obesity among African-American boys between 2006 and 2010.[70]

The city of Chicago created an initiative called Active Living Logan Square, which sponsors Open Streets events where roads are shut down to provide safe places for urban Hispanic communities to engage in physical activity. Part of the program's success has been attributed to the use of culturally competent social media by bilingual planners and community members.

New York City's Healthy Bodega Initiative recruited over 1,000 bodegas (small grocery stores usually in Hispanic communities) to increase low-fat milk, fruit, and vegetable availability and published promotional materials to encourage consumers to buy healthier products. Low-fat milk consumption increased by 45%, fruit by 32%, and vegetables by 26% at participating stores.[71]

Silver Lining: Healthy Hunger-Free Kids Act and 2015–2020 Dietary Guidelines

In 2010, Congress passed the Healthy Hunger-Free Kids Act, which instructed the USDA to develop higher nutrition standards for its core child-nutrition programs based on recommendations from the Institute of Medicine. This act allowed the USDA to make reforms to school breakfast and lunch programs for the first time in over 30 years.[72] Specifically, the USDA was instructed to double the amount of fruit served at breakfast; increase the quality of vegetables at lunch, including dark green and orange varieties; limit the amount of potatoes that can be served as a vegetable to twice per week; transition to whole grains after two years; reduce sodium in lunch by 53% over the course of ten years; reduce saturated fat to less than 10% of all calories served in a week; and require all chocolate milk to be fat-free. Although a spending bill blocked some of these requirements, overall the act was a major accomplishment for child nutrition.[73]

Another major breakthrough was the 2015–2020 edition of *Dietary Guidelines for Americans*. Every five years, the Dietary Guidelines Advisory Committee submits a scientific report summarizing the body of evidence on nutrition. For the first time, they recommended a whole-foods, plant-based diet high in vegetables, fruits, whole grains, low- or non-fat dairy, legumes, seafood, and nuts, and low in red and processed meats, sugar-sweetened

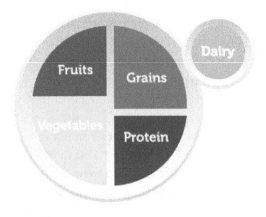

products, and refined grains.[74] This federally appointed panel of nutritional experts is highly influential and helps set standards for school lunches, subsidized food programs, and other programs for children and pregnant women. Thus, the panel's recommendations will help enact future policies to ensure Americans eat healthier than they have been to-date. The FDA also updated the Nutrition Facts label requirements for packaged foods in hopes that consumers would make informed decisions in accordance with the 2015–2020 Dietary Guidelines. By July 26, 2018, food manufacturers will be required to highlight calories per servings as well as calories per package to encourage moderation; remove calories from fat because the type of fat was found to be more important; adjust the serving size so it reflects the amount consumers actually eat; declare grams and percent daily value for added sugars (to help limit consumption) in addition to vitamin D and potassium (to help increase consumption); update daily values for nutrients like sodium, dietary fiber, and vitamin D consistent with the 2015–2020 Dietary Guidelines; and provide a more in-depth explanation of daily values in general.

Conclusion

In sum, the obesity epidemic is complex, and the interventions to create a healthier America need to be equally multifaceted. Personal accountability, health education, public policy, public health initiatives, and equitable communities for all are crucial steps in fighting obesity in America today.

Case Study

Benjamin is the first child of Annalise and Dimitri. When Benjamin was born, he weighed ten pounds, four ounces and was a happy, healthy baby boy. His mother, Annalise, worked at a job that did not guarantee paid maternity leave, so she continued working after childbirth. Due to her busy schedule, Annalise decided to formula feed Benjamin because breastfeeding proved too time-consuming. As Benjamin grew older, Annalise found that he was very food motivated. During his early childhood, Annalise would simply give Benjamin a snack whenever he was upset, and then he would stop crying. At the time, Annalise kept only healthy food in the house because she was trying to lose weight, so Benjamin ate healthy food as well. Benjamin's favorite snacks were pitted cherries, pears, yogurt, and bologna. By age six, Benjamin had two younger siblings, and it became more difficult for Annalise to afford whole foods. Benjamin started craving junk foods like fried chicken, potato chips, and juice that he saw advertised on television instead of his old favorites.

By age eight, his BMI jumped from the 85th percentile to the 95th percentile. During Benjamin's annual check-up, his pediatrician encouraged Annalise to pay closer attention to Benjamin's caloric intake and suggested she sign him up for a sport to increase his physical activity. Benjamin said that he would like to try lacrosse. At first, he thought it was fun, but he had a hard time keeping up with the other boys. One day during practice, Benjamin's teammate came up to him and asked, "Have you ever realized how fat you are?" Benjamin didn't answer and never returned to practice after that day. Throughout elementary and middle school, Benjamin continued to be bullied by his peers and struggled to make friends. Snacking on French fries and orange soda became a source of comfort when he came home from a stressful day at school. Benjamin started to neglect his studies and picked up video-gaming instead. By age 12, Benjamin's family had grown from a family of three to a family of seven. Annalise was struggling to maintain her own weight and simply did not have the time or energy to motivate Benjamin. Dimitri was barely ever home.

Then, at the beginning of his freshman year, the football coach came up to Benjamin during P.E. and asked him if he would ever consider joining the team. Benjamin declined, saying team sports were not for him, but the coach told Benjamin he thought he had serious potential as a defensive lineman. Benjamin was tired of feeling lonely, so he decided to try out. He struggled at first, just like in lacrosse, but the freshman football team was much more welcoming. He felt like he was making connections, which motivated him to keep working out. By his senior year, Benjamin was performing at a college level at six feet, five inches tall and 315 pounds. He still loved the calorie-dense foods served in the cafeteria, like buffalo chicken wings, nachos, and pizza, but he was exercising on a daily basis and felt good about himself for the first time. He established a community with his teammates, stopped playing videogames, and put more effort into his school work. When he graduated, he accepted a football scholarship at a Division 1 school. His family was very proud of him.

Everything was going well until the summer after his sophomore year when his best friend on the team died in a drunk-driving accident. Benjamin became clinically depressed and quit the team. Instead of conditioning in the weight room, he spent his free time isolated in his dorm room binging on junk food. Second semester of his junior year, Benjamin left school because he was doing so poorly. After treatment, he slowly reincorporated back into college life. Benjamin eventually graduated at age 22, weighing 400 pounds.

Although he struggled to find work at first, he ultimately landed a job at a manufacturing company. Benjamin befriended some of his co-workers and started playing basketball with them after work. He was slow but enjoyed feeling like he was part of something again. At 25, Benjamin was diagnosed with type 2 diabetes, hyperlipidemia, hypertension, and kidney disease. Benjamin took this news as a wake-up call and attempted to make some lifestyle changes. Benjamin exercised when he could but did not monitor his blood glucose levels or diet; old habits die hard. After six years, he started insulin, but often missed doses when he was out with his friends. On his 31st birthday, he went to the doctor to discover that his cholesterol was at a higher level, and he had a number of other obesity-related complications to add to the list. Sadly, at the age of 42, Benjamin passed away as a result of a massive heart attack.

Notes

1 Preamble to the Constitution of the World Health Organization as adopted by the International Health Conference, New York, 19–22 June, 1946; signed on 22 July 1946 by the representatives of 61 States (Official Records of the World Health Organization, no. 2, p. 100) and entered into force on 7 April, 1948.

2 Jensen, M. D., Ryan, D. H., Apovian, C. M., Ard, J. D., Comuzzie, A. G., Donato, K. A., ... & Loria, C. M. (2014). 2013 AHA/ACC/TOS guideline for the management of overweight and obesity in adults: A report of the American College of Cardiology/American Heart Association Task Force on Practice Guidelines and the Obesity Society. *Journal of the American College of Cardiology, 63*(25_PA).

3 Fight your bulge with brains. (n.d.). Retrieved January 19, 2017, from http://www.menscience.com/Fight-Your-Bulge-with-Brains-_ep_106.html

4 Obesity and overweight. (2016, June). Retrieved January 19, 2017, from http://www.who.int/mediacentre/factsheets/fs311/en/

5 Skelton, J. A., Cook, S. R., Auinger, P., Klein, J. D., & Barlow, S. E. (2009). Prevalence and trends of severe obesity among U.S. children and adolescents. *Academic Pediatrics, 9*(5), 322–329.

6 De Onis, M., Blössner, M., & Borghi, E. (2010). Global prevalence and trends of overweight and obesity among preschool children. *The American Journal of Clinical Nutrition, 92*(5), 1257–1264.

7 Childhood obesity facts. (2016, December 22). Retrieved January 19, 2017, from http://www.cdc.gov/obesity/data/childhood.html

8 Brener, N. D., Kann, L., Shanklin, S., Kinchen, S., Eaton, D. K., Hawkins, J., & Flint, K. H. (2013). Methodology of the youth risk behavior surveillance system—2013. *Morbidity and Mortality Weekly Report Recommendations and Reports* (Centers for Disease Control and Prevention), *62*(1), 1–20.

9 Healthy People 2020. (n.d.). Washington, DC: U.S. Department of Health and Human Services, Office of Disease Prevention and Health Promotion. Retrieved 10 January, 2017.

10 Koh, H. (2014, May 9). Healthy places, healthy people: A progress review on nutrition and weight status, & physical activity. Retrieved January 19, 2017, from https://www.cdc.gov/nchs/ppt/hp2020/hp2020_nws-and_hp_progress_review_presentation.pdf

11 Rossi, C. (2013, June 24). Is obesity a disease? *Prevention.* Retrieved January 19, 2017, from http://www.prevention.com/health/health-concerns/debate-obesity-disease

12 Mullin, G. E., Cheskin, L. J., & Matarese, L. E. (2014). *Integrative weight management: A guide for clinicians.* New York: Springer Science Business Media.

13 Lifshitz, F. (2008). Obesity in children. *Journal of Clinical Research in Pediatric Endocrinology, 1*(2), 53–60. http://doi.org/10.4008/jcrpe.v1i2.35

14 Woods, S. C., Schwartz, M. W., Baskin, D. G., & Seeley, R. J. (2000). Food intake and the regulation of body weight. *Annual Review of Psychology, 51*(1), 255–277.

15 Sam, S. (2007). Obesity and polycystic ovary syndrome. *Obesity Management, 3*(2), 69–73. http://doi.org/10.1089/obe.2007.0019

16 Obesity. (n.d.). Retrieved January 19, 2017, from http://www.healthcentral.com/obesity/encyclopedia/heart-disease-introduction-4003707/causes/

17 Collins, J. C., & Bentz, J. E. (2009). Behavioral and psychological factors in obesity. *The Journal of Lancaster General Hospital, 4*(4), 124–127.

18 Alfredo, M. J., Enriquez, L., Moreno-Aliaga M. J., Marti, A. (2009). Genetics of obesity. Public *Health Nutrition, 12*(1), 136.

19 Staffieri, J.R. (1967) A study of social stereotype of body image in children. *Journal of Personality and Social Psychology. 7*(1):101–104. Retrieved from http://pediatrics.aappublications.org/content/101/Supplement_2/518#ref-2

20 Richardson, S.A., Goodman, N., Hastorf, A.H., Dornbusch, S.M. (1961). Cultural uniformity in reaction to physical disabilities. *American Sociological Review. 26*:241–247. Retrieved from http://pediatrics.aappublications.org/content/101/Supplement_2/518#ref-1

21 Kaplan, K.M. and Wadden, T.A. (1986) Childhood obesity and self-esteem. *Journal of Pediatrics. 109*:367–370; Sallade, J. (1973) A comparison of the psychological adjustment of obese vs. non-obese children. *Journal of Psychometric Research. 17*:89–96. Retrieved from http://pediatrics.aappublications.org/content/101/Supplement_2/518#ref-8

22 Stunkard, A., and Burt, V. (1967). Obesity and the body image. II. Age at onset of disturbances in the body image. *American Journal of Psychiatry. 123*:1443–1447. Retrieved from http://pediatrics.aappublications.org/content/101/Supplement_2/518

23 Consequences of obesity. (n.d.). Retrieved January 19, 2017, from http://frac.org/initiatives/hunger-and-obesity/what-are-the-consequences-of-childhood-overweight-and-obesity/

24 Wallen, K.C., Reither, E.N., Haas, S.A., Meier, A.M. (2005). Overweight, obesity, and health-related quality of life among adolescents: the National Longitudinal Study of Adolescent Health. *Pediatrics. 115*:340–347.

25 Flegal, K. M., Williamson, D. F., Pamuk, E. R., & Rosenberg, H. M. (2004). Estimating deaths attributable to obesity in the United States. *American Journal of Public Health, 94*(9), 1486–1489.

26 Consequences of obesity. (n.d.). Retrieved January 19, 2017, from http://frac.org/initiatives/hunger-and-obesity/what-are-the-consequences-of-childhood-overweight-and-obesity/

27 Finkelstein, E. A,, Trogdon, J. G., Cohen JW, Dietz W. Annual medical spending attributable to obesity: payer- and service-specific estimates. *Health Aff (Millwood).* 2009; 28:w822–31.

28 Consequences of Obesity. (n.d.). Retrieved January 19, 2017, from http://frac.org/initiatives/hunger-and-obesity/what-are-the-consequences-of-childhood-overweight-and-obesity/

29 Ramachenderan, J., Bradford, J., & Mclean, M. (2008). Maternal obesity and pregnancy complications: a review. *Australian and New Zealand Journal of Obstetrics and Gynaecology, 48*(3), 228–235.

30 Haskell, W. L., Lee, I. M., Pate, R. R., Powell, K. E., Blair, S. N., Franklin, B. A., ... & Bauman, A. (2007). Physical activity and public health: Updated recommendation for adults from the American College of Sports Medicine and the American Heart Association. *Circulation, 116*(9), 1081.

31 Corpas, E., Harman, S., & Blackman, M. (1993). Human growth hormone and human aging. *Endocrinology Review, 14*, 20–39.

32 Halliday, J. A., Palma, C. L., Mellor, D., Green, J., & Renzaho, A.M. (2014). The relationship between family functioning and child and adolescent overweight and obesity: A systematic review. *International Journal of Obestetrics, 38*(4), 480–93.

33 Duncan, D. T., Hansen, A. R., Wang, W., Yan, F., & Zhang, J. (2015). Change in misperception of child's body weight among parents of American preschool children. *Childhood Obesity*, *11*(4), 384–393.

34 Portion Sizes and Obesity. (2013, February 13). Retrieved January 19, 2017, from http://www.nhlbi.nih.gov/health/educational/wecan/news-events/matte1.htm

35 Nutrition fact sheet. (2012, May). Retrieved January 19, 2017, from http://www.centerforfood-safety.org/files/nutrition_fact-sheet.pdf

36 Portion sizes and obesity. (2013, February 13). Retrieved January 19, 2017, from http://www.nhlbi.nih.gov/health/educational/wecan/news-events/matte1.htm

37 Rolls, B. J., Morris, E. L., & Roe, L. S. (2002). Portion size of food affects energy intake in normal-weight and overweight men and women. *The American Journal of Clinical Nutrition*, *76*(6), 1207–1213.

38 Nutrition fact sheet. (2012, May). Retrieved January 19, 2017, from http://www.centerforfood-safety.org/files/nutrition_fact-sheet.pdf

39 Nutrition fact sheet. (2012, May). Retrieved January 19, 2017, from http://www.centerforfood-safety.org/files/nutrition_fact-sheet.pdf

40 Nutrition fact sheet. (2012, May). Retrieved January 19, 2017, from http://www.centerforfood-safety.org/files/nutrition_fact-sheet.pdf

41 Cohen, D. A., & Babey, S. H. (2012). Contextual influences on eating behaviors: Heuristic processing and dietary choices. *Obesity Reviews: An Official Journal of the International Association for the Study of Obesity*, *13*(9), 766–779. http://doi.org/10.1111/j.1467–789X.2012.01001.x

42 Hari, V. (2014, November 19). Just because this Kraft food is "easy" doesn't mean you should eat it! Retrieved January 19, 2017, from http://foodbabe.com/2014/11/19/just-because-this-kraft-food-is-easy-doesnt-mean-you-should-eat-it/

43 Nutrition fact sheet. (2012, May). Retrieved January 19, 2017, from http://www.centerforfood-safety.org/files/nutrition_fact-sheet.pdf

44 McFarland, J. (2001). Insufficient FDA resources: Levelling the playing field and reducing fraud by altering incentives. Digital Access to Scholarship at Harvard. Retrieved from http://nrs.harvard.edu/urn-3:HUL.InstRepos:8852104

45 Klesges, R. C., Shelton, M. L., & Klesges, L. M. (1993). Effects of television on metabolic rate: Potential implications for childhood obesity. *Pediatrics*, *91*(2), 281–286.

46 Causes of obesity. (2012, July 13). Retrieved January 19, 2017, from http://www.nhlbi.nih.gov/health/health-topics/topics/obe/causes

47 The weight of the nation. (2012, May). *HBO*. Retrieved January 18, 2017, from http://theweigh-tofthenation.hbo.com/watch/main-films/Consequences

48 Wang, Y., & Beydoun, M. A. (2007). The obesity epidemic in the United States—gender, age, socioeconomic, racial/ethnic, and geographic characteristics: A systematic review and meta-regression analysis. *Epidemiologic Reviews*, *29*(1), 6–28; National health and nutrition examination survey. (2008). U.S. Department of Health and Human Services, Centers for Disease Control and Prevention, National Center for Health Statistics.

49 Understanding the connections: Food insecurity and obesity (Rep.). (2015, October). Retrieved January 18, 2017, from Food Research and Action Center website: http://frac.org/wp-content/uploads/frac_brief_understanding_the_connections.pdf

50 Understanding the connections: Food insecurity and obesity (Rep.). (2015, October). Retrieved January 18, 2017, from Food Research and Action Center website: http://frac.org/wp-content/uploads/frac_brief_understanding_the_connections.pdf

51 Wang, Y., & Beydoun, M. A. (2007). The obesity epidemic in the United States—gender, age, socioeconomic, racial/ethnic, and geographic characteristics: A systematic review and meta-regression analysis. *Epidemiologic Reviews*, *29*(1), 6–28; National health and nutrition examination survey. (2008). U.S. Department of Health and Human Services, Centers for Disease Control and Prevention, National Center for Health Statistics.

52 Wang, Y., & Beydoun, M. A. (2007). The obesity epidemic in the United States—gender, age, socioeconomic, racial/ethnic, and geographic characteristics: A systematic review and meta-regression analysis. *Epidemiologic reviews*, *29*(1), 6–28; National health and nutrition examination survey. (2008). U.S. Department of Health and Human Services, Centers for Disease Control and Prevention, National Center for Health Statistics.

53 Ver Ploeg, et al. (2009). *Access to affordable and nutritious food: Measuring and understanding food deserts and their consequences—report to Congress.* Washington, DC: U.S. Department of Agriculture, Economic Research Service.

54 Koball, H., & Douglas-Hall, A. (2004, September). Rate of children in low-income families varies widely by state. National Center for Children in Poverty.

55 Understanding the connections: Food insecurity and obesity (Rep.). (2015, October). Retrieved January 18, 2017, from Food Research and Action Center website: http://frac.org/wp-content/uploads/frac_brief_understanding_the_connections.pdf

56 Harris, J., Shehan, C., Gross, R., Kumanyika, S., Lassiter, V., Ramirez, A., & Gallion, K. (2015, August). Food advertising targeted to Hispanic and black youth: Contributing to health disparities (Rep.). Retrieved January 18, 2017, from UCONN Rudd Center for Food Policy and Obesity website: http://www.uconnruddcenter.org/files/Pdfs/272–7%20%20Rudd_Targeted%20Marketing%20Report_Release_081115%5B1%5D.pdf

57 Harris, J., Shehan, C., Gross, R., Kumanyika, S., Lassiter, V., Ramirez, A., & Gallion, K. (2015, August). Food advertising targeted to Hispanic and black youth: Contributing to health disparities (Rep.). Retrieved January 18, 2017, from UCONN Rudd Center for Food Policy and Obesity website: http://www.uconnruddcenter.org/files/Pdfs/272–7%20%20Rudd_Targeted%20Marketing%20Report_Release_081115%5B1%5D.pdf

58 Harris J. L. (2010) Fast food facts: Evaluating fast food nutrition and marketing to youth. Rudd Center for Food Policy and Obesity. (http://stateofobesity.org/disparities/blacks/)

59 Harris, J., Shehan, C., Gross, R., Kumanyika, S., Lassiter, V., Ramirez, A., & Gallion, K. (2015, August). Food advertising targeted to Hispanic and black youth: Contributing to health disparities (Rep.). Retrieved January 18, 2017, from UCONN Rudd Center for Food Policy and Obesity website: http://www.uconnruddcenter.org/files/Pdfs/272–7%20%20Rudd_Targeted%20Marketing%20Report_Release_081115%5B1%5D.pdf

60 Harris-Lovett, S. (2015, August 13). Junk food ads on TV tend to target African American and Latino youth. *Los Angeles Times.* http://www.latimes.com/science/sciencenow/la-sci-sn-junk-food-advertising-racial-disparity-20150812-story.html

61 Wang, Y., & Beydoun, M. A. (2007). The obesity epidemic in the United States—gender, age, socioeconomic, racial/ethnic, and geographic characteristics: A systematic review and meta-regression analysis. *Epidemiologic Reviews, 29*(1), 6–28; National health and nutrition examination survey. (2008). U.S. Department of Health and Human Services, Centers for Disease Control and Prevention, National Center for Health Statistics.

62 Understanding the connections: Food insecurity and obesity (Rep.). (2015, October). Retrieved January 18, 2017, from Food Research and Action Center website: http://frac.org/wp-content/uploads/frac_brief_understanding_the_connections.pdf

63 The weight of the nation. (2012, May). *HBO*. Retrieved January 18, 2017, from http://theweightofthenation.hbo.com/watch/main-films/Consequences

64 Wang, Y., & Beydoun, M. A. (2007). The obesity epidemic in the United States—gender, age, socioeconomic, racial/ethnic, and geographic characteristics: A systematic review and meta-regression analysis. *Epidemiologic Reviews, 29*(1), 6–28; National health and nutrition examination survey. (2008). U.S. Department of Health and Human Services, Centers for Disease Control and Prevention, National Center for Health Statistics.

65 111   Let's move. (n.d.). Retrieved January 19, 2017, from http://www.letsmove.gov/learn-facts/epidemic-childhood-obesity

66 Supplemental nutrition assistance program (SNAP). (2014, November 20). United States Department of Agriculture, Food and Nutrition Service. Retrieved January 19, 2017, from http://www.fns.usda.gov/snap/short-history-snap

67 Women, infants, and children (WIC). (2016, December 14). United States Department of Agriculture, Food and Nutrition Service. Retrieved January 19, 2017, from http://www.fns.usda.gov/wic/women-infants-and-children-wic

68 SNAP. (n.d.). Retrieved January 19, 2017, from http://frac.org/wp-content/uploads/2011/06/SNAPstrategies.pdf

69 Women, infants and children. (2013, December). United States Department of Agriculture, Food nd Nutrition Service, Office of Policy Support. Retrieved January 19, 2017, from http://www.fns.usda.gov/sites/default/files/WICPC2012_Summary.pdf

70 Wang, Y., & Beydoun, M. A. (2007). The obesity epidemic in the United States—gender, age, socioeconomic, racial/ethnic, and geographic characteristics: A systematic review and meta-regression analysis. *Epidemiologic Reviews, 29*(1), 6–28; National health and nutrition examination survey. (2008). U.S. Department of Health and Human Services, Centers for Disease Control and Prevention, National Center for Health Statistics.

71 Dannefer, R., Williams, D. A., Baronberg, S., & Silver, L. (2012). Healthy bodegas: Increasing and promoting healthy foods at corner stores in New York City. *American Journal of Public Health, 102*(10), e27–e31. http://doi.org/10.2105/AJPH.2011.300615

72 S. Res. 111–296, 111th Cong., 156 U.S. G.P.O. (2010) (enacted).

73 The weight of the nation. (2012, May). *HBO*. Retrieved January 18, 2017, from http://theweightofthenation.hbo.com/watch/main-films/Consequences

74 United States Department of Health and Human Services (2015). *Dietary guidelines for Americans, 2015–2020*. Washington, DC: U.S. Government Printing Office.

Figure Sources

1 Figure 3.1: Copyright © 2016 Depositphotos/elenabs.

2 Figure 3.2: Source: https://commons.wikimedia.org/wiki/File:BMIBoys.pdf.

3 Figure 3.3: Copyright © Jks111 (CC BY-SA 3.0) at https://upload.wikimedia.org/wikipedia/commons/2/2d/Body_Fat_Caliper.png.

4 Figure 3.4: Copyright © cosmed (CC BY-SA 3.0) at https://upload.wikimedia.org/wikipedia/commons/3/3d/Adult_body_composition_through_air_displacement_plethysmography.jpg.

5 Figure 3.5: Source: https://www.cdc.gov/obesity/data/prevalence-maps.html.

6 Figure 3.6: Source: https://www.cdc.gov/obesity/data/prevalence-maps.html.

7 Figure 3.7: Source: https://www.cdc.gov/obesity/data/prevalence-maps.html.

8 Figure 3.8: Source: https://www.cdc.gov/obesity/data/prevalence-maps.html.

9 Figure 3.9: Source: https://commons.wikimedia.org/wiki/File:Medical_complications_of_obesity.png.

10 Figure 3.10: Copyright © U.S. Department of Agriculture (CC by 2.0) at https://commons.wikimedia.org/wiki/File:Michelle_Obama_Lets_Move_2nd_anniversary_tour_February_9,_2012.jpg.

11 Figure 3.11: Source: https://www.choosemyplate.gov.

CHAPTER FOUR

Diabetes

Coauthors:
Sue K. Adams, Ph.D., Contributor: Meredith Rose, L.S.W.

@AmDiabetesAssn

Diabetes is a chronic disease, which means that people often have it for the rest of their lives, and it has no cure. According to the Centers for Disease Control, 29 million people, or 9.3% of Americans, have diabetes.[1] Statistically, that means that out of a class of 100 people, we would expect nine to 10 people to have diabetes! Although 21 million are diagnosed, an estimated 8 million people are undiagnosed and silently live with the symptoms. With so many people diagnosed with the disease, there is a very large economic cost. In 2012, the direct medical costs associated with having diabetes was $176 billion. and the indirect costs associated with loss of work, disability, and premature death were $69 billion. That is a grand total of $245 billion to treat diabetes. Diabetes is the seventh leading cause of death in the United States, although that may be an underestimation. By the end of this chapter, you will learn about the three different types of diabetes, symptoms of diabetes, best management practices, and the impact of diabetes on individuals, families, and the community.

What Is Diabetes?
In order to understand the symptoms and effects of diabetes on the body, it is important to understand the diabetic process. Simply put, diabetes mellitus is a metabolic disorder in which a person's body does not properly process and use the energy that is provided in food. When a person eats, food travels down to the stomach, where it is digested and broken down into sugars (i.e., glucose). Glucose is the body's primary source of energy and largely comes from carbohydrates.

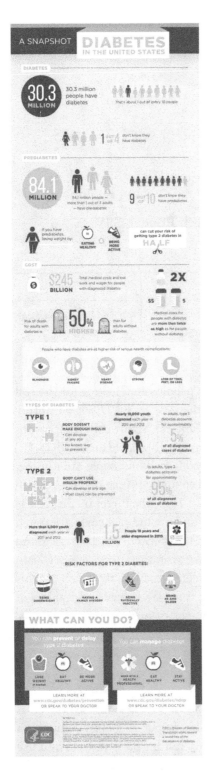

FIGURE 4.1   **A Snapchot of Diabetes in the United States**

Once broken down, glucose enters the bloodstream and is then referred to as blood glucose or blood sugar. In someone who does not have diabetes, blood glucose stimulates the pancreas to secrete the hormone, insulin. Once insulin is secreted into the bloodstream it acts like a key and unlocks cells, allowing cells to absorb sugar from the blood and use that sugar as energy. Without energy at the cellular level, a person would not be able to engage in any activities–no texting, exercising, or even breathing. If the body does not have an immediate need for the glucose, it is stored in the muscles or liver as glycogen, to be used at a later point in time.

In people with diabetes, two biological processes do not function properly, depending on the specific type of diabetes. In the first type, a person's body may not make enough insulin to be able to effectively process the glucose. In the second type, people may become insulin resistant to the point where their cells do not respond to the insulin that is produced. In both conditions, blood sugar cannot be converted into energy, and glucose lingers in the bloodstream with detrimental long-term effects. When a person has too much glucose in the blood, it is called *hyperglycemia*. Conversely, when a person has abnormally low glucose in their blood, it is called *hypoglycemia*, or insulin shock. The only way to know for sure if blood glucose is too high or low is to test the blood. In general, symptoms of hypoglycemia happen quickly and are very uncomfortable and potentially dangerous. Symptoms include shakiness, nervousness, sweating, chills, confusion, fast heartbeat, lightheadedness, and seizures among others. Perhaps you know someone who drinks 15–20 grams of orange juice or gobbles some jelly beans when he or she is hypoglycemic? That is because the person is trying to increase glucose levels. We will discuss the symptoms of hyperglycemia in more depth later in the chapter.

Prediabetes
Another concern is the number of Americans who are prediabetic. Prediabetes is when blood glucose levels

are elevated, but not yet high enough to be diagnosed with diabetes. Even though "pre" makes it sounds like it is not yet a problem, do not be fooled. Between 2009 and 2012, 37% of U.S. adults ages 20 and older were prediabetic (that is every one in three people, and 51% of those aged 65 and older).[2] When added to the existing statistics, a whopping 86 million Americans are either diabetic or prediabetic. Just imagine what the economic cost alone would be for Americans if people who are prediabetic become diabetic? Furthermore, no significant health disparities exist among groups–that is, people in all racial and ethnic groups have equal amounts of prediabetes. Alarmingly, however, although there are equal rates of prediabetes across all groups of people, individuals from racial and ethnic minority groups are more likely to go on to develop diabetes. Why might that be? The answer is complex but may have something to do with the fact that most people with prediabetes can get their glucose levels back into the normal range with increased exercise and proper nutrition. Factors such as economics, access to health care services, and discrimination may play a role in a person's inability to reverse prediabetes.

Health Disparities in Diabetes

Significant racial/ethnic health disparities exist in diabetes. Across all racial groups in the U.S., Native Americans/Alaskan Natives experience the highest rates of diabetes. In fact, 15.9% of Native American/Alaskan Native adults over the age of 20 have diagnosed diabetes, and AI/AN adults are over twice as likely to have diagnosed diabetes than whites. This is followed by Africans Americans, with 13.2% of black adults over the age of 20 having diagnosed diabetes, and black adults are over 70% more likely to have diagnosed diabetes than whites. Also, 12.8% of Latino adults over the age of 20 have diagnosed diabetes, and Latinos are 70% more likely to have diagnosed diabetes than whites. In Asian populations, 9% of adults over the age of 20 have diagnosed diabetes, and Asians are 20% more likely to have diagnosed diabetes than whites. Only 7.6% of whites in the U.S. over the age of 20 have diagnosed diabetes.[3]

Health disparities in diabetes are caused by a confluence of factors very similar to those discussed in the obesity chapter. In the U.S., low-income populations are more likely to develop diabetes.[4] Low socioeconomic status increases the likelihood of poverty, reduced access to healthy food, obesity, hazardous home environments, and stress, all of which are associated with diabetes.[5] Low socioeconomic status is also related to poorer glycemic control, more diabetes-related complications, and higher mortality rates in minority populations.[6, 7]

Healthy People 2020

Healthy People 2020 includes 20 objectives to improve diabetes health and wellness. The objectives fall into these categories: Reducing the numbers of new cases; reducing the death rate among people with diabetes; reducing the rate of diabetes-related amputations; improving glycemic control, lipid control, and blood pressure in people with diabetes; increasing doctor's visits, including dental and foot visits; and increasing preventive behaviors and formal education in patients with diabetes. Between 2010 and 2020, the national goal is to improve outcomes by 10%.

The Three Types of Diabetes

Now that we understand the overall impact of diabetes in the U.S., let's spend some time going into some detail to help you understand the three types of diabetes.

Types of Diabetes	Description
Type 1 Diabetes	Occurs from a failure of the pancreas to produce insulin. Individuals with Type 1 diabetes require daily insulin injections.
Type 2 Diabetes	Occurs when the pancreas does not produce enough insulin to control glucose levels, or the cells do not respond appropriately to insulin. Individuals with Type 2 diabetes can often manage the disease with a low glucose diet and exercise, although some require insulin injections.
Gestational Diabetes	Occurs when the body of a pregnant woman does not secrete enough insulin to control the glucose levels in her and her fetus's bodies. Pregnant women with gestational diabetes can often manage the disease with a low glucose diet and exercise, although some require insulin injections.

FIGURE 4.2   The three types of diabetes

Type 1 Diabetes

Type 1 diabetes, also known as juvenile diabetes, is an autoimmune disorder, an immune reaction that cannot be prevented. For unknown reasons, which likely include a combination of autoimmunity, genetics, and environmental factors, the body attacks the beta cells in the pancreas. Beta cells are responsible for creating insulin, and without them the body is unable to create and secrete insulin. Therefore, the sugar in a person's blood cannot be used as energy at the cellular level. People with type 1 diabetes are dependent on synthetic insulin and require daily insulin injections.

In children less than ten years old, the highest rates of diagnosis continue to be for type 1 diabetes, with non-Hispanic white children more often diagnosed than children from other groups. In 2008–2009, 18,436 children were diagnosed with type 1 diabetes. Type 1 diabetes makes up approximately 5% of all cases of diabetes.[8]

Type 2 Diabetes

In type 2 diabetes, the pancreas makes insulin, but for some reason, the body's cells no longer respond to it and do not unlock to absorb the glucose for energy. They become resistant to the insulin. Alternatively, some people produce insulin but not enough to allow the cells to get the glucose out of the blood. In either scenario, the extra glucose is left to accumulate in the bloodstream, and the body's cells are starved of energy.

In the United States, approximately 28 million people are diagnosed with type 2 diabetes, and it accounts for 90 to 95% of all people who have diabetes.[9] Although type 2 diabetes is greatly influenced by lifestyle factors, type 2 diabetes also appears to have a strong genetic component. If a parent has type 2 diabetes, children are more likely to be diagnosed with diabetes during their lifetime. Twin studies have also shown that if an identical twin has type 2 diabetes, the chance of the other twin also being diagnosed is 75% (as opposed to a 50% chance in type 1 diabetes).[10] However, one major difference between type 1 and type 2 diabetes is the role of lifestyle factors as risk factors for developing the disease. Being overweight, getting too little exercise, and eating diets high in saturated fat and sugar all contribute to type 2 diabetes.

Type 2 diabetes was once considered a disease that mostly developed during adulthood. Alarmingly, as rates of obesity increase, we are also seeing increased rates of diagnoses among children and adolescents. In 2008–2009, 5,089 children and adolescents under the age of 19 were diagnosed with type 2 diabetes.[11] Similar to the health disparity statistics in adults, the highest rates of these diagnoses were in American Indian/Alaska Natives, non-Hispanic black, and Hispanic children and adolescents.

Gestational Diabetes

The third but less commonly known form of diabetes is gestational diabetes. Gestational diabetes occurs only during pregnancy, with approximately 9% of pregnant women developing this condition every year. For these pregnant women, their bodies do not produce enough insulin or use the insulin they do produce efficiently, causing their blood sugar to rise. Although the specific reason why some women develop gestational diabetes is unknown, researchers suspect that a hormone made by the placenta (i.e., placental lactogen) plays a role in causing gestational diabetes.[12] Although the hormones in the placenta help the baby to grow, they also block the mother's ability to utilize insulin in her own body, and she develops insulin resistance. The glucose builds up in her blood, leading to many of the symptoms of diabetes such as fatigue and excessive urination. Interestingly, once the mother gives birth to both the baby and the organ that nourishes the baby, the placenta, gestational diabetes almost always disappears shortly thereafter. Half of all women, however, who had gestational diabetes, develop type 2 diabetes later in life,[13] so women should remind their health care providers to check her blood glucose levels every few years. Some factors put certain women at risk for developing gestational diabetes, including pregnancies in women over the age of 25, being overweight before pregnancy, having a family history of diabetes, having previously given birth to a baby who weighed more than nine pounds or the mother herself weighed more than nine pounds at birth, and being non-white.

All pregnant women who receive regular prenatal care will be tested for gestational diabetes between the 24th and 28th week of pregnancy. The mother is given an oral glucose tolerance test in which she drinks a very sugary beverage (which tastes like stale soda), and her blood glucose levels are monitored an hour later to check if her body is effectively utilizing the glucose. If the woman fails the test, she will be asked to take a three-hour challenge in which technicians monitor her blood glucose levels three hours after she ingests the drink. If she fails that test, she is diagnosed with gestational diabetes. This type of test is necessary because many of the symptoms of diabetes are very common during pregnancy (e.g., running to use the bathroom every hour and feeling like one needs to take a nap every 20 minutes).

The Symptoms of Diabetes

Many symptoms of diabetes range in severity. It is important to remember that diabetes is a systemic disease; that is, excess blood sugar affects *every* part of the body—the blood, the cells, the nerves, the saliva, and even the urine. To provide a visual courtesy of Dr. Mehmet Oz, think of excess blood sugar as shards of glass that make tiny abrasions throughout the body. Virtually no part of the body escapes the damaging effects of glucose, although some parts of the body are more prone to injury. As the glucose makes tiny abrasions throughout the body, it will develop scar tissue and an eventual loss of functioning.

Remember that we mentioned that eight million people are undiagnosed with diabetes? The primary reason is because the symptoms of diabetes can be quite general, and many people (or health care providers) may not associate them with elevated blood glucose levels.

Here is a list of common symptoms in individuals with hyperglycemia:

Frequent Urination
People with diabetes may urinate more than ten times per day and have full bladders each time. This is because the kidneys work overtime to filter the excess glucose out of the bloodstream. The excess sugar absorbs water from the body, thus leading to many trips to the bathroom.

Feeling Very Thirsty
As the excess sugar absorbs water, the body can become very dehydrated. Gallons of water per day may not fulfill the thirst of someone with diabetes.

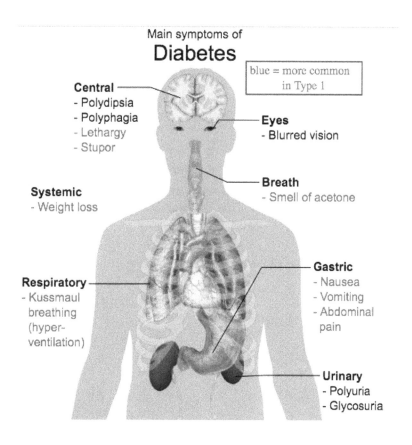

Main symptoms of
Diabetes

blue = more common
in Type 1

Central
- Polydipsia
- Polyphagia
- Lethargy
- Stupor

Eyes
- Blurred vision

Breath
- Smell of acetone

Systemic
- Weight loss

Gastric
- Nausea
- Vomiting
- Abdominal pain

Respiratory
- Kussmaul breathing (hyper-ventilation)

Urinary
- Polyuria
- Glycosuria

FIGURE 4.3   The main symptoms of Diabetes

Fatigue and Weakness
When cells cannot get enough energy, the person will start to feel lethargic and tired.

Blurry Vision
High levels of sugar pull fluid from the lenses of the eyes, which can result in the inability to focus. Also, the shards of glucose can damage the optic nerve making it harder to see.

Slow-healing Cuts, Bruises, and Infections
Excess sugar makes it difficult for the white blood cells to fight off infections. Therefore, cuts and scrapes can take longer to heal and may be more prone to developing infections.

Numbness and Tingling in the Extremities
The shards of glucose damage all nerves but especially nerves in the extremities where blood can pool due to gravity. People with this type of nerve damage may experience numbness, tingling, or burning in the hands and feet. Numbness may also make it harder for a person to feel if he or she gets a cut on the body. Not knowing to take proper care of the wound site could also lead to infection or, at the extreme, amputation of toes, feet, or legs.

Sweet-Smelling Urine and Saliva
Since glucose travels throughout the body, and the kidneys work extra hard to expel it through urine, a person with diabetes may have sweet-smelling urine. This puts women at increased risk for yeast infections. Also, extra-sweet saliva can also lead to dental issues and tooth loss resulting from tartar, gingivitis, and cavities.

Weight Gain or Loss
When the body's cells are starved of energy, the body begins to break down fat and muscle for energy, resulting in weight loss. Conversely, when cells are starved of energy, a person may eat more to compensate, thus resulting in weight gain.

The Long-Term Effects of Diabetes on the Body and Mind
As we have discussed, diabetes is a systemic disease. Because the underlying mechanism works through the blood system, all parts of the body, including the brain, are affected. Below, we will discuss some of the ways that high blood sugar impacts specific areas of the body.

Neuropathy
Neuropathy is nerve damage. All of that extra glucose in the body causes nerve damage, leading signals to misfire or never reach the brain. Here are some examples of common nerve damage:

- When the nerves in the bladder are damaged, it may be difficult to sense when the bladder is empty. People may not empty their bladders completely, leading to urinary tract infections.
- When the nerves in the penis are damaged, men may have difficulty achieving and maintaining an erection. Women may also experience pelvic nerve damage, making it difficult to achieve orgasm.
- The blood vessel that feeds the retina of the eye can also be damaged, leading to blurriness, swelling, vision loss, or blindness. This is called retinopathy.

Chronic Kidney Disease
Kidneys are the body's filtration system, where toxins are filtered from the blood, converted into urine, and then excreted from the body. With diabetes, the kidneys work in overdrive to clear the blood of extra glucose. Over time, the kidneys can become taxed, begin to fail, and not be able to clear your blood of toxins.

Diabetes and Cardiovascular Disease (CVD)
We do not have a chapter in this book dedicated to heart disease and, therefore, will spend some time here discussing what cardiovascular disease is and how it is affected by diabetes. Shockingly, at least 65% of diabetics die from heart attack or stroke, as CVD is the leading

cause of premature death amongst people with diabetes.[14] The primary reason for this is because many people who are diabetic also have high blood pressure, high cholesterol, and are overweight, all of which are risk factors for CVD. Glucose also makes the fat and cholesterol in the body stickier and more likely to stick to blood vessel walls and cause the arteries to narrow.

Myocardial Infarction, otherwise known as a heart attack, is when the blood flow to the heart is severely reduced or completely blocked. Remember how we mentioned earlier that glucose acts like shards of glass? These shards of glass can knick the walls of the arteries and veins, causing scar tissue to form. These buildups, in addition to the buildup of fatty deposits on the arterial ways, can break off and form a blood clot. When the blood clot blocks blood to the heart, the heart muscle can suffer permanent damage or death. Similarly, strokes occur when the blood clots block blood flow to the brain, and pulmonary embolisms occur when blood clots block blood flow to the lungs. Here is a list of the symptoms of heart attack and stroke:

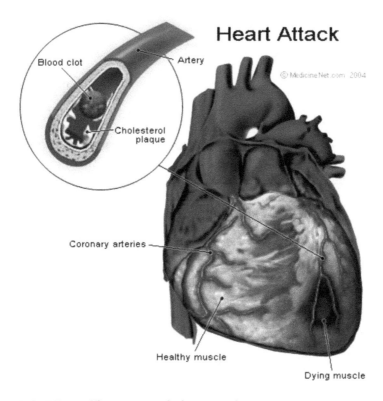

FIGURE 4.4   The anatomy of a heart attack

Heart Attack
- Pressure/pain in the chest that can radiate down the arm
- Pressure in the back, shoulders, neck, arms, and jaws (especially in women): *Please tell the women in your life to seek medical care if they are feeling pain in these areas.*

This is a primary symptom for women but is often disregarded because it is more subtle than the symptoms of heart attack in men.

- Shortness of breath
- Lightheadedness
- Fainting
- Sweating
- Nausea
- Fatigue

Common Heart Attack Symptoms	
Women	**Men**
Arm, neck and **jaw** pain	Chest pain or tightness; back, shoulder, neck and arm pain
Heartburn-like feelings	Heartburn-like feelings
Nausea or vomiting	Nausea or vomiting
Cold Sweat	Sweating
Extreme fatigue	Shortness of breath

FIGURE 4.5   Common heart attack symptoms in females versus males

*If a person experiences neuropathy, it is possible that he or she will have a "silent heart attack," one he or she cannot feel because nerves in the heart are damaged.

Stroke
- Weakness or numbness in face, arm, or leg
- Weakness in one side of the body (depending on what side of the brain the clot lands)
- Confusion
- Difficulty speaking
- Vision impairment
- Trouble balancing
- Sudden and severe headaches

Case Vignette
When I was 15 years old, I witnessed my grandfather's stroke. It was Christmas morning, and my grandfather was sitting on the couch after we had just finished eating our traditional Christmas breakfast. As my grandfather went to stand up, he suddenly fell back on

the couch. The right side of his body "gave out." He couldn't stand, walk, lift his arm or smile, but he could speak enough to tell us to call 911. Considering what had just happened, he seemed OK. However, once he arrived at the hospital, he had the "big" stroke. Often, heart attacks and strokes occur in sequence. A mini episode is followed by the bigger and more severe episode. In my grandfather's case, the second stroke was debilitating. Due to a dislodged blood clot, his brain cells were starved of blood, and he lost the ability to use the right side of his body, as well as his ability to speak. He was given five years to live due to the severity of his symptoms. He went through physical therapy, which was grueling and frustrating for someone who was so independent, and from that day on he relied on others to care for him, although he did gain more independence over time. It was also an incredibly difficult time for my grandmother, as my grandfather had just retired, and they had plans to travel and do the things they were not able to when they were younger. My grandfather ultimately passed away from stroke-related complications; specifically, he developed pneumonia from food going down to his lungs as a result of the paralysis of his throat muscles. However, my grandfather lived every day to the fullest and lived ten years longer than expected!

Gestational Diabetes and "Fat" Babies

For women who develop gestational diabetes, there are concerns for both the mother and the baby. The primary concern in the developing fetus is Macrosomia, otherwise known as "fat" baby. A baby diagnosed with macrosomia weighs more than eight pounds, 13 ounces at birth. Babies that weigh more than nine pounds, 15 ounces are particularly vulnerable for a number of complications. These babies are larger birth weight because the extra glucose in the mother's blood crosses the placenta. Although the fetus's pancreas produces extra insulin to try to use the glucose, all of the extra energy eventually gets stored as extra fat, thus increasing the baby's weight.[15]

A larger baby is likely to have larger shoulders and body fat at birth, making it harder to move through the mother's pelvis and birth canal. These babies may get stuck in the birth canal and sustain birth injuries such as broken collar bones or nerve damage, or require the use of vacuum devices or forceps to aid in delivery. If the baby is too large, the mother may be required to have a cesarean section. Additionally, the mother may be at risk for developing excessive uterine bleeding or genital tract lacerations. Although childbirth often requires deviating from the birth plan, these mothers may experience anxiety, depression, or even trauma as a result of the complications related to childbirth.

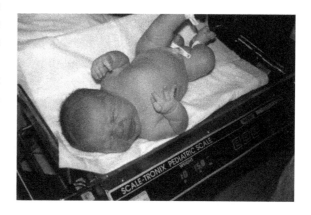

FIGURE 4.6   "Large" baby with Macrosomia

Macrosomia also puts babies at risk for having lower-than-normal blood sugar (due to the extra insulin secreted by the baby's pancreas), breathing problems, and jaundice (a yellowish hue in the baby's skin), and it has also been linked to increased rates of obesity, type 2 diabetes, and metabolic syndrome later in life (i.e., higher blood pressure, high blood sugar, and excess body fat around the midsection which can lead to heart disease later in life).[16] Although this illustrates the importance of getting a healthy start to life, being born with macrosomia does not mean that the child will undoubtedly experience these problems later.

Psychosocial Effects of Diabetes

Receiving a diagnosis of diabetes can be a shock to anyone. As with any disease, the ways that people cope can range from "I can do it!" to "why is this happening to me?" to "I can't handle this." Diabetes management can take an emotional toll, and the severity of its impact on mental and emotional health can depend on a number of factors including support systems, a person's confidence in his or her ability to manage the disease, personality, economic resources, and access to health care. However, it is also important to note that fluctuations in blood sugar throughout the day can also make someone feel anxious, feel tired, have a loss of appetite, or have trouble sleeping, all of which are symptoms of larger mental health concerns.

Depression

It has been well documented that individuals with diabetes experience increased rates of depression. Statistically, 11–31% of people with diabetes are also diagnosed with depression or experience increased depressive symptoms.[17] Some people experience short bouts of depression while others experience chronic sadness and despair, which impacts their ability to function on a daily basis. If a person is unable to get out of bed and function, it is less likely that he or she will be able to adequately monitor blood sugar and take insulin and/or medications. Someone who is depressed may eat more, causing him or her to gain weight and have even more dysregulated blood sugar. Some people with diabetes may also get overwhelmed by the constant management of the disease and lose hope about the future. Others may be in denial about their diagnosis and, therefore, may not engage in diabetes management because they do not believe that they have a problem. Still others may become annoyed, furious, and/or sad that they cannot do simple, everyday things that most people take for granted, like eating a slice of birthday cake.

Anxiety

Diabetes can also cause anxiety, as it is a complicated disease to manage. People may worry about the long-term complications associated with diabetes and wonder how many years they have before they lose a leg or go blind. They may worry about the financial strain that the disease puts on their family. It is stressful to think that one cannot send a child to camp or buy the family healthy food because money must be spent on medications. These people may feel out of control of their bodies, like their bodies have betrayed them and are not working "the way they should." Interpersonally, people may be concerned that others will not understand their diagnosis and will not be able to relate to what they are experiencing. This may lead to isolation from others. It is important for health care providers to assess for depression and anxiety and for patients to have open and honest communication about how they are feeling.[18] A referral to a mental health clinician who specializes in working with individuals with chronic illness may also become an important component of the treatment plan. Taking back control over the disease is vital for the psychological well-being of people with diabetes.

Diabetes Across Development

Family Management

As is the case with most chronic diseases, children and adolescents require support from their caregivers and family members to properly manage the disease. Support can take different forms depending on the child's level of responsibility and maturity. In young children, parents are often responsible for the majority of diabetes management and have to either administer the regimen or remind the child when to measure glucose, take medications, etc. In preschoolers, simple explanations for how the insulin shots keep them healthy often suffice. In school-aged children, parents should take the child's lead in how much they want to independently manage. Although parents may have the best of intentions, sometimes children feel like they are constantly being nagged. As children get older and can take on more responsibility for their diabetes management, it may be difficult for parents to "let go." They may worry that the child will forget to do something important and may check up on them too often. Finally, siblings may also begin to feel jealous or resentful that so much attention is being given to the child with diabetes. Families can be intense, especially when there is a fear about a child's safety, but the hope it is that children and parents find a way to work together to manage diabetes and reduce tension in the family.

Childhood: Working With Schools

Sending children to school to manage their diabetes without the help of a primary caregiver can be a very stressful experience, especially for parents who have younger children or newly diagnosed children. Luckily, as children approach adolescence they generally take more control over their medical management and are able to provide safe and reliable self-care for their diabetes. Regardless, however, of where the child and family are in the course of the disease, families and schools should work together to make sure the child's diabetes is well managed throughout the school day. Children with diabetes may benefit from having written accommodations under the federal disability law, such as a Section 504 plan or an Individualized Education Plan. As part of this accommodation, the parents, school staff, and pediatricians should create a written action plan. In fact, parents can request a Diabetes Medical Management Plan from their child's health care provider, which outlines instructions for checking glucose levels throughout the day, how to treat hypo- and hyperglycemia, how and when to deliver insulin, meal planning, and planning for emergencies.[19] Since there is no one-way to treat and manage diabetes, written instructions are essential for consistent and effective treatment of diabetes at school. The *American Diabetes Association* even offers free webinars for parents and teachers at

http://www.diabetes.org/living-with-diabetes/parents-and-kids/diabetes-care-at-school/safe-at-school-webinars.html.

Adolescence

As children get older, other issues arise. For example, children and adolescents may feel like they are different from their friends, leading to feelings of isolation or embarrassment. They may experience activity restrictions (e.g., they may not be able to sleep over friend's houses because their friend's parents do not feel comfortable giving insulin shots). During adolescence, there are competing needs, and teens tend to want independence when it comes to food, fun, and relationships. Adolescents may start to resent their disease, rebel against their parent's rules by not taking insulin, or use insulin inappropriately (e.g., as a way to control weight). All of these actions come at the expense of caring for diabetes and overall health. Additionally, alcohol, drug use, and sex can have an immediate effect on low blood sugar and make it hard to take insulin, leading to a potentially dangerous situation. Ideally, adolescents with diabetes should stay away from alcohol and drugs. If they do engage in risky behavior, they should wear a medical ID bracelet and let others know of their condition. What if they are embarrassed by their disease or do not want to disclose their personal health status to their friends? As you can see, living with diabetes is complex, and people do the best they can to make their way through.

Older Adulthood

With more than 25% of people with diabetes over the age of 65,[20] diabetes in older adults is a substantial driver of the epidemic in the U.S. The incidence of diabetes increases through the age of 65, at which time it appears that the rates level off. Older adults have the highest rates of a number of short- and long-term effects of diabetes, including amputations, heart disease, visual impairment, and kidney failure. Older adults are also twice as likely to have emergency room visits for hypoglycemia.[21]

As a result of the impact that diabetes has on older adults, the American Diabetes Association has outlined specific guidelines for this population, specifically: 1) older adults with good cognitive functioning and who are in good general physical health should receive diabetes care similar to younger adults; 2) if older adults are not in good physical and cognitive health, their blood sugar goals can be adjusted to be a bit more lax; 3) other cardiovascular risk factors and diseases should be treated to help avoid diabetes complications; and 4) regular screenings should be conducted for diabetes complications, paying particular attention to complications that could lead to functional impairment (e.g., nerve damage or foot wounds).[22] These recommendations suggest that diabetes care in older adults should be tailored to the individual person, be a bit more flexible than we would expect for younger adults, and achieve the goal of helping to maintain the ability to function independently and live full lives.

Treatments and Prevention Programs: What Can Individuals, Families, and Communities Do to Help?

Given the prevalence of diabetes diagnoses in the United States, interventions require a multidisciplinary approach to treatment that supports the whole person and involves community efforts to combat the disease. Treatment strategies range from medical strategies to behavioral health interventions to community-based prevention and intervention programs. The specific combination of strategies used largely depends on the type of diabetes present. We will spend some time reviewing these strategies.

Medical Strategies

Medical strategies, such as insulin shots, pumps and pills, are important components of diabetes treatment, especially for people whose bodies do not make insulin and have type 1 diabetes. These folks rely on injecting insulin into their bodies to help their cells use glucose as energy. Insulin injections are administered multiple times per day into a person's fatty tissue. Luckily, modern syringes have a special coating making them less painful. Insulin can also be injected via pump. The pump is connected to a small needle that is placed in fatty tissue in the abdomen and taped in place. Insulin is slowly pushed into the body throughout the day, and the person can push a button for extra insulin before he eats. The pump may be preferred for those who are afraid of needles but needs to be changed and cleaned every few days. Technology is also moving toward allowing people to measure their blood glucose levels via a device that is synced to a smart phone (called a Continuous Glucose Monitoring device). Via a small needle similar to the pump, the device will monitor blood glucose levels throughout the day and alert the person via their phone when their blood glucose levels begin to drop or rise. The phone will also be able to calculate how much insulin should be injected via the pump. Finally, oral medications are often used for Type 2 diabetes, especially if diabetic symptoms are not controlled with diet and exercise. Oral medications do carry risks of side effects, such as constipation, diarrhea, cramping, nausea, and headaches, amongst others. Finally, people with diabetes should also regularly visit the ophthalmologist to check their eyes, as well as their dentists to check their teeth and gums.

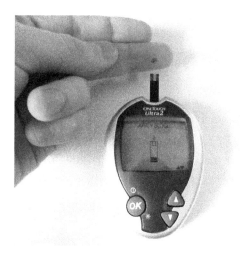

FIGURE 4.7   **Blood Glucose Monitor**

Behavioral Strategies

As with many illnesses, proper diet and exercise are essential for controlling diabetes. Eating in diabetes means following a healthy and balanced diet. The goal is to stay away from processed foods, refined sugars, and excess salt while increasing healthy foods like fruits, vegetables, and whole grains. It is common to work with a registered dietician so that a person can develop meal plans that fit their lifestyle, schedule, and food preferences, which will increase the chances that the person will actually stick to the plan. Daily exercise is also very important because a) our bodies are made for moving, b) exercise can build muscle mass which will process more glucose, and c) exercise makes your body's cells more sensitive to insulin which will reduce glucose from your blood. For both Type 1 and 2 diabetes, people may require specific instructions on when and how to exercise, as well as measuring blood glucose levels before exercise. For instance, a person who has Type 1 diabetes may be hypoglycemic (i.e., too little blood glucose) and will need to eat a snack before exercising so that he or she has enough energy to sustain exercise. Conversely, if a person is hyperglycemic (i.e., too much blood glucose) he or she may need to wait to exercise. Interestingly, Type 2 diabetes can sometimes be completely controlled and reversed by diet and exercise. Overall, exercise is part of the doctor's orders, so people with diabetes should find ways to stay active.

National Diabetes Prevention Programs

Many of the federally-funded prevention and intervention efforts are funded by the Centers for Disease Control's Division of Diabetes Translation or the American Diabetes Association (e.g., Diabetes Camp, Step Out: Walk to Stop Diabetes). Others, however, are grass-roots efforts developed by concerned citizens and communities.

The National Diabetes Prevention Program

The National Diabetes Prevention Program (NDPP) is a partnership among public and private community organizations, health insurance companies, health care organizations, employers and government agencies to promote lifestyle changes for people at risk for Type 2 diabetes. The key component of this program is that community agencies work together to offer The Lifestyle Change Program.[23] Either in-person or via online classes, people are taught strategies to increase physical activity, reduce weight, manage stress, and stay committed to a behavior-change plan. The Centers for Disease Control approves and monitors these well-designed and effective programs, because if the CDC is going to provide funding for programs offered to the public, it is important to have data to prove that the programs work.

The Native Diabetes Wellness Program

The Native Diabetes Wellness Program is part of the Center for Disease's Control Division of Diabetes Translation and is an example of a multifaceted and culturally sensitive approach to working with communities disproportionately affected by diabetes. The mission of this wellness program is to work with community partners to address health inequities that affect Native Americans, while respecting both Native and Western science. This program utilizes a strong cultural history of storytelling to educate children and families about wellness and diabetes prevention. The program publishes a series of Eagle Books which can be downloaded free of charge by parents or community members, and teaches about diabetes management and prevention through the lens of traditional Native American characters, such as the main character named Rain That Dances and his friends, Thunder Cloud, Little Hummingbird, and Simon, as well as traditional folk art illustrations.[24] The program is also

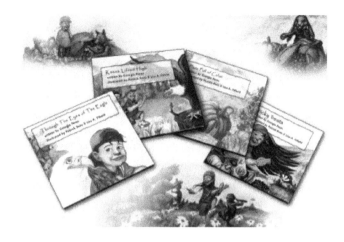

FIGURE 4.8   Photos of Eagle Books from the Native Diabetes Wellness Program

working to make systemic changes by restoring access to local, healthy, and traditional foods and physical activity to promote wellness. As we learned in the health disparities section, poverty, food, and diabetes are very closely related.

Conclusion

Diabetes is a complex disease which requires knowledge and discipline to control. For some, diabetes develops at a young age and without warning. For others, diabetes develops gradually and is related to lifestyle issues that affect bodies over many decades. Although diabetes might be considered a disease of personal responsibility, it is imperative to acknowledge the influence that genetics, culture, socioeconomic status, poverty, and access to health care have on the development of the disease. Diabetes can be difficult to manage and affects individuals, families, and communities, but many people with diabetes find a way to thrive and live happy, fulfilling, and healthy lives.

When Lara was born, her parents moved to the United States from Ethiopia. Growing up in an underprivileged community in West Philadelphia was difficult. After Lara's father left her mother at the age of five, her mother worked endlessly to be able to feed her five children and provide them with the tools for a successful future. With five children, little outside support, and a home in an area considered to be a food desert (an urban area where there is a struggle to obtain affordable, high quality, healthy foods), Lara's mother resorted to fast food. The family lived off meals high in saturated fats and sugars. When Lara turned 18, she was asked to leave home. With no money to afford the necessities for survival, she moved into an emergency housing shelter for individuals and families experiencing homelessness. Lara became increasingly concerned with her weight. She weighed 200 pounds and was unable to access healthy foods. Lara's weight continued to rise while living in emergency housing and being served foods with no nutritional benefit. Three months after moving into the emergency housing shelter, Lara noticed that she was urinating every 30–60 minutes and could not control her thirst. She was also too fatigued to go out and look for jobs. Her case manager became concerned with her condition and encouraged Lara to go to the emergency room. Lara agreed. At this point, Lara had blurry vision and could hardly walk due to numbness in her feet.

Lara was nervous when she entered the emergency room. After explaining her symptoms to the health care professionals, they decided to do a blood test to measure insulin and C-peptide, an insulin-related protein. The team immediately suspected that this might be a case of diabetes. In Type 2 diabetes, the insulin and C-peptide levels will be normal or elevated but are typically low in Type 1 diabetes. When Lara was informed of her diagnosis, she remembered that her father also had Type 2 diabetes. The health care team discussed with her that this was a common disease to inherit, but her eating habits and lack of physical activity were the main factors behind her diagnosis. It is possible that Lara had this illness for years without noticing the symptoms. The nurses suspected that the stress of residing in the emergency housing shelter might have heightened her symptoms.

The health care professionals discussed a treatment plan with Lara. They informed her how important it was for her to make lifestyle changes, including dietary adjustments and an exercise routine. Weight loss and healthy food choices can make a drastic difference in the underlying problem of Type 2 Diabetes, insulin resistance. Lara was informed that she would have to lower her caloric, carbohydrate, and fat intake by using portion control. This did not seem feasible for Lara, as she did not have much of a choice in her food options living in a shelter with minimal resources. This was not the only obstacle. Lara would have to check her blood sugar at least four times per day, as well as take medication to assist her insulin in working properly. She pleaded with the health care team about how unfair it was that she grew up poor and never had a choice in her diet. With all of the challenges already in Lara's life, Type 2 diabetes management would be an obstacle.

Notes

1 National diabetes statistics report, 2014. (2014). National Center for Chronic Disease Prevention and Health Promotion, Division of Diabetes Translation. Retrieved January 18, 2017, from https://www.cdc.gov/diabetes/pdfs/data/2014-report-estimates-of-diabetes-and-its-burden-in-the-united-states.pdf

2 Tuso, P. (2014). Prediabetes and lifestyle modification: Time to prevent a preventable disease. *The Permanente Journal*, *18*(3), 88–93. http://doi.org/10.7812/TPP/14–002

3 Statistics about diabetes. (2016, December 12). American Diabetes Association. Retrieved January 20, 2017, from http://www.diabetes.org/diabetes-basics/statistics/

4 Robbins, J. M., Vaccarino, V., Zhang, H., & Kasl, S.V. (2000). Socioeconomic status and diagnosed diabetes incidence. *Diabetes Research and Clinical Practice*, *68*, 230–236pmid:15936465

5 Everson, S. A., Maty, S. C., Lynch, J. W., Kaplan, G.A. (2002). Epidemiologic evidence for the relation between socioeconomic status and depression, obesity, and diabetes. *Journal of Psychosomatic Research, 53*, 891–895pmid:12377299

6 Chaturvedi, N., Jarrett, J., Shipley, M. J., & Fuller, J.H. (1998). Socioeconomic gradient in morbidity and mortality in people with diabetes: Cohort study findings from the Whitehall Study and the WHO Multinational Study of Vascular Disease in Diabetes. *British Medical Journal, 316,* 100–105pmid:9462313

7 Weng, C., Coppini, D. V., & Sönksen, P. H. (2000). Geographic and social factors are related to increased morbidity and mortality rates in diabetic patients. *Diabetes Medicine, 17,* 612–617.

8 Statistics about diabetes (2006). American Diabetes Association. Retrieved from http://www.diabetes.org/diabetes-basics/statistics/?referrer=https://www.google.com/.

9 Santos-Longhurst, A. (2014, September 8). Type 2 diabetes statistics and facts. *Healthline*. Retrieved January 17, 2017, from http://www.healthline.com/health/type-2-diabetes/statistics

10 The genetics of diabetes. (2014, March 12). American Diabetes Association, Diabetes Stops Here. Retrieved January 17, 2017, from http://diabetesstopshere.org/2014/03/12/the-genetics-of-diabetes/

11 Hamman, R. F., Bell, R. A., Dabelea, D., D'Agostino, R. B., Dolan, L., Imperatore, G., Saydah, S. (2014). The search for diabetes in youth study: Rationale, findings, and future directions. *Diabetes Care*, *37*(12), 3336–3344. http://doi.org/10.2337/dc14–0574

12 Gestational diabetes causes. (2014, April 25). Mayo Clinic. Retrieved January 17, 2017, from http://www.mayoclinic.org/diseases-conditions/gestational-diabetes/basics/causes/con-20014854

13 After diabetes during pregnancy, healthy diet linked to reduced type 2 diabetes risk. (2012, October 9). National Institutes of Health. Retrieved January 17, 2017, from https://www.nih.gov/news-events/news-releases/after-diabetes-during-pregnancy-healthy-diet-linked-reduced-type-2-diabetes-risk

14 Diabetes, heart disease, and stroke. (2014, February). National Institute of Diabetes and Digestive and Kidney Diseases, U.S. Department of Health and Human Services. Retrieved January 18, 2017, from https://www.niddk.nih.gov/health-information/diabetes/overview/preventing-problems/heart-disease-stroke

15 Fetal macrosomia. (2015, April 16). Mayo Clinic. Retrieved January 18, 2017, from http://www.mayoclinic.org/diseases-conditions/fetal-macrosomia/basics/definition/con-20035423

16 Fetal Macrosomia. (n.d.). Birth Injury Guide. Retrieved January 17, 2017, from http://www.birthinjuryguide.org/birth-injury/causes/fetal-macrosomia/

17 Katon, W. J. (2008, November). The comorbidity of diabetes mellitus and depression. U.S. National Library of Medicine, National Institutes of Health. Retrieved January 30, 2017, from http://www.ncbi.nlm.nih.gov/pmc/articles/PMC2717744/

18 Gupta, D. S. (2014, April 24). The emotional effects of diabetes. *Everyday Health*. Retrieved January 30, 2017, from http://www.everydayhealth.com/hs/type-2-diabetes-live-better-guide/sanjay-gupta-emotional-effects

19 Diabetes care in the school and day care setting. (2012, January). American Diabetes Association. Retrieved January 18, 2017, from http://care.diabetesjournals.org/content/35/Supplement_1/S76.full

20 National diabetes fact sheet: General information and national estimates on diabetes in the United States, 2011. Atlanta, Georgia, U.S. Department of Health and Human Services, Centers for Disease Control and Prevention, 2011.

21 Diabetes public health resource. (n.d.). Centers for Disease Control and Prevention. Available from www.cdc.gov/diabetes. Accessed 27 September 2012.

22 American Diabetes Association. (2012). Standards of medical care in diabetes—2012. *Diabetes Care, 35*, (Suppl. 1):S11-S63.

23 Lifestyle change program details. (2016, January 14). National Diabetes Prevention Program, Centers for Disease Control and Prevention. Retrieved January 18, 2017, from https://www.cdc.gov/diabetes/prevention/lifestyle-program/experience/index.html

24 Eagle books. (2015, May 05). Native Diabetes Wellness Program, Centers for Disease Control and Prevention. Retrieved January 18, 2017, from https://www.cdc.gov/diabetes/ndwp/eagle-books/index.html

Figure Sources

1 Figure 4.1: Source: https://www.cdc.gov/diabetes/pdfs/library/socialmedia/diabetes-infographic.pdf.

2 Figure 4.3: Source: https://commons.wikimedia.org/wiki/File:Main_symptoms_of_diabetes.svg.

3 Figure 4.4: Copyright © ravindra gandhi (CC BY-SA 2.0) at https://www.flickr.com/photos/gandhiji40/395241000.

4 Figure 4.6: Copyright © Andwhatsnext (CC BY-SA 3.0) at https://commons.wikimedia.org/wiki/File:New-baby-boy-weight-11-pounds.jpg.

5 Figure 4.7: Copyright © David-i98 (CC BY-SA 3.0) at https://en.wikipedia.org/wiki/File:Blood_Glucose_Testing.JPG.

6 Figure 4.8: Source: https://govbooktalk.files.wordpress.com/2013/03/cdc-eagle-book-series.jpg.

CHAPTER FIVE

Autism Spectrum Disorders

Author:
Sue K. Adams, Ph.D.

@autismspeaks

During my clinical training in a sleep clinic, I had a 13-year-old male who came to see me for sleep problems. As we started talking about his sleep needs, he brought up that many of his sleep problems were a result of sensory issues, such as feeling like the sheets were uncomfortable on his body and hearing every car drive by outside the house. This is very common for children with autism. He also described that he was one of three brothers, all of whom were diagnosed with autism. His autism was mild, and his brother had severe autism. I will never forget his description, however, of the difference between him and his brother. "My brothers are blissfully unaware," he said, "they do not want to fit in with others. They do not even realize that they are being left out. For me, I desperately want to fit in with my peers, but I can't figure out how to." This was an eloquent and poignant illustration of how autism affects individuals very differently depending on the severity of the disorder. Each person with autism is unique. Their symptoms are unique. Many professionals in the field view the autism epidemic as a public health emergency—and perhaps the largest childhood epidemic in history.

What Is Autism?
Autism Spectrum Disorder (ASD) refers to a broad group of neurodevelopmental disorders. The term *spectrum* refers to the presence of a wide range of symptoms, skills, and severity of disability. Individuals are often classified as either high functioning or low functioning depending on the severity of symptoms. The term *neurological* disorder indicates many distinct anomalies in the brain and central

nervous system that are associated with the disorder. The classification as a *developmental* disorder refers to the fact that the symptoms develop over time. Many children appear to be typically developing infants and toddlers, and around the age of two or three there is a significant shift in the way they interact with the world. For other children, however, their parents may observe them to be different from other children in infancy. They may become overly focused on certain toys or objects, rarely make eye contact or fail to babble with their caregivers. Over time, these symptoms evolve and often include difficulty with social interactions, verbal and nonverbal communication, the use of repetitive behaviors, and restricted activities and interests. A person does not "outgrow" autism and will have these symptoms for life. As you will see below, there is a wide range of what social impairment and communication might look like depending on the person's severity level. Although many of the examples discussed in the section below sound very reminiscent of typical child behavior, it is important to note that children with ASD will often engage in these behaviors at a higher frequency and will continue to use these behaviors beyond the age at which they will be outgrown by typically developing children.

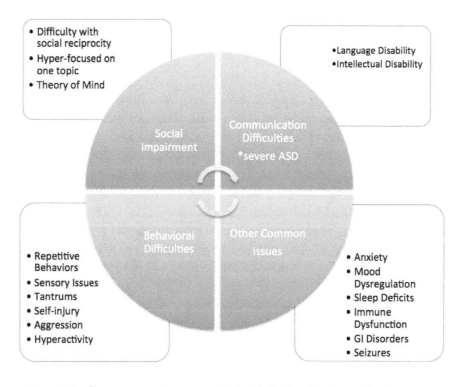

FIGURE 5.1   Common symptoms associated with Autism Spectrum Disorders

Social Impairment

For many people with ASD, social interactions are difficult. The give-and-take nature, or social reciprocity, necessary for social communication and interactions can be particularly challenging. People with ASD may be hyper-focused on discussing one topic and may not be able to read others' verbal and nonverbal cues that it is time to change the subject. They may have difficulty understanding other people's thoughts and feelings, which can lead to the appearance of a lack of empathy for others. The ability to put oneself in someone else's shoes and understand their perspective is called "Theory of Mind" and is a core difficulty with ASD.[1] Additionally, people with ASD may not understand how to play or socially engage with others and may find themselves isolated from groups, sometimes by choice—and sometimes not. Children with ASD may have difficulty responding to their name and may interact with others only to achieve a specific goal (for instance, asking for a cookie).

Communication Difficulties

On one end of the spectrum, some people with ASD have profound disability and no speech. Others may have delayed speech and language skills, often repeating the same phrases (called *echolalia*) or appearing to say things that are incoherent and unrelated to the conversation at hand.[2] Still others may have very fluent and articulate speech and language skills, but their speech may sound flat, robotic, or sing-song-like in tone and cadence. While speaking, people with ASD often have difficulty attending to non-verbal cues such as gestures, body language, and tone of voice. They may also have difficulty using the appropriate nonverbal cues while they are communicating with others, such as making eye contact or sensing when others are disinterested in their conversation.

Repetitive Behaviors

Repetitive behaviors include any behavior, movement, object, or pattern with which one is engaged beyond what one would typically expect for a person that age. For instance, many toddlers engage in hand and arm flapping, rocking from side to side, twirling, or self-injurious behaviors such as head banging as a way to soothe emotional and neurological dysregulation. They may be overly preoccupied with specific objects or parts of objects such as vacuums or wheels on a truck. Young children with ASD may line toys up in a row, rather than playing with them as intended (e.g., lining up books rather than bringing them to an adult for reading). Many people with ASD are also very rule and routine bound and thrive on doing the same thing at the same time every day. Disruptions to these routines can be very difficult to handle and lead to emotional outbursts. Additionally, people with ASD may have a different way of perceiving sensory input from their environments and may be hyper- or hypo-reactive to their environment. For instance, they may be indifferent to pain or extreme temperatures, may not be able to tolerate certain loud sounds or textures, or have a fascination with smelling, touching, or watching certain objects. The feel of a seam in a sock may be difficult to tolerate, the person may have trouble tuning out background noise that others very naturally tune out while focusing on tasks, or light touch may be physically painful to the person.

Other Symptoms

Some individuals with autism also experience a variety of specific symptoms that are not necessary for diagnosis but important to address in treatment. For instance, people with autism also tend to have gross motor difficulties, such as extreme clumsiness, an atypical gait (or way of walking), and a head tilt. Also, there is a high co-occurrence of autism and gastrointestinal issues such as leaky gut and food sensitivities. Food sensitivities can lead to feeling sluggish, bloating, gas, and inflammation, and the most common food sensitivities are to gluten, which is found in wheat, and casein, which is found in milk. Similarly, leaky-gut syndrome occurs when the stomach is less able to break down proteins and absorb them into the body.[3] The excess proteins eventually break down the lining of the stomach, allowing toxins to more easily enter into the bloodstream. As a result, elimination diets that eliminate certain foods from consumption may help people with autism to feel better on a day-to-day basis but do not cure autism.

Health Disparities in Autism

The rates of ASD diagnoses have dramatically increased in the past decade. Currently, the Centers for Disease Control estimate that one in 68 children in the United States has ASD.[4] This is in contrast to the 2007 rates, when it was estimated that one in 150 children had autism. Health disparities include a significant gender disparity, with ASD 4.5 times more common in boys than girls. Most children with ASD are diagnosed after the age of four, despite the fact that diagnoses can be made as early as two years old. Though ASD diagnoses occur in every racial and ethnic group and across all socioeconomic levels, white children are more likely to be identified as having ASD than black or Hispanic children. However, we cannot necessarily conclude that rates are lower in minority populations, as many issues may affect diagnostic rates across groups. For instance, although black and Hispanic children are diagnosed with ASD less often than whites,[5] they are diagnosed with other comorbid disorders such as conduct disorder or attention deficit/hyperactivity disorder at a higher rate. Black children are also diagnosed with ASD at later ages than white children.[6] Several factors lead to these disparities, including inadequate screening procedures, slow response to parental concerns, delayed access to services, or misdiagnosis.

Diagnostic Issues

Many researchers believe that the rates cited above are underestimates of the number of children with autism. The Centers for Disease Control calculates its rates by collecting data from school systems on the children who have the diagnosis and/or qualify for services.[7] However, many children who have not yet started elementary school or are homeschooled are not included in these estimates. Additionally, clinicians are much better at diagnosing autism than they were decades ago. Many cases that were previously diagnosed as *mental retardation* or other developmental disorders are being reclassified as autism, which partially accounts for the differences in diagnosis rates since the 1980s.[8] Finally, the social stigma around autism has decreased, and parents may be more likely to have their children tested and diagnosed.[9] Much more diagnostic testing is taking place due to the increased demand resulting from more awareness of autism.

Healthy People 2020

Given the increasing public health concern of ASD, Healthy People 2020 recently added ASD as a ten-year health objective. The overarching goal is to "increase the proportion of young children with an autism spectrum disorder and other developmental delays who are screened, evaluated, and enrolled in early intervention services in a timely manner."[10] More specifically, Healthy People 2020 aims to increase the proportion of children who are screened and have their first evaluation by the age of three, and increase the proportion of children enrolled in special education services by the age of four. Early detection of the disorder is essential to effective and often free treatment before the age of three.

Developmental Screening

A short developmental screening is often the first step in identifying if children have delays in their development. Most often a child's pediatrician will ask the parent to answer the CHADDIS, which is made up of questions about how the child learns, speaks, behaves and moves, and the pediatrician will also assess these skills in a face-to-face visit.[11] Regular developmental screenings occur at nine months, 18 months, and 24 or 30 months. Children who have other risk factors for ASD, including prematurity, may require additional screenings.

Comprehensive Diagnostic Evaluation

If a pediatrician believes that a child requires further assessment and diagnosis for a possible ASD diagnosis, the child will be referred for a comprehensive diagnostic evaluation. This evaluation is typically conducted either by a developmental pediatrician, child psychologist, child psychiatrist, or child neurologist. It includes an observation of the child's behavior and development, interviews with the primary caregivers, and screenings for other potential medical issues. If a child meets ASD criteria after this evaluation, he or she will receive a formal diagnosis. Diagnosis is necessary to ensure that the child will receive proper services and treatment as he or she moves through school-aged years. Unfortunately, there are often long wait lists for testing, as many children need testing and not enough qualified clinicians are available to meet the demand. This results in a delay between symptoms presentation and diagnosis.

What Puts a Person at Risk for Developing Autism?

Risk Factors

A number of risk factors have been identified that put people at higher risk of having children with autism. It is not necessarily the number or level of toxins in the body that cause distress but the ability of the immune system to tolerate the toxins. Furthermore, risk factors do not cause autism but rather set the tipping point for when the exposure to the risk factors tips the barrel.

Some of the major risk factors for ASD include: [12]

1. Sex: Boys are four times more likely than girls to develop autism.
2. Preterm babies: Babies born before 26 weeks of pregnancy have a higher risk of developing autism.
3. Paternal Age: Fathers over the age of 40 are more likely to pass on genetic mutations to their offspring.
4. Maternal Health: Mothers who have health issues during pregnancy are at increased risk for their children developing autism. Health conditions include obesity, smoking, and type 1 diabetes, among others.
5. Close age of siblings: Children who are born less than one year apart are three times more likely to develop autism than those born three to five years apart.
6. Exposure to environmental pollution during pregnancy: Chronic exposure to environmental pollutants during pregnancy, such as pesticides, insecticides, and road pollution, has been associated with increased rates of autism.

Although there is no known, single cause of ASD, researchers are working tirelessly to identify the "perfect storm" of events that occur in a person's brain and lead to the development of ASD over time. Below, we will present some of the proposed causes for autism, acknowledging that no one factor that has been proven to cause autism.

Theorized Causes of Autism

Genetics

Current evidence suggests that multiple genes on different chromosomes influence the expression of ASD symptoms. It appears that a person must have several different gene abnormalities for autism to occur. This is supported by identical twin studies that suggest that if one identical twin has autism, the likelihood of the other developing it was as high as 90%. Interestingly, though, fraternal twins also have a likelihood of both developing autism (10–20%).[13] Since fraternal twins share only approximately 50% of their genes but share virtually the same environment, this leads us to believe that nurture is an important component in developing autism. Gene expression for certain genes is influenced by factors such as environmental exposure to toxins both inside and outside the womb.

Brain Structures

Functional magnetic resonance imaging (fMRI) has identified that people with autism have differences in brain development in several regions of the brain. These brain changes could occur at conception due to genetic defects, could occur early in utero, or very early in infancy.[14] More specifically, people with autism have larger brains (especially in the right hemisphere) and, therefore, larger head circumferences after birth. The theory is that these individuals do not experience normal synaptic pruning, which is the process

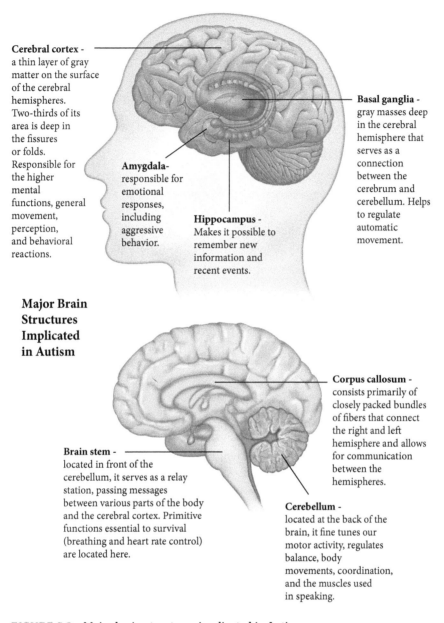

Cerebral cortex - a thin layer of gray matter on the surface of the cerebral hemispheres. Two-thirds of its area is deep in the fissures or folds. Responsible for the higher mental functions, general movement, perception, and behavioral reactions.

Amygdala- responsible for emotional responses, including aggressive behavior.

Hippocampus - Makes it possible to remember new information and recent events.

Basal ganglia - gray masses deep in the cerebral hemisphere that serves as a connection between the cerebrum and cerebellum. Helps to regulate automatic movement.

Major Brain Structures Implicated in Autism

Corpus callosum - consists primarily of closely packed bundles of fibers that connect the right and left hemisphere and allows for communication between the hemispheres.

Brain stem - located in front of the cerebellum, it serves as a relay station, passing messages between various parts of the body and the cerebral cortex. Primitive functions essential to survival (breathing and heart rate control) are located here.

Cerebellum - located at the back of the brain, it fine tunes our motor activity, regulates balance, body movements, coordination, and the muscles used in speaking.

FIGURE 5.2   Major brain structures implicated in Autism

where extra neurons and synaptic connections die to help improve the efficiency of the stronger neural pathways. These brain changes could also be a major factor as to why one third of individuals with autism also have a seizure disorder.[15] Extra neurons appear to be concentrated in the following areas of the brain:

1.   The *limbic system*, which houses the amygdala and regulates emotions and behaviors, as well as the sense of smell.

2. The *cerebellum*, which controls cognitive skills such as thinking, language, and attention, as well as motor skills.
3. The *prefrontal cortex*, which controls executive functioning such as decision making and emotion regulation.
4. The *brain stem*, which controls the sense of balance and movement through space.

Extreme Maleness Theory

According to Dr. Simon Baron-Cohen,[16] abnormally high levels of testosterone in the womb are causing infants' brains to be hyper-male. Specifically, Baron-Cohen hypothesizes that if male babies are exposed to higher-than-normal levels of testosterone at 18 weeks of pregnancy, they will develop hyper-male symptoms such as extreme systematizing and a lack of female-typical traits such as empathizing. Although this theory accounts for why more boys develop autism than girls, it does not account for other traits that are typically male dominant and that boys with autism have trouble with, such as gross motor skills and coordination.

Mirror Neuron System

Studies in monkeys have shown that a pathway in the brain, called the Mirror Neuron System (MNS), is linked to imitating the movements, gestures, facial expressions, and actions of others. Some fMRI studies have also found this system is active in humans and helps us to understand other's actions and goals (that is, empathy). Children with ASD have difficulty imitating another person's actions and facial expressions. Researchers hypothesize that dysfunction in the MNS may be a major factor in the development of ASD.[17]

Environmental Triggers

Although exposure toxins early in life can be harmful, a mother's exposure to toxins while pregnant appears to be a factor in the development of autism. (We are not mother blaming here. In fact, a theory of autism in the 1950s was that emotionally distant and "frigid" moms, also known as "refrigerator mothers," caused autism. How awful is that?) All pregnant mothers should be aware of environmental toxins during pregnancy and take steps to wash produce, avoid exposures to strong fumes, avoid cigarette smoke, limit the use of personal care products with strong scents or artificial ingredients, and talk with their health care provider about the medications they are taking, especially valproic acid (prescribed for seizures) and thalidomide (prescribed for inflammatory disorders).[18]

Vaccines

What you are about to read is very important. In 1988, a British researcher and physician by the name of Andrew Wakefield published a journal article in a well-respected, peer reviewed journal, *The Lancet*. Using a sample of 12 children, Wakefield and his colleagues concluded that there was a link between autism, bowel disease, and the MMR (Mumps, Measles and Rubella) vaccine. Wakefield also did a number of press conferences and called for the MMR vaccine to be halted until further research could be conducted. This press conference spurred the anti-vaccination movement that has gained momentum over the past few decades. Over time, researchers in the field who attempted to recreate his findings were unsuccessful, leading to a more systematic review of his initial study. After a lengthy investigation that spanned two decades, it was concluded that Wakefield "changed and misreported results in his research, creating the appearance of a possible link with autism," and the journal article was retracted.[19] Dr. Wakefield lost his medical license in England but is now the owner and director of an autism research center in Austin, TX. Since then, researchers have not been able to substantiate the claims that the MMR vaccine leads to autism. Some have hypothesized that a preservative found in vaccines, called thimerosal, may lead to autism. However, countries that have removed thimerosal from vaccines continue to see an increase in autism, which is the opposite of what would be expected if it caused autism.[20] Yet others argue that it is not the actual vaccines that cause the problem but rather that children get too many vaccines at one time and too early in life. To examine this, researchers examined the records of over 1,000 children, specifically paying attention to when they received their first-year vaccines.[21] The researchers concluded that the timing of vaccines in the first year did not lead to any significant differences in speech, memory, achievement, coordination, behavior regulations, or intellectual functioning at the ages of 7–10 years old. They concluded that the current vaccination schedule is safe. Parents must decide for themselves and need to understand the information, as well as history of the vaccine debate, to be fully informed.

Autism Across Development

Much of what we have reviewed about Autism is based on extensive research in children. As adolescents age into adulthood, more research must be conducted to understand the developmental characteristics of autism across the lifespan. In the following section, we will review specific psychosocial challenges for children, adolescence, and adults with autism.

Childhood and Adolescence

Bullying is a challenge for children and adolescents, and particularly so for those with autism. It has been estimated that 63% of teenagers with autism were victims of bullying, which is a rate three times higher than those without autism.[22] Bullying can occur for a number of reasons. Adolescents with autism may appear different in the way they dress and care for their hygiene. They may appear clumsy at times, may continue to talk about their favorite topics when others have lost interest, and may have repeated meltdowns in class. Also, people with autism are very rule bound and may challenge their peers or teachers when they perceive others to be breaking the rules. Since we know that bullying is related to increased depression, anxiety, somatic symptoms, such as stomachaches and headaches, and suicide, it is important that schools offer anti-bullying interventions to help promote acceptance of differences and empathy for others.[23]

The transition to adolescence is a tumultuous time for most young people. An adolescent with high functioning autism may become painfully aware that he is different from his peers. Despite a longing to fit in, he may have difficulty navigating the social landmines of adolescence, resulting in an increase in depression, anxiety, or other mental health disorders.[24] As tension, conflict, and confusion increases, there may also be an increase in aggressive or externalizing behaviors. Conversely, however, adolescents with autism may find themselves challenged to learn new social skills and improve interactions with others. Additionally, children with autism need to be taught appropriate boundaries across different contexts. For instance, the way to interact with a parent is different than the way to interact with a teacher, which is different than the way to interact with a stranger. Sadly, those with intellectual disabilities are at greater risk of being victims of sexual abuse. Children and adolescents need to be taught about consent in sexual relationships, the meaning of "no," and how to reach out to trusted adults when they are in trouble.[25] Mental health therapists and school counselors are professionals who can offer a safe place to learn and practice new social skills and boundaries individually or in a group setting.

Another developmental milestone that requires thoughtful care is puberty. Even the most well meaning parents of typically developing adolescents can have a hard time talking about sex. Adolescents with autism will require additional support to help them understand the physical changes that are happening in their bodies. For instance, boys may be seeing an increase in erections or nighttime ejaculations, and they must understand that this is a normal part of growing up. Girls will be developing breasts and starting their menstrual cycle, which could be very scary without information about what is happening to their bodies. Hygiene must also be addressed and taught, as adolescents begin to sweat more which leads to body odor and acne. Additionally, adolescents with autism must be taught about "public versus private." Running around naked in one's bedroom (with the blinds down) is appropriate, but running around naked outside the home is not appropriate. Masturbation is a normal part of sexual self-discovery but can only be done in the privacy of the home and not at school. These conversations will need to be explicit and clear.[26]

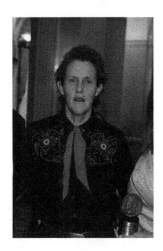

FIGURE 5.3   **Temple Grandin: Autism Advocate**

Young Adulthood

Although the transition to college or work may not be an option for adolescents with lower-functioning autism, many others will go on to college and employment. The statistics show that approximately 55% of students with autism are employed two years after graduating high school, and 35% attend college.[27] It can be helpful to assist young adults to find majors or employment that correspond with their interests. For instance, if they are interested in computers or gaming, computer science might be a good fit. Transition planning before the adolescent graduates high school can help facilitate a smooth path to post-secondary education or employment. Many great resources can guide parents and young adults through the transition to adulthood, such as author, spokesperson, and professor with autism, Temple Grandin.

Adulthood

As a generation of adolescents with autism transitions into adulthood, many questions remain about how to fully integrate adults with autism into the workplace. The promising news is that multiple researchers have found that the symptoms of people with high functioning autism tend to improve or get "toned down" in adulthood. The areas that show particular improvement into adulthood are social and daily living skills, repetitive behaviors, and emotional reciprocity.[28] However, many people with low-functioning autism continue to remain functionally impaired and require continued caregiving throughout their lifetimes. Overall, the goal is to support individuals to be able to obtain employment and live independently with a partner/spouse should they choose to do so. One study conducted by the Interactive Autism Network (IAN) found that over half of high-functioning adults with autism were employed and living with a spouse.[29] The main reason why people reported not having a job was because they were afraid that the workplace would be too challenging for them given their diagnosis. Moreover, individuals with high-functioning autism may need support, encouragement, and/or social skills training to practice how to make friends and acquaintances, although joining clubs related to specific interests is a good start. Community support is an essential component to helping people with autism thrive into adulthood, but more resources are needed to provide services to meet the needs of this population.

Family Dynamics

The moment that a child is diagnosed with autism is indelibly etched into the mind of his or her parent. A tremendous amount of grief accompanies the diagnosis. Parents may grieve the image of a typically developing child who met all of his developmental, educational, and social expectations with ease. They may grieve the loss of the child who was hitting all of his developmental milestones and then suddenly one day began losing his skills. Imagine what it would feel like to be a parent whose child grins and says, "I love you," and then one day no longer speaks? Parents may also feel confused and scared about what lies ahead for their child. Without a doubt, autism is a disease the affects the entire family. Families experience emotions such as shock and disbelief that this is happening to their child, denial that their child has autism, anger and rage that this is happening to their child, depression resulting from the challenge of daily caretaking, guilt that they did something to cause the disorder, shame and embarrassment about what others think about their child's behavior, fear about what will happen to their child as he gets older, and isolation from others. However, they may also experience significant hope that their child's behavior is improving and acceptance of the situation as time progresses. Significant challenges lie ahead, and the family must cope with the loss of what they envisioned and now live within the reality of what is. They must learn "a new normal."

Caregiving for a child on the spectrum can be very stressful for couples. They must learn to navigate the daily stress, fatigue, and decision making associated with having a child with autism. Often, one partner may be further along in the grief cycle than the other, leading to stress and conflict in how they emotionally react to the situation. The thought of planning for the child's future (e.g., who will care for the child, pay for his or her needs, etc. after the parents pass away) can feel overwhelming. Couples must try their best to focus on their relationship, identify a division of responsibility to which both partners agree, and attend counseling if needed. When support is not available, primary caregivers often experience increased daily hassles, life stress, and depression.[30] Similarly, it can be difficult for typically developing siblings to cope with the disorder. They may be jealous that their sibling requires so much attention, or they may be embarrassed by their sibling's behavior in public. If their parents are stressed, this stress can trickle down to their relationship with the siblings. It may also be difficult to live with a sibling who is not interested in playing or spending time together. However, siblings of children with autism tend to become incredibly empathetic, show compassion for others, and develop a strong sense of responsibility.[31]

The Role of Individuals, Families, and Communities in Promoting Autism Interventions

There is no cure for autism. Therefore, the most effective and encouraging treatments are those that help to manage the symptoms associated with ASD. Below, we will briefly describe the most effective treatments.

Applied Behavior Analysis

Applied Behavior Analysis (ABA) is a treatment supported by research to be effective for managing ASD symptoms and is currently considered the "gold standard" treatment for autism.[32] ABA, which was created by Dr. Ole Ivar Lovaas, is based on B.F. Skinner's behavioral principles of reinforcement and operant conditioning (i.e., every behavior has an antecedent and a consequence and can be shaped by reinforcement). In ABA, a trained therapist breaks down behaviors to the most basic parts and consistently rewards the child for approximating and completing those parts. For instance, take the example of teaching a child to make eye contact with adults. First, you might reward the child for looking in the general direction of the person speaking by giving him or her a Cheerio. After that skill is mastered, the child would earn a Cheerio for turning his or her head, then for looking somewhere on the person's face, and then in his or her eyes. If a skill is done incorrectly (e.g., turning away from the adult rather than toward him or her) the incorrect behavior is ignored. In ABA, the therapist breaks down the component parts of behavior for each skill that the child needs to master,

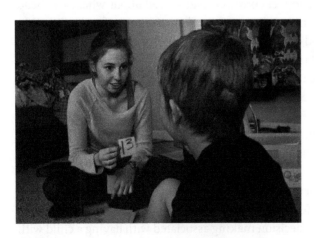

FIGURE 5.4 **A young boy with Autism and his therapist engaging in Applied Behavior Analysis (ABA)**

ranging from social interactions to academic learning to activities of daily living such as using the toilet. When done correctly and in its purest form, ABA is an intensive program requiring 30–40 hours per week of therapy, first in the home, then at school, and finally generalized to the community (e.g., teaching the child how to behave in the grocery store). There are many different forms of ABA, all tailored to children of different age ranges. Children in ABA make considerable gains in all areas, and it is amazing to watch their progress over time!

Early Intervention

Early Intervention, or EI, is a free service offered to children who are under the age of three and have been diagnosed with some sort of developmental delay or health condition that affects their development. These children are evaluated by a team of specialists, including speech and language therapists, occupational therapists, physical therapists, developmental specialists, registered nurses, social workers, and mental health clinicians, and the team decides what skills require attention. The team creates an Individualized Family Service Plan, which outlines the goals for the child's development and how they will be achieved. On a regular basis, therapists come to the home and work with the child to improve his or her skills and to also educate the family in how to support the child's progress throughout the week. Early Intervention has been shown in research to significantly improve a child's development in the early years and beyond.[33]

Medication

While there is not a medication that will cure ASD, medications can be used to treat the behavioral excesses (i.e., behaviors that a person does too much of) or behavioral deficits (i.e., behaviors that a person does too little of). For instance, if a person with ASD is experiencing anxiety and depression, he or she may be prescribed antidepressant or anxiolytic medications. If a person has trouble sleeping, he or she may be prescribed a sleeping medication. If a person experiences seizures, he or she will likely be treated with an anticonvulsant medication. At times, antipsychotic drugs may be prescribed, as they can be effective in controlling extreme behavioral excesses.[34]

Picture Exchange Communication System (PECS)

Most people who have worked with young children have had the opportunity to use a picture-exchange system. PECS uses picture symbols to allow a person to communicate by teaching the person to exchange picture symbols to ask questions and have conversations. PECS are also widely used to display the routine for the day so that the routine can be followed without the need to read words.[35] Since some children with ASD lack language, PECS are used to facilitate communication.

Sensory Integration Therapy

Since many people with ASD experience difficulty processing and integrating sensory information, sensory integration therapy helps rewire the person's brain to be able to tolerate different types of lights, noises, and touch. A trained occupational therapist will work with the child to increasingly challenge the child to immerse himself in new sensory environments by using carefully selected games that challenge the child but do not stress him to the point of panic.[36]

Alternative Therapies

Aside from the mainstream treatment described above, many alternative treatments can be used in combination with Applied Behavior Analyses. For instance, many people with autism benefit from Equine Therapy, or horse riding therapy. Equine Therapy helps foster emotional bonds with the horse, work on cognitive and language skills by interacting with the trainer, and helps improve balance and spatial orientation. It's also fun! Another promising type of therapy is Virtual-reality Training Programs. These programs project the face of the person with autism onto an avatar. The therapist and one or two others have avatars that help to teach social skills for specific situations such as going on a job interview or a date.[37]

Community Action Programs—Autism Speaks

Although many community action programs exist in different communities, perhaps the most well known is Autism Speaks. Established in 2005 by Bob and Suzanne Wright, grandparents of a child with autism, Autism Speaks is the world's leading organization dedicated to researching both causes and treatment for ASD, advocating for the needs of individuals with ASD and their families, working toward creating policy that protects the rights of individuals with ASD, and working toward finding a cure for the disease.[38] Autism Speaks also initiates significant fundraising efforts to be able to fund these endeavors.

Autism Speaks engages in community-level advocacy in a variety of ways. Its website provides legal resources and health care insurance information for families. The organization also participates in state and federal initiatives. For example, at the state level, the organization advocates for legislative reform such as the Achieving a Better Life Experience (ABLE) reform, which allows families to set up tax-exempt savings accounts for disability-related expenses, or laws allowing families to access health insurance to cover the costs of Applied Behavior Analysis. At the federal level, Autism Speaks has advocated for laws that allow funding to help children with autism through increased education and prevention programs targeted at caregivers, to increase access to Career and Technical Education training and job opportunities for young adults with autism, and to promote reforms that provide formal education to caregivers for how to locate services to care for loved ones with autism. To become involved in this organization or for more information, please visit www.autismspeaks.org.

Individual with Disabilities Education Act

All children with disabilities are covered under the *IDEA* (Individual with Disabilities Education) *Act*.[39] This act ensures that all children have access to "free and appropriate education." While a child or adolescent is in school and covered by IDEA, it is important

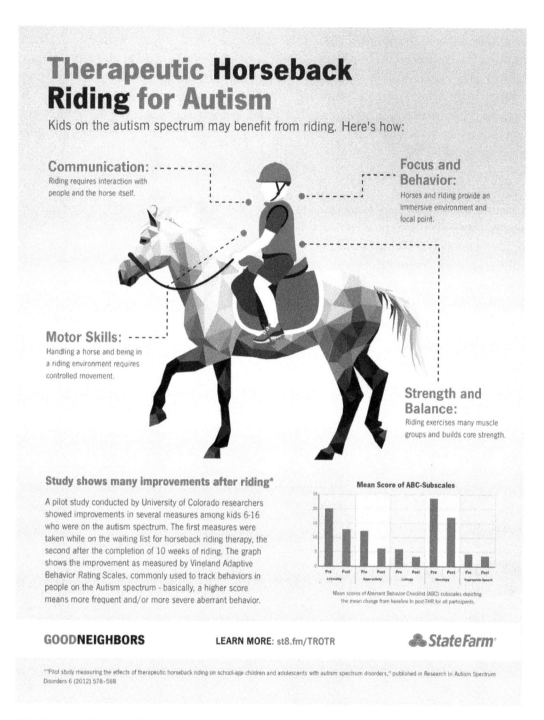

Therapeutic Horseback Riding for Autism

Kids on the autism spectrum may benefit from riding. Here's how:

Communication:
Riding requires interaction with people and the horse itself.

Focus and Behavior:
Horses and riding provide an immersive environment and focal point.

Motor Skills:
Handling a horse and being in a riding environment requires controlled movement.

Strength and Balance:
Riding exercises many muscle groups and builds core strength.

Study shows many improvements after riding*

A pilot study conducted by University of Colorado researchers showed improvements in several measures among kids 6-16 who were on the autism spectrum. The first measures were taken while on the waiting list for horseback riding therapy, the second after the completion of 10 weeks of riding. The graph shows the improvement as measured by Vineland Adaptive Behavior Rating Scales, commonly used to track behaviors in people on the Autism spectrum - basically, a higher score means more frequent and/or more severe aberrant behavior.

Mean Score of ABC-Subscales

Mean scores of Aberrant Behavior Checklist (ABC) subscales depicting the mean change from baseline to post-THR for all participants.

GOODNEIGHBORS   LEARN MORE: st8.fm/TROTR   🍀 *State Farm*

*"Pilot study measuring the effects of therapeutic horseback riding on school-age children and adolescents with autism spectrum disorders," published in Research in Autism Spectrum Disorders 6 (2012) 578–588

FIGURE 5.5   Benefits of therapeutic horseback riding for Autism

to use it to teach necessary life skills, such as self-regulation and organizational skills. These skills will be required as the adolescent moves into adulthood, but free services are harder to access after graduation from high school. Although the federal government originally pledged to subsidize 40% of the cost of each student with a disability, IDEA funding has continued to drop over the past two decades. The federal government currently funds only 11 to 16% per student with a disability, depending on level of poverty within the district. Decreased funding, coupled with high special education teacher turnover and sometimes inadequately trained paraprofessionals, leads to a system where people try their best, but sometimes their best does not meet the needs of each individual student.

Insurance Benefits

Learning to navigate the health care system becomes an increasingly important part of autism management. Parents will find themselves immersed in a world of learning their rights and responsibilities, as well as figuring out how to access services. Contacting local autism support groups can be very helpful, as well as learning about Medicaid benefits, eligibility of services for people with developmental disabilities, and eligibility for Supplemental Security Income (SSI) to help supplement the cost of treatment. Also, did you know that currently private insurance companies can choose whether to cover autism related treatment? Advocacy groups are working tirelessly to make mandatory coverage a federal mandate.

Conclusion

Autism Spectrum Disorder is a developmental disability that causes changes in how people communicate, behave, act, and learn. Autism has a profound effect on the individual, as well as on parents, siblings, teachers, and communities. Although autism can never be cured, a variety of treatment options are available to improve functioning. Community advocacy groups also do important work to increase awareness, therapeutic programs, and funding for research.

Case Study

The following is a letter to a teacher, written from a mother. The purpose of this letter is for you to understand how parents of a child with autism feel and think upon sending their children to school.

Dear Teacher:

My 12-year-old son will be beginning the new year in your classroom. He is a smart, funny, and responsible child. He excels in science and math, but like all kids, he also struggles in some areas. His biggest struggle is that he has been diagnosed with autism.

At the beginning of every school year I am unsure if I should meet with you in advance to tell you about his diagnosis. Every year, I decide to let you form your own opinions of him.

And every year, I get a call a few weeks into the school year to discuss his "issues." Yes, he does have issues. He is extremely literal and requires precise instruction and feedback. If your directions or feedback are unclear, he will not know how to follow them. He needs extra time in subjects such as English and Social Studies because those subjects can be illogical. My son has difficulty focusing and is easily distracted. He also has few, if any friends, and feels very lonely on a daily basis.

All of these issues have been addressed in my son's 504 plan, and you have very clear suggestions for how to deal with my son. Some teachers are great about reading and applying his 504; others are not. I hope that you are the former. Instead of viewing my child as being "a complete distraction," "an attention seeker," or viewing me as "an overbearing mother," I hope that you are one of the teachers who tries to understand what it is like to be my son. To be a child who wants to learn but whose brain won't allow him to focus and learn in the traditional way. To be a child who wants to have friends but whose brain can't figure out how to say socially appropriate things and seems to often start fights with his peers. To be a child who, as he gets older, develops different quirks and moves further away from fitting in with his peers.

Your daily interactions will teach him that he is valued, and your daily interactions will shape the way that our family interacts when he arrives home from a long and overwhelming day. Your daily interactions will also be watched by his peers and will set the tone for the way that other kids will interact with him and other children like him. Thank you for remembering that he is a good boy, and he is someone's son—my son—and I will be forever grateful for the empathy, compassion, and patience that you show him on a daily basis.

Yours truly,
Noah's Mom

Notes

[1] Karim, K., Ali, A., & O'Reilly, M. (2014). *A practical guide to mental health problems in children with ASD*. London: Jessica Kingsley.

[2] National Institute on Deafness and Other Communication Disorders (2012). *Autism spectrum disorder: communication problems in children* (NIH Publication No. 97–4315). Washington, DC: U.S. Government Printing Office.

[3] Coury, D. L., Ashwood, P., Fasano, A., Fuchs, G., Geraghty, M., Kaul, A., Mawe, G., Patterson, P., and Jones, N. (2012). Gastrointestinal conditions in children with autism spectrum disorder: Developing a research agenda. *AAP News & Journals Gateway*, 130. doi:10.1542/peds.2012-0900N

[4] Christensen, D.L., Baio, J., Van Naarden Braun, K., et al. (2016). Prevalence and characteristics of autism spectrum disorder among children aged 8 years—Autism and developmental disabilities monitoring network, 11 sites, United States, 2012. *MMWR Surveillance Summaries*. 65(No. SS-3): 1–23.

5 Mandell, D. S., Wiggins, L. D., Carpenter, L. A., Daniels, J., DiGuiseppi, C., Durkin, M. S., & Shattuck, P. T. (2009). Racial/ethnic disparities in the identification of children with autism spectrum disorders. *American Journal of Public Health*, *99*(3), 493–498.

6 Mandell, D. S., Wiggins, L. D., Carpenter, L. A., Daniels, J., DiGuiseppi, C., Durkin, M. S., & Shattuck, P. T. (2009). Racial/ethnic disparities in the identification of children with autism spectrum disorders. *American Journal of Public Health*, *99*(3), 493–498.

7 Centers for Disease Control and Prevention. (2015). Estimated prevalence of autism and other developmental disabilities following questionnaire changed in the 2014 national health interview survey. Retrieved from https://www.cdc.gov/nchs/data/nhsr/nhsr087.pdf

8 Miller, J. S., Bilder, D., Farley, M., Coon, H., Pinborough-Zimmerman, J., Jenson, W., McMahon, W. M. (2013). Autism spectrum disorder reclassified: A second look at the 1980s Utah/UCLA autism epidemiologic study. *Journal of Autism and Developmental Disorders*, *43*(1), 200–210. http://doi.org/10.1007/s10803-012-1566-0

9 Liu, K., King, M., & Bearman, P. S. (2010). Social influence and the autism epidemic. *American Journal of Sociology*, *115*(5), 1387–1434.

10 CDC estimates 1 in 68 children has been identified with autism spectrum disorder. (2014). Centers for Disease Control and Prevention. Retrieved January 16, 2017, from https://www.cdc.gov/media/releases/2014/p0327-autism-spectrum-disorder.html

11 Marks, K. P., Glascoe, F. P., & Macias, M. M. (2011). Enhancing the algorithm for developmental-behavioral surveillance and screening in children 0 to 5 years. *Clinical Pediatrics*, *50*(9), 853–868. doi:10.1177/0009922811406263

12 Autism spectrum disorder. (2014). Mayo Clinic. Retrieved January 16, 2017, from http://www.mayoclinic.org/diseases-conditions/autism-spectrum-disorder/basics/risk-factors/con-20021148

13 Hallmayer, J., Cleveland, S., Torres, A., Phillips, J., Cohen, B., Torigoe, T., & Lotspeich, L. (2011). Genetic heritability and shared environmental factors among twin pairs with autism. *Archives of General Psychiatry*, *68*(11), 1095–1102.

14 Autism spectrum disorder fact sheet. (2015, September). National Institute of Neurological Disorders and Stroke. Retrieved January 16, 2017, from https://www.ninds.nih.gov/Disorders/Patient-Caregiver-Education/Fact-Sheets/Autism-Spectrum-Disorder-Fact-Sheet

15 Virtual reality training improves social skills and brain activity. (2014). *Autism Speaks*. Retrieved from https://www.autismspeaks.org/science/science-news/virtual-reality-training-improves-social-skills-and-brain-activity

16 Baron-Cohen, S. (2002). The extreme male brain theory of autism. *Trends in Cognitive Sciences*, *6*(6), 248–254.

17 Shannon, J.B. (2011). Autism and pervasive developmental disorders sourcebook (Health Reference). Second Edition. Detroit, MI: Omnigraphics, Inc.

18 Centers for Disease Control (2015). *Thimerosal in vaccines*. Retrieved from http://www.cdc.gov/vaccinesafety/Concerns/thimerosal/index.html

19 Deer, B. (2009). MMR doctor fixed data on autism. *The Sunday Times* (London).

20 Centers for Disease Control (2015). *Thimerosal in vaccines*. Retrieved from http://www.cdc.gov/vaccinesafety/Concerns/thimerosal/index.html

21 Smith, M. J., & Woods, C. R. (2010). On-time vaccine receipt in the first year does not adversely affect neuropsychological outcomes. *Pediatrics*, *125*(6), 1134–1141.

22 Anderson, C. (2014). IAN research report: Bullying and children with ASD. Interactive Autism Network. Retrieved from http://www.iancommunity.org/cs/ian_research_reports/ian_research_report_bullying

23 New study finds bullying causes significant short-term emotional and physical consequences for children with autism. (2013). Kennedy Krieger Institute. Retrieved from https://www.kennedykrieger.org/overview/news/study-finds-bullying-causes-significant-short-term-emotional-physical-consequenses-for-children-with-autism

24 Autism spectrum disorder. (2016). National Institute of Mental Health. Retrieved from http://www.nimh.nih.gov/health/topics/autism-spectrum-disorders-asd/index.shtml#part_145442

25 Sicile-Kira, C. (2014, May 05). Autism life skills: 10 essential abilities for children with ASD. Education.com. Retrieved January 16, 2017, from http://www.education.com/reference/article/autism-life-skill-ten-essential-abilties-ASD/

26 Sicile-Kira, C. (2014, August 7). Autism & modern love. Autism College. Retrieved January 16, 2017, from http://autismcollege.com/blog/tag/puberty/

27 Shattuck, P. T., Narendorf, S. C., Cooper, B., Sterzing, P. R., Wagner, M., & Taylor, J. L. (2012). Postsecondary education and employment among youth with an autism spectrum disorder. *Pediatrics*, peds-2011.

28 McGovern, C. W., & Sigman, M. (2005). Continuity and change from early childhood to adolescence in autism. *Journal of Child Psychology and Psychiatry*, *46*(4), 401–408.

29 First look: Data on adults on the autism spectrum. (2009). Interactive Autism Network. Retrieved from https://iancommunity.org/cs/ian_research_reports/adults_on_the_autism_spectrum_september_2009

30 Quintero, N., & McIntyre, L. L. (2010). Sibling adjustment and maternal well-being: An examination of families with and without a child with an autism spectrum disorder. *Focus on Autism and Other Developmental Disabilities*, *25*(1), 37–46.

31 Sicile-Kira, C. (2015, October 23). The affects of autism in families and in partner relationships. Retrieved January 17, 2017, from http://autismcollege.com/blog/2015/07/27/the-affects-of-autism-in-families-and-in-partner-relationships-3/

32 Applied Behavior Analysis (ABA). (2012). Autism Speaks. Retrieved January 17, 2017, from https://www.autismspeaks.org/what-autism/treatment/applied-behavior-analysis-aba

33 Overview of early intervention. (2014, March). Center for Parent Information & Resources. Retrieved January 17, 2017, from http://www.parentcenterhub.org/repository/ei-overview/

34 Madden, J., Lakoma, M., Lynch, F., Rusinak, D., Owen-Smith, A., Coleman, K., & … Croen, L. (2017). Psychotropic medication use among insured children with autism spectrum disorder. *Journal of Autism & Developmental Disorders*, *47*(1), 144–154. doi:10.1007/s10803–016-2946–7

35 Alsayedhassan, B., Banda, D. R., & Griffin-Shirley, N. (2016). A review of picture exchange communication interventions implemented by parents and practitioners. *Child & Family Behavior Therapy*, *38*(3), 191–208. doi:10.1080/07317107.2016.1203135

36 Schaaf, R. C., Hunt, J., & Benevides, T. (2012, September). Occupational therapy using sensory integration to improve participation of a child with autism: A case report. *American*

Journal of Occupational Therapy. Retrieved January 17, 2017, from http://ajot.aota.org/article.aspx?articleid=1851609

37 Kandalaft, M. R., Didehbani, N., Krawczyk, D. C., Allen, T. T., & Chapman, S. B. (2012). Virtual reality social cognition training for young adults with high-functioning autism. *Journal of Autism and Developmental Disorders*, *43*(1), 34–44. doi:10.1007/s10803-012-1544-6

38 Community Grants. (2014). Autism Speaks. Retrieved January 17, 2017, from https://www.autismspeaks.org/families-and-adults/grants/community-grants

39 IDEA—Building the legacy of IDEA 2004. (n.d.). Retrieved January 17, 2017, from http://idea.ed.gov/explore

Figure Sources

1 Figure 5.2: Source: https://commons.wikimedia.org/wiki/File:Autismbrain.jpg.

2 Figure 5.3: Copyright © Peabody Awards (CC by 2.0) at https://commons.wikimedia.org/wiki/File:Temple_Grandin_Peabody_Awards_2011.jpg.

3 Figure 5.4: Source: https://media.defense.gov/2012/Apr/18/2000160075/670/394/0/120416-F-LR006-016.JPG.

4 Figure 5.5: Copyright © Research in Autism Spectrum Disorders (CC by 2.0) at https://c1.static flickr.com/8/7485/15163072864_463c907f39_b.jpg.

CHAPTER SIX

Alzheimer's disease

Coauthors:
Genevieve Dash, M.S., Sue K. Adams, Ph.D., Sarah W. Feldstein Ewing, Ph.D.

@ alzheimerssoc

We all know someone who has a bad memory: a friend who always forgets what time to meet for coffee, a coworker who has to make lists to remember what needs to be done, or a grandparent who tells the same story repeatedly. Short-term memory can decline with age, and older adults may begin to forget things as simple as the content of a conversation from earlier in the day. Often times, these lapses in memory are explained away by statements such as "It's normal for old people to forget things." At what point does forgetfulness cross the line to disease? For many families, it is when safety issues arise. For others, it is when there is a crisis so serious that it cannot be ignored. The following chapter offers an overview of Alzheimer's disease. By the end of this chapter, you will be familiar with the causes of Alzheimer's disease, what the symptoms of Alzheimer's look like, how the disease is diagnosed and treated, and the broad implications of the disease for the individual, the family, and society. You will also be introduced to the reciprocal relationships between Alzheimer's and genetics, environment, and social issues.

What Is Alzheimer's Disease?

You may have heard of Alzheimer's referred to as "old timer's" disease, as it is most often a disease of old age. The symptoms, however, of Alzheimer's are not a normal part of aging. When memory and cognitive impairment begin to interfere with daily functioning, it may cause impairment to a point at which it is a diagnosable disease in need of medical attention. With Alzheimer's disease, memory and other *cognitive skills*, or the basic mental processes such as thinking, reasoning, and memory that are used in daily life, become impaired. Because Alzheimer's is *degenerative* and progressively causes irreversible damage to the brain, these skills can degrade to a point at which the tasks of daily living are unmanageable for the afflicted individual, and he or she becomes dependent on others for care.

Alzheimer's is a major public health concern, and it is estimated that 5.1 million adults in the United States have Alzheimer's disease, with someone developing Alzheimer's every 66 seconds. It is the sixth-leading cause of death in the United States and the third-leading cause of death among older adults, behind heart disease and cancer. In 2015, Alzheimer's cost the U.S. approximately $236 billion, and the cost is estimated to skyrocket to $1 trillion by 2050[1].

Health Disparities

Some people may be more likely to be diagnosed with Alzheimer's due to existing *health disparities* that cause the disease to differentially impact particular groups based on inequalities in access to health care across racial, ethnic, and socioeconomic groups. Different cultural groups, however, have different ideas about the progression of normal aging, which can make assessment of Alzheimer's difficult. Another challenge that arises is the ability to perform objective tests of cognitive functioning across a population with hugely discrepant levels of educational attainment.

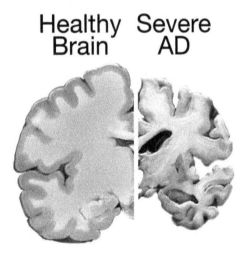

Healthy Severe
Brain AD

FIGURE 6.1 **Healthy brain vs. brain with severe Alzheimer's Disease**

Age

Alzheimer's is a disease of age. Those aged 65 and older are disproportionately affected by Alzheimer's, simply by the nature of the disease itself. Four percent of individuals under the age of 65, 15% of individuals aged 65–74 years, 43% of individuals aged 75–84 years, and 38% of individuals aged 85 years or older have Alzheimer's disease.[2] Of concern is the notable growth of the elderly population in the U.S. over time, which leads to Alzheimer's becoming an intensified public health issue. According to the U.S. Census, the percentage of the U.S. population accounted for by individuals age 65 and over is at an all-time high and is expected to continue increasing. This places 13% of the country's people at increased risk of Alzheimer's.[3]

Race

It appears as though there are differences in the etiology, onset, and presentation of Alzheimer's across different racial and ethnic groups. Age of onset of Alzheimer's is significantly earlier in Latinos than in non-Hispanic whites and African Americans. Latinos diagnosed with Alzheimer's also demonstrate lower levels of cognitive performance than non-Hispanic whites and African Americans; African Americans also show lower performance than non-Hispanic whites. While there are differences between the racial and ethnic groups in level of educational attainment, the differences in cognitive performance remain even when controlling for education. This demonstrates that individuals identifying as non-white seem to fare worse with respect to cognitive decline due to Alzheimer's. Latinos also seem to experience the most severe symptoms of dementia as compared to African Americans and non-Hispanic whites. Interestingly, the APOE-ε4 risk gene (which you will read about shortly) does not seem to be associated with Alzheimer's in Latinos, while this is known to be a risk gene and is associated with Alzheimer's in African Americans and non-Hispanic whites. Overall, Hispanics and African Americans are more likely to be diagnosed with Alzheimer's than non-Hispanic whites, and these minority groups are also more likely to experience more severe symptoms.[4] In addition, the rate of preventable hospitalizations in Hispanic and Latino adults with diagnosed dementias (34.2%) were approximately one and half times the rate of those in non-Hispanic white adults with a diagnosed dementia (23.7%) according to Healthy People 2020. The cause of these differences is not clear, and a number of factors including income, diet, health care access, cognitively stimulating work, and other environmental factors may be responsible.

Gender

Women bear the burden of Alzheimer's diagnoses in the United States, making up about two-thirds of all cases. This may be due to women having longer lifespans and, therefore, having increased exposure to the risk factor of old age. However, women seem to experience more severe symptoms and decline more rapidly than men do.

In addition to experiencing higher rates of diagnosis and more severe symptoms, women disproportionately bear the burden of caregiving for individuals with Alzheimer's. A vast majority of those caring for family members with Alzheimer's are women, and they experience the effects of stress, depression, and anxiety that come with filling that role. Women are also less likely to receive the benefits of social care and support when they themselves have Alzheimer's, as they are more likely to be living without a spouse and tend to receive less time in the care of family and friends.

Income and Education

Income and education are often presented together, and socioeconomic status and educational attainment are strongly related. Individuals with lower educational attainment appear to be at higher risk for Alzheimer's; it may be the case that higher socioeconomic status and higher educational attainment are protective factors in brain shrinkage and cognitive decline in early Alzheimer's. One theory suggests that lower levels of educational attainment lead to lower socioeconomic status, which increases the likelihood of poor nutrition and decreased accessibility to health care. These factors would increase the risk for development of Alzheimer's. It has also been hypothesized that higher levels of education lead to more neural connections in the brain, which build a "cognitive reserve" that creates resilience and the ability to compensate for deterioration. Similarly, other theories suggest that individuals with higher levels of education are also more likely to have more mentally stimulating jobs, which strengthen neural connections and cognitive abilities that protect against Alzheimer's.[5]

These disparities also impact individuals who have already been diagnosed. The rate of preventable hospitalizations in adults with diagnosed dementias with family incomes at 100–199% of the poverty threshold (30.7%) were more than one and half times the rate of those whose family incomes were at or above 400% of the poverty threshold (18.8%). Perceived income inadequacy is also related to depression and anxiety in caregivers for those with Alzheimer's.[6]

Social Environment

It has been shown that extent of social ties and networks modify the relationship between Alzheimer's disease and cognitive decline. It seems to be the case that elderly individuals with more extensive social networks experience the negative effects of Alzheimer's to a lesser extent than those who are less socially engaged. It can become increasingly challenging for individuals with Alzheimer's to maintain social relationships, as cognitive abilities steadily decline and social interactions become increasingly confusing and frustrating.

Healthy People 2020

According to Healthy People 2020, only about half of people with Alzheimer's have been diagnosed. Given the potential public health impact, a number of health objectives have been identified by Healthy People 2020 as goals to work toward over the next few years and likely over the next decade. Objectives include reducing the costs of caring for those living with Alzheimer's, reducing the Alzheimer's morbidity, increasing the rates of diagnosis, reducing symptoms through improved medical management, reducing the rate of co-morbid conditions (e.g., depression), decreasing preventable hospitalizations that could be treated in an outpatient setting, and supporting family and caregivers of those with Alzheimer's.

Symptoms and Diagnosis of Alzheimer's

It can be challenging to differentiate declines in memory that are part of normal aging from declines that may be caused by Alzheimer's. Specific areas of cognitive decline that may signal the onset of Alzheimer's include regular and consistent troubles with word-finding, visiospatial challenges, and impaired reasoning and judgment. More definitive symptoms of Alzheimer's include significant problems in attention, executive function, learning and memory, language, perception, motor skills, and/or social cognition. This leads to observable impairment in attention, abstract thinking, problem solving, short-term memory, speech, responsiveness to surrounding environment, and processing of social information.

Signs are objective characteristics of a disease that are observable by others, and *symptoms* are subjective feelings of disease or illness that are perceived and reported by the person experiencing them. The most well-known and recognizable symptom of Alzheimer's is memory loss. This can lead to secondary symptoms of disorientation, challenges in attentiveness and planning, decline in short-term memory, and decreased language capabilities. As the disease progresses, cognitive symptoms become more pronounced, and mood and behavioral signs and symptoms begin to become more apparent.

The *Alzheimer's Association* provides a list of the 10 most common signs and symptoms of Alzheimer's. Most of these are related to the cognitive declines that lead to the most significant impairment due to Alzheimer's. *Cognitive* symptoms include:

- disruptive memory loss that leads to forgetfulness of important events and requesting the same information repeatedly,
- misplacing items,
- difficulty in problem solving and concentrating, and
- challenges with daily tasks such as driving familiar routes.

Symptoms of *disorientation* are also a red flag, such as losing track of the day and passage of time, difficulty understanding spatial relationships and judging distance, and getting lost. Another symptom that indicates the presence of Alzheimer's symptoms is *language trouble*, such as struggling with finding a particular word. Also *social and mood changes* can indicate the onset of Alzheimer's. These include poor judgment, social withdrawal, and mood changes to become more suspicious, depressed, or anxious.

Stages and Progression

Alzheimer's begins to impact the brain and body before symptoms are present. Biological changes due to Alzheimer's begin to occur and continue through development of Alzheimer's. In *preclinical*, or *presymptomatic*, Alzheimer's, biological changes related to the progression of Alzheimer's are occurring in the body. Symptoms have yet to reach clinical levels and may or may not be apparent to the individual. In *mild cognitive impairment due to Alzheimer's*, some memory and thinking abilities are impaired to an extent noticeable to the individual and those around them, but symptoms do not inhibit daily functioning. Finally, in *dementia due to Alzheimer's*, cognitive decline increases to a point at which daily functioning is impaired.

Dementia is a general term for the loss of cognitive functions such as thought, memory, and reasoning that is severe enough to cause distress or impairment in daily life. Over time, neural connections decline, and impairment increases. People living with Alzheimer's are at greater risk for frequent injury, financial difficulty, and personal challenges that impact the individual, his or her family and friends, and society as a whole. Depending on the age at which they were diagnosed, those with Alzheimer's typically live for about four to eight years after diagnosis, but can survive much longer—up to 20 years in some cases. Alzheimer's is the most common form of dementia and accounts for 60 to 80% of cases. There are, however, many other causes of dementia such as Parkinson's Disease, strokes, brain

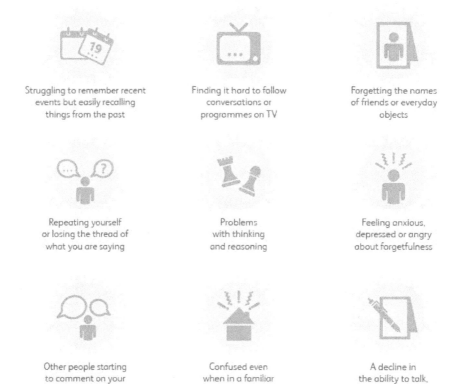

Recognising the signs and symptoms of dementia

Only 41% of people with dementia receive a diagnosis. Dementia affects everyone in different ways, but you should seek help from your GP if your memory is not as good as it used to be and especially if you notice the following signs and symptoms.

Struggling to remember recent events but easily recalling things from the past

Finding it hard to follow conversations or programmes on TV

Forgetting the names of friends or everyday objects

Repeating yourself or losing the thread of what you are saying

Problems with thinking and reasoning

Feeling anxious, depressed or angry about forgetfulness

Other people starting to comment on your forgetfulness

Confused even when in a familiar environment

A decline in the ability to talk, read or write

FIGURE 6.2   **Symptoms and signs of Alzheimer's can vary from person to person. Alzheimer's is a disease which falls under the broad category of Dementia—a syndrome that affects cognitive processes**

tumors and infections, sleep disorders, chronic alcohol use disorder, vitamin deficiencies, and side effects of certain medications.

Three-stage Model of Alzheimer's Severity

The Alzheimer's Association developed a three-stage model for Alzheimer's that describes the course of the disease once it has become symptomatic. The disease progresses through *mild*, *moderate*, and *severe* stages as degeneration progresses and cognitive capacity declines. These stages account for the progression of the disease in someone who has dementia due to Alzheimer's.

Mild Stage

The first stage is *mild, or early-stage, Alzheimer's*, in which some memory and thinking abilities are impaired to an extent noticeable to the individual and others, but symptoms do not inhibit daily functioning. Diagnosis typically occurs in this stage, as memory loss and cognitive decline become apparent. Many people in this stage are able to retain the ability to participate in work and social activities but may repeat questions and take longer to perform daily tasks and notice themselves forgetting familiar words or where they placed a personal belonging. This might include minor errors such as putting keys in the sugar bowl, forgetting the name of a newly introduced person, or struggling to find the right word. While these errors may be thought of as relatively minor, as we have all likely had similar experiences, these types of errors can be indicative of the development of cognitive impairment if they become increasingly frequent.

Moderate Stage

The second and longest stage is *moderate, or middle-stage, Alzheimer's*, which can last for many years. Damage in areas of the brain controlling language, reasoning, sensory processing, and conscious thought occurs during the moderate phase of Alzheimer's. Symptoms occurring in the mild phase get worse, as memory impairment and confusion become more severe. Forgetfulness increases, leading to mood symptoms of frustration and anger. In this phase, individuals may struggle to complete tasks of daily living and self-care such as dressing, and they may be unable to learn new things or cope with unfamiliar situations. Other symptoms that occur in this stage include forgetting personal history, struggling to recognize familiar people, disorientation to time, changes in sleep patterns, and social withdrawal. In this stage individuals with Alzheimer's may wander aimlessly, become lost and not know the day or time, wear odd clothes if dressing without assistance, and become paranoid or suspicious about those around them. Repetitive behaviors, such as wringing the hands and shredding tissues, can also occur. Many of the symptoms of paranoia and delusion may be due to inability to orient to day and time or to recognize familiar faces. Imagine how fearful you might be if you suddenly did not know where you were, and you were surrounded by people you thought were strangers but all knew your name.

Severe Stage

In *severe, or late stage, Alzheimer's*, brain tissue shrinks as plaques and tangles spread throughout the brain. Some people may lose the ability to respond to their environment, making communication difficult or impossible. They may also require full-time care due to difficulty with walking, sitting, and eating, and they may eventually lose control of all movement. In some advanced cases of severe Alzheimer's, speech is completely impaired, and individuals are fully dependent on others for their care; they may be rendered almost or completely immobile. In this stage, individuals require around-the-clock care and are completely disoriented. They are likely bedridden, living only with assistance from a caretaker. Alzheimer's is a *terminal disease*, meaning that those who have the disease will die from it unless they die from something else first.

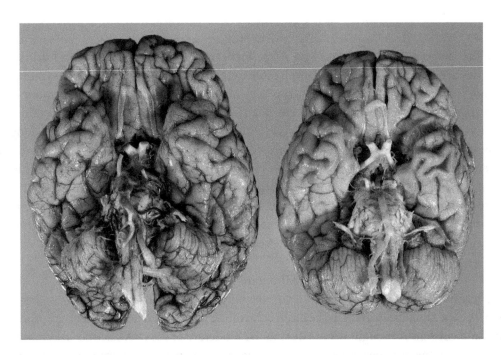

FIGURE 6.3   A healthy brain (left) and the brain of a person with Alzheimer's (right)

What Causes Alzheimer's Disease?

Alzheimer's primarily impacts adults over the age of 65, although about 5% of those diagnosed with the disease are in their 40s or 50s. Those who begin experiencing symptoms when they are younger have *early onset Alzheimer's,* while those who begin experiencing symptoms when they are over 65 have *late onset Alzheimer's.* Clearly, these forms of Alzheimer's differ in the typical age of the person when they begin to experience symptoms and also differ in *etiology,* or the cause, of the disease. The cause of Alzheimer's disease is not completely understood, although some genetic mutations are identifiable in a minority of cases. Early-onset Alzheimer's is typically caused by these genetic mutations. Late-onset Alzheimer's, which is the most common, is thought to be caused by a number of complex changes in the brain that occur over a long period of time (some research indicates decades) and are influenced by genetic, environmental, and lifestyle factors which are discussed below.

Genes

Scientists have found that genes play a role in the development of Alzheimer's disease and have even discovered specific genes that may be culprits. One of these genes is a *deterministic gene* and another is a *risk gene.*

Deterministic genes are a causal factor in the development of disease and typically guarantee that the carrier of that gene with develop the disease. In the case of Alzheimer's, variations in the genetic coding of three particular proteins have been linked to development of the disease. These proteins are the *amyloid precursor protein (APP), presenilin-1 (PS-1),* and *presenilin-2 (PS-2)* proteins. When Alzheimer's is directly caused by the biologically inherited variation in coding of these proteins, it is referred to as *"Autosomal Dominant Alzheimer's Disease (ADAD)"* or *"Familial Alzheimer's Disease (FAD)."* While FAD is uncommon and accounts for only about 5% of all Alzheimer's cases worldwide, it can affect multiple generations of family members and cause symptoms to show as early as a person's 30s with symptoms almost guaranteed to appear by age 60.

Risk genes, on the other hand, make it more likely that the carrier of the gene will develop a disease, but do not guarantee that he or she will have it. Forms of the apolipoprotein E (APOE) gene have been implicated in late-onset Alzheimer's. The three common types of the APOE gene are APOE-ε2, APOE-ε3, and APOE-ε4; risk of Alzheimer's is associated with the APOE-ε4 form of the gene. One form of the APOE gene is inherited from each parent. This means that the risk for developing Alzheimer's is higher in those who inherit the ε4 form of the APOE gene, and even higher in those who inherit two APOE-ε4 forms (one from each parent). While the ε4 form of the APOE gene increases risk of developing Alzheimer's and late onset of the disease, it does not guarantee that the person carrying it will develop Alzheimer's. However, it is estimated that 20–25% of people carrying this gene will develop Alzheimer's, and people without the APOE-ε4 gene can also develop Alzheimer's due to other risk factors.

Changes in the Brain

Genes, environment, and lifestyle all have an effect on whether or not someone will develop Alzheimer's, and these factors lead to physical changes in the brain that cause the symptoms of Alzheimer's. The changes that occur are progressive and degenerative, meaning that they continue to get worse over time, and the damage that occurs is permanent.

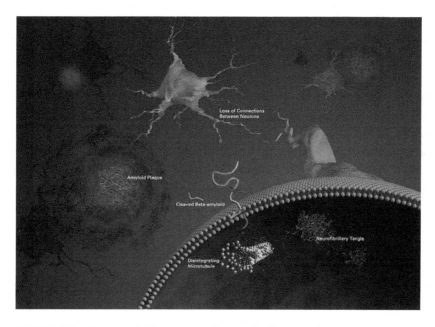

FIGURE 6.4   Beta-amyloid plaques and neurofibrillary tangles

Alzheimer's symptoms are directly caused by abnormal clumps in the brain made of a sticky protein called *beta-amyloid*. These clumps are called *beta-amyloid plaques*, and they inhibit cell transmission by blocking synapses. You can think of them like clumps of sticky proteins that block the path between the two synapses. When synapses are blocked, cells have no way of communicating with each other, and they become disabled. The plaques may even trigger immune system responses that lead to inflammation and destruction of disabled cells.

Bundles of fibers, called *neurofibrillary tangles*, that are caused by *tau protein* deposits in the brain are also a cause of Alzheimer's symptoms. Tau proteins are part of the transportation system in the brain, and they help stabilize the cell structure so that molecules can be transported efficiently. During the progression of Alzheimer's, the tau protein collapses and gets tangled. The tangles kill the synapses from the inside—think of it like roots of a tree growing inside the neuron. The tangles then cause the structure to collapse and make it so that molecules can no longer be transported throughout the brain, which leads to cell death.

As Alzheimer's progresses, connections between nerve cells, or *neurons*, are lost. This inhibits the transmission of messages between different parts of the brain and between the brain and body. The *hippocampus*, the part of the brain associated with memory, appears to be the first area of the brain that is affected. This structure of the brain is a crucial component in consolidating new information and encoding it into memories to be stored in the brain. Alzheimer's causes the hippocampus to shrink, which leads to impairment in storing new memories and, at least partially, explains the symptoms of memory loss that are associated with Alzheimer's. The hippocampus is part of *the limbic system*, which plays a large role in regulating emotion and memory formation. Alzheimer's causes the *cerebral cortex* to shrivel, which leads to impairment in cognitive skills such as thought and memory. The cortex is a hallmark of the mammalian brain. The brain's outer layer is made of cell bodies and plays a role in many processes associated with consciousness, such as attention and awareness, thought and language, and memory and perception. As Alzheimer's progresses, the *ventricles*, which are spaces within the brain that are filled with cerebrospinal fluid, grow larger. This enlargement has been proposed as a diagnostic measure of Alzheimer's, since it is a biological marker of changes in the brain that occur due to the progression of the disease.

Understanding how Alzheimer's impacts the brain can help to better understand some of its symptoms. Different parts of the brain are associated with different cognitive and behavioral skills, so changes in particular areas of the brain can be implicated in specific areas of decline.

Risk Factors
Thinking back to the beginning of this book, remember that a *risk factor* is something that makes someone more likely to develop a disease, infection, or injury. Risk factors for Alzheimer's include an array of personal, genetic, and environmental factors.

One risk factor is *family history*. The risk of developing Alzheimer's is higher for those who have a biological family member (e.g., parent, sibling, child) with the disease, and risk increases with the number of family members who develop Alzheimer's. This may be due to both genetic and environmental factors that are shared within families.

Risk of Alzheimer's drastically increases with *age*. Approximately one in nine people age 65 or older has Alzheimer's, and approximately one in three people age 85 or older has the disease. Despite these high prevalence rates, Alzheimer's is *not* a normal part of aging, and it is not well understood why risk increases with age.

Various *lifestyle factors* influence the appearance of Alzheimer's. Diet, activity level, socialization, and cognitive engagement can play a role in the development of Alzheimer's. High blood pressure, heart disease, stroke, diabetes, high cholesterol, and other conditions that can be exacerbated by an unhealthy lifestyle have been identified as risk factors. Some evidence indicates that eating a healthy, balanced diet, exercising regularly, having social support and engaging in social activities, and engaging in mentally stimulating activities may help reduce the risk of developing Alzheimer's.

Individuals with *Down syndrome* are at increased risk for developing Alzheimer's. Down syndrome is a congenital disorder caused by the presence of an extra copy of chromosome 21, which carries the gene that creates the amyloid plaques that lead to the abnormal brain clumps that characterize Alzheimer's. In addition, a number of other genes that are involved in aging and are associated with the increased risk of developing Alzheimer's are located on chromosome 21.

Other Potential Causes

Genes, environment, and lifestyle contribute to the likelihood of developing Alzheimer's, and plaques and tangles are part of the changes in the brain that cause symptoms of Alzheimer's. There are, however, other potential causes of Alzheimer's disease. These health events can greatly impact the likelihood of developing Alzheimer's.

Head trauma or injury has been linked to the development of Alzheimer's. Risk is increased when the trauma was recurring and/or there was a loss of consciousness due to trauma. It has been found that the plaques associated with Alzheimer's can be detected in the brain just hours after a traumatic brain injury, such as a concussion. For example, professional football players are exposed to head injury, and it is not uncommon for them to be diagnosed with a concussion. Some players sustain numerous concussions over the course of their career, which may make for a dramatic game but cause increasing harm and risk for cognitive impairment and Alzheimer's. One study on traumatic brain injury in retired football players found that players with three or more concussions were five times more likely to have cognitive impairment and three times more likely to report significant memory problems.[7] Other accidents due to sports such as biking, skateboarding, and snowboarding are common causes of concussions.

Heart health and function can directly impact the brain, since the heart transports 20–25% of the body's blood to the brain with each beat. The brain uses 20% or more of the oxygen and energy carried by the body's blood supply, making heart function an important player in the health of the brain.

Infections such as those from the herpes simplex virus have been linked to Alzheimer's. It has been found that reactivated herpes simplex greatly increases the likelihood of developing Alzheimer's.[8]

Some of these risk factors, such as family history and age, cannot be reduced or controlled. Others, such as diet and exercise, are factors that can be adjusted and improved as a means of reducing risk. It appears that the best ways to reduce the risk of developing Alzheimer's include maintaining a healthy diet and exercise, increasing mental stimulation, and avoiding head injuries.

Diagnostic Criteria and Methods

The diagnostic process begins when an individual or his or her friends and family begin to experience or observe abnormal changes in behavior and ultimately make the decision to seek professional consultation. Specific signs and symptoms help health care professionals recognize and diagnose Alzheimer's disease. These are included in the *diagnostic criteria*, or the items required to make a diagnosis, and include gradual impairment in learning new information, recalling new information, and the presence of other cognitive issues. A physician would assess the patient using a variety of methods, including individual and family interview, physical exams, neurological exams, behavioral and cognitive tests of memory, a Mini Mental Status Exam (MMSE), and imaging techniques such as computed tomographs (CT), magnetic resonance imaging (MRI), and positron emission tomography (PET). Definite Alzheimer's, however, can only be diagnosed upon examining the brain in an autopsy, so it can only be truly diagnosed after death.

Biopsychosocial Perspective of Alzheimer's

Biological

Alzheimer's affects the body in a number of different ways. Physical deterioration begins in the brain and begins to impact bodily functions as decline continues over time. As Alzheimer's progresses, it impacts basic bodily functions such as swallowing and toileting. This biological deterioration has an impact on a person's independence and dignity, making it an important consideration in terms of examining well being. In addition, circulation is impacted as blood pressure decreases, making hands feel cold and lips and nails appear blue. Skin over bony areas of the body may redden, and sores may develop, particularly in areas in contact with bedding. Body fluids and secretions may build up in the lungs and/or the back of the throat, and breathing may sound congested with an irregular rate of breath. Sleepiness may increase and awareness of pain decreases. Fever may appear, and the person may need to cool down with the help of a caregiver. Vision may become blurred, and sensitivity to noise and lights may increase. Though Alzheimer's is a disease of the brain, it compromises the integrity of the sufferer's body over time and leads to significant biological deterioration.

Psychological

Despite the many cognitive changes associated with Alzheimer's, feelings and emotions remain intact throughout its progression. Individuals may experience issues with identity and feel like they are not the same person as they were before. They may also experience discomfort in disclosing their diagnosis and may feel disappointed by the reactions of some friends and family. This can lead to feelings of anxiety, frustration, and loss, and feelings of isolation may arise. Withdrawal and isolation are not uncommon, and individuals experiencing milder Alzheimer's may experience depression, apathy, and anxiety. Engaging in social relationships can become more challenging as symptoms worsen, and engaging in conversation becomes increasingly difficult. This can lead to isolation and depression. Some individuals may feel shame or depression as they see themselves as a burden to family members or friends for whom they were once a caretaker.

Social

Individuals with Alzheimer's may become increasingly withdrawn as their symptoms progress. This is in part due to the difficulty that social situations can present in light of the symptoms Alzheimer's causes. Because language skills can be impaired, socializing may be unappealing and challenging. Alzheimer's can also impact intimate relationships with partners and spouses. The new dynamic of being more dependent on a partner may also lead to feelings of anger or resentment targeted at that person. Desire for physical intimacy may change and decrease due to depression brought on by diagnosis or by side effects of medications taken to manage symptoms.

The Role of Individuals, Families, and Community in Alzheimer's Management

Family Functioning

Alzheimer's disease not only impacts the individual suffering from it but also alters the lives of those around them. At a certain point, patients lose the awareness that they are no longer participants in their own lives, but their family members have the agonizing task of watching their loved ones fade away. Family systems and roles can change dramatically as a member of the group begins to decline, and other members take on new responsibilities. Changes and disruption in these roles, on top of the already existing strain of having a terminally ill family member, can cause

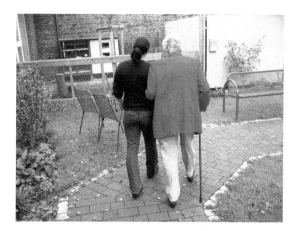

FIGURE 6.5 **Caregivers play a vital role in the day to day management of Alzheimer's Disease**

tension and conflict in the family system. Because each family manages conflict differently, the impact of Alzheimer's on the family system can vary greatly.

Role Changes

As someone progresses through the stages of Alzheimer's, his or her familial role is likely to change. Individuals with Alzheimer's may be left out of family decision making and long-term planning for important future decisions. Families may have important conversations and may make important decisions without the individual's presence or input. Many individuals are not even told about their diagnosis. As symptoms progress, the individual becomes less capable of functioning independently. These changes may lead to family members making decisions about the individual discontinuing driving, loss of employment and breadwinner status, and loss of ability to make personal financial decisions. Dependence may also include needing others to help fulfill needs of daily functioning.

Pearce[9] proposes that much of dealing with stressful role changes within the family system involves framing a "new normal." While members of a family may have perceived themselves as intact, rational, and functional before the introduction of Alzheimer's, they may now see themselves as stressed, crazy, or out of control. These feelings can be reframed as normal reactions in the context of the situation, removing the panic and anxiety about the changes occurring in the family system. Part of these changes also includes integrating self-care for the family members of an individual with Alzheimer's. Family members may begin to feel guilty about doing things for themselves or not constantly prioritizing their family member with Alzheimer's. Self-care can be reframed as something that is necessary to being an adequate caregiver and helping to restructure the family into a community of care and shared responsibility. Pearce also recognizes that a diagnosis of Alzheimer's in the family and the role changes it causes can lead to major disruption in the values, perceptions of role, secrets, and rules (both spoken and unspoken) within the family. Members of the same family may bring very different values and perspectives on how to deal with an Alzheimer's diagnosis, which can cause rifts and identity confusion within families who perceived themselves as being more similar to each other than they really are.

Conflict

A majority of families that have a member experiencing symptoms of dementia experience family conflict, as the emotional and practical burdens of caring for a family member with these symptoms can cause major changes in the family system. This conflict tends to be most severe among siblings and can be related to disagreements over the needs and capabilities of the care recipient, financial issues, the delegation of caretaking responsibilities, and even rivalries from childhood. Differing opinions on caretaking needs, decision making, and utilization of resources can cause significant tension among family members. Lieberman and Fisher[10] found that the best method to avoid family conflict is to assign caretaking and decision making responsibilities to a single family member and allow for some input from other family members. Unsurprisingly, this study also found that families that utilize positive conflict resolution skills are more effective in providing assistance to their family member with Alzheimer's.

Caregivers

Those caring for individuals with Alzheimer's are often spouses or family members. Caring for an individual with Alzheimer's incurs financial, social, and emotional burdens. Considerations for care range from day-to-day issues such as completion of daily tasks to higher-level issues such as restructuring of family roles and to lifestyle changes such as placement in a permanent care facility. It comes as no surprise that caregivers are at increased risk for developing depression and anxiety as a result of their caregiving demands and the emotional toll of the disease. Watching your parents slip away and no longer remember who you are, not being able to sleep because you must watch your loved one overnight, or having to balance watching an aging parent while also caring for your own children are stressors that cause significant pileup. Perhaps the saddest of all is that the caregiver's loved one will never get better even if he or she does everything right.

Caregivers are often family members, typically spouses or adult children of the individual for whom they are caring. This creates a change in the power dynamic of the relationship, as a marriage becomes less egalitarian or an adult child assumes a parental role over their mother or father. The quality of the caregiver relationship in these situations is, unsurprisingly, related to the quality of the relationship between the caregiver and the individual with Alzheimer's. Family caregivers who reported good relationships with the person they are caring for before the onset of the disease also reported lower feelings of burden and reactivity to behavioral symptoms, as well as better problem solving and communication.[11] This indicates that familial caregivers who had more positive relationships with the people they are caring for may be more resilient in their roles as caregivers, despite the challenges they face with the changes occurring within their family system. In addition, caregivers are more likely to experience anxiety and depression when their relationship with the person with Alzheimer's is poor, and the person with Alzheimer's tends to exhibit more behavioral problems when they sense that their caregiver is becoming distant.[12]

Children and Adolescents

Children and adolescents who have close relationships with parents, grandparents, or loved ones who develop Alzheimer's can experience an array of emotions. These include sadness about the changes that are happening, hurt when their name is forgotten, confusion about why the person acts differently, fear that the disease will get worse, frustration with repeated questions, jealousy for the amount of time given to their loved one, embarrassment about their loved one's behavior, and guilt for feeling all of the feelings listed above. Caregivers can help the child manage his or her emotions by having honest conversations about the disease, normalizing emotions, providing them education and information about the disease, and providing opportunities for the child to be able to talk about his or her feelings. Online resources are also available for parents who need a place to start the conversation.

Maria Shriver has developed a series of videos for the HBO Alzheimer's Project called *Grandpa: Do You Know Who I Am?* to teach children and adolescents a variety of tools for coping with Alzheimer's.

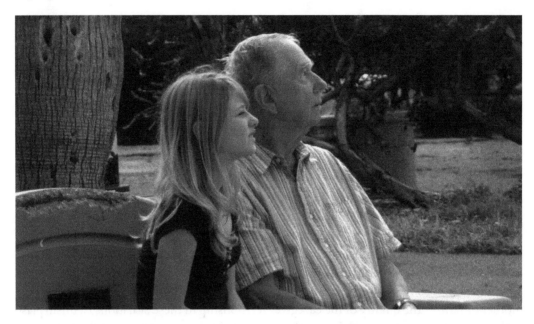

FIGURE 6.6   A photo from the HBO documentary—*Grandpa: Do You Know Who I Am?*

Effective Treatments for the Management of Alzheimer's

Medication

Currently, there is no cure for Alzheimer's. However, symptoms can be managed in a number of ways. The treatment for Alzheimer's will vary depending on stage, severity, and symptom presentation. Treatment in the earlier stages of Alzheimer's focuses on reducing agitation and providing memory aids, and treatment in the late stages of Alzheimer's focuses on managing daily tasks of feeding and bathing. A number of FDA-approved drugs can be used to treat Alzheimer's. These drugs work by regulating *neurotransmitters*, which are the chemicals that transmit messages between neurons; this helps manage some of the symptoms affecting thinking, memory, communication, and behavior, but they do not do anything to inhibit the progression of the disease. Rivastigmine (Exelon®), and galantamine (Razadyne®) are used to treat mild to moderate Alzheimer's, and Memantine (Namenda®) is used to treat moderate to severe Alzheimer's. Donepezil (Aricept®) can be used to treat symptoms of mild, moderate, or severe Alzheimer's.

Behavioral symptoms also manifest with the progression of Alzheimer's disease. These include wandering, sleep disruption, and aggression. Both medication and behavior skills training can be used to manage these symptoms. As these symptoms can be stressful for both the patient and the caregiver, treating these symptoms eases some of the challenges of coping with the disease.

Therapy

Some methods of therapy are used to help increase cognitive engagement and memory. These include music therapy, which includes singing and music relaxation exercises, and reminiscence therapy, in which the individual is shown pictures and other items that are familiar to them as a means of aiding their recall. Caregivers and family may also be involved in the therapeutic experience with the Alzheimer's patient.[13] Occupational therapy that integrates both caregiver and patient well being as therapeutic goals has also been implemented successfully, such that the individual with Alzheimer's has a higher quality of life, and their caregivers feel less burden.[14] According to the Alzheimer's Association, these therapies have not been demonstrated to be particularly effective but could potentially be useful in reducing the symptoms of depression and anxiety that accompany Alzheimer's. Participation in group activities (i.e., adult day care) and support groups may also be effective ways of improving mood and mental health in individuals with Alzheimer's. Specialized support groups help caregivers handle the stress of caretaking by providing an outlet where they can discuss their experiences, share concerns and tips, and receive emotional support from other people going through similar experiences. A variety of support groups exist for caregivers, including in-person and online groups, as well as groups for caretakers whose loved ones are in different stages of Alzheimer's.

Behavior Skills Training

Caregivers of those with Alzheimer's may engage in skills training to learn how to effectively handle the behavioral symptoms of Alzheimer's. These symptoms include aggression, agitation, confusion, repetitive behavior, suspicion, wandering, and trouble sleeping. Caregivers are taught about the common reasons for negative behaviors in Alzheimer's patients, including pain, overstimulation, and confusion. Caregivers are taught to identify the behavior and examine its reason and function, including assessing potential triggers and outcomes of the behavior. They are also taught specific responses to various problem behaviors. Next, they are taught to take steps to find potential solutions to a problem that may be causing the behavior by assessing the needs of the person for whom they are caring, how to adapt their environment to resolve the problem, and changing personal reactions to the behavior. Caregivers are also encouraged to try a variety of different responses to the behavior and examine how their responsiveness helped or hindered resolution of the problem behavior.

Specialists

Alzheimer's may require specialized care given the particular population within which this disease commonly occurs. Health and lifestyle complications in elderly individuals may require special attention. Given this consideration, an array of medical specialization focuses on providing specialized care for older individuals experiencing complications associated with age. *Geriatricians* are medical doctors who specialize in work with elderly populations and have specialized knowledge of the unique needs of aging individuals. *Geriatric psychiatrists* specialize in preventing and treating mental disorders in elderly people and can provide specialized treatment to those with cognitive disabilities resulting from Alzheimer's. Because Alzheimer's is a disease that directly impacts the brain, medical professionals who specialize in treating and managing brain disorders may also be integrated into a care plan. *Neurologists* specialize in neurological disorders, such as Alzheimer's, that are the result of dysfunction in the body's nervous system. This includes problems in the brain, spine, and nerves that cause cognitive and behavioral symptoms. *Neuropsychologists* specialize in treating individuals with injuries or diseases of the brain that manifest in cognitive and mental disability.

Cultural Barriers in Treatment

It is important to note that in many cultures the idea of psychotherapy and mental health disorders are stigmatized, and the stigma sometimes extends to Alzheimer's. For instance, African Americans, Latinos, and Asians tend to talk to family first about the symptoms of the disease. Sometimes family is supportive, but at other times the family's response may be driven by fear (e.g., fear that the disease is contagious). Research suggests that white families often feel comfortable speaking with their health care providers about symptoms; Chinese families seek information privately from regional health centers as to avoid information about the disease getting out to their community; black families often turn to religious leaders, and Latino families turn to friends and Spanish-speaking community members. Many of these communication patterns and preferences are deeply rooted in collectivist approaches emphasizing the importance of family responsibility for caregiving. However, they are also informed by patterns of institutional racism, dismissal of symptoms by health care providers, and perceived disrespect by health care providers who are culturally insensitive.[15] Efforts to provide culturally-sensitive health care will help to overcome some of these barriers for diverse families.

Alzheimer's Advocacy Efforts

Legal Issues

An important part of planning for Alzheimer's is legal care. Early planning allows the person with Alzheimer's to be involved with communicating wishes for long-term care, financial planning of how finances and property will be used or distributed, planning for health care, and naming a person who will be authorized to make decisions on the patient's behalf. This planning will happen with the assistance of a lawyer and helps guide the family as the patient loses the ability to make rational legal decisions.

National Advocacy Groups

The Alzheimer's Association is a leading volunteer health and advocacy organization whose mission is to provide care and support for all people affected by Alzheimer's and other types of dementia. The Alzheimer's Association organizes research, clinical care efforts, and social/emotional support at the global, national and local levels. Its primary fundraiser, the Walk to End Alzheimer's, occurs in over 600 communities across the United States and has funded over $350 million in research for finding a cure for Alzheimer's. The association's website (www.alz.org) is a treasure trove of resources that help people obtain education, find clinical trials and community supports, read about advancements in research, and learn about current advocacy efforts at the federal, state, and local levels.

The Alzheimer's Association's efforts led to a major legislative victory with the passing of The National Alzheimer's Project Act (NAPA) into law in 2011. NAPA requires the following efforts: 1) coordination of research and services across all federal agencies, 2) accelerated development of treatment that would prevent, halt, or reverse Alzheimer's, 3) improvement of early diagnosis and coordination of care and treatment, 4) improvement of outcomes for ethnic and racial minority populations, and 5) coordination with international organizations to fight Alzheimer's on a global level. These efforts will be achieved by increasing the financial commitment to Alzheimer's research and expanding public awareness of Alzheimer's by providing unpaid family caregivers with free education, outreach, and support.[16] The hope is that collaborating agencies will work toward common goals and more quickly find a cure for Alzheimer's, while also supporting caregivers who are the frontlines of care.

Conclusion

Throughout this chapter, you have been introduced to the symptoms, causes, diagnosis, and social implications of Alzheimer's. While we are continually learning more about this disease, there is still much to find out about the causes of Alzheimer's and why it develops and progresses the way that it does. These developments are crucial to the public health of the United States, given the rapidly aging population of this country. We must also remember the emotional, financial, and physical demands that caregivers experience when providing care to loved ones with Alzheimer's. Support must be provided that improves the quality of life for individuals experiencing this disease, as well as for their friends, families, and caregivers.

Case Study

Dorothy, a 71-year-old woman who lives with her husband Russell, is a high school graduate and worked as a secretary until her retirement six years ago; presently, she volunteers at her community center teaching art classes four days a week. She has always lovingly cared for her husband, three children and six grandchildren—cooking and cleaning, providing childcare for her grandchildren, and maintaining the home and finances. She has a past medical history of arthritis and high blood pressure, but past neurological exams have been normal. Dorothy's maternal father was diagnosed with Alzheimer's and passed away at age 81. Dorothy visits her primary care physician for a routine appointment and mentions that her husband urged her to come in because he has observed some recent changes in her memory. She reports that she sometimes forgets where she puts her keys and mixes up the names of family members. Dorothy's doctor performs physical and neurological exams, finding nothing abnormal other than mildly high blood pressure; Dorothy scores 27 on the Mini Mental Status Exam (MMSE).

Dorothy returns to her doctor the next year for an annual checkup accompanied by Russell, who reveals that Dorothy had been resistant to coming to the doctor because she was convinced that the appointment was not until next month. The doctor asks Dorothy, who has been quiet and withdrawn since she arrived, about the mix up. She seems confused and struggles to find the words she is looking for, but she ultimately jokes that "old people don't need to care about time." Her doctor performs an individual and family interview with Dorothy and Russell, which reveals that Dorothy has been frequently misplacing items, struggling to remember names of family members, and getting lost on her way to the community center and other familiar places; Russell reports that he has noticed a decline in her memory and is worried about her and that a volunteer who works with Dorothy at the community center called him about recent changes in Dorothy's functioning. Dorothy's children are also concerned about her memory. On numerous occasions Dorothy forgot to pick up her grandchildren from school, and one grandchild came home frightened because "grandma was driving on the wrong side of the road." The doctor also notices Dorothy struggle with finding the word she is looking for and keeping track of the conversation—she repeated some of the same information twice. Dorothy's doctor administers the MMSE, on which she scores 25, and makes a note of possible dementia. He orders blood tests to rule out other causes of dementia.

Within eight months, Dorothy has abandoned her volunteer work due to her memory impairments; she is struggling to remember routine tasks that need to be done, as well as names of recent acquaintances and content of conversations. She is increasingly reliant on Russell to assist her with managing routine tasks, such as paying bills and cooking meals. She often becomes disoriented and is unsure of the day or time, and her mood has become increasingly depressed and agitated. She no longer provides regular childcare for her grandchildren because she appears to get easily overwhelmed by the kids. Russell reports that Dorothy will become easily frustrated and lash out at him, her children, and the grandchildren. This is uncharacteristic of her personality, as she has always been a very patient person. She scores 24 on the MMSE, and her doctor orders imaging tests, which show mild hippocampal shrinkage. Dorothy is diagnosed with probable Alzheimer's disease. Her doctor advises that she should engage in a support group for individuals with Alzheimer's and other memory-loss problems.

One year later, Dorothy has become increasingly secluded and isolated. She takes medication to alleviate her symptoms, as well as medication to help her disrupted sleep. She rarely leaves the house because of her symptoms, as she becomes easily lost and cannot remember her address or phone number. She no longer performs any routine tasks such as cooking or cleaning and has severe impairment of short-term memory. Her family safety-proofed her house after finding her cutting up curtains, blinds, phone cords, and photo albums with scissors. She often repeats questions, forgets recent conversations, and becomes spatially disoriented in her home. While she is able to maintain personal hygiene, she needs assistance in dressing and other tasks. Russell has also enrolled her in an adult day care facility once a week, where she engages in recreational activities and receives therapy.

Within 18 months, Dorothy is under constant supervision. Her husband hired a caretaker to assist him with meeting Dorothy's daily needs, which include incontinence and behavioral problems. Two of Dorothy's children were not supportive of this, as they felt their father should be saving money and not squandering it on help that they could provide. Dorothy's third child does not visit often, as it is "too depressing," and his young children are very sad and hurt that their grandmother does not recognize them. Dorothy often wanders aimlessly and is extremely disoriented. While she can recall some memories from her childhood, she has lost much of the detail of her personal history and repeats the same story over and over. She is unable to recognize familiar people and introduces herself to her grandchildren each time she sees them. Over time, Dorothy loses the ability to walk, communicate, and respond to her environment. She struggles to eat on her own and requires constant care and supervision. She remains in bed, requiring assistance to meet all of her survival needs. Dorothy's husband used most of his savings to care for Dorothy and will continue to deplete his savings until she passes away. Sadly, Russell's health is also declining, and he often expresses that he does not want to live without the love of his life, Dorothy.

Notes

1 Alzheimer's Association. (n.d.). Retrieved from http://www.alz.org/

2 Hebert, L. E., Weuve, J., Scherr, P. A., & Evans, D. A. (2013). Alzheimer's disease in the United States (2010–2050) estimated using the 2010 census. *Neurology, 80*(19), 1778–1783.

3 The older population: 2010. (2011) 2010 Census Briefs. Retrieved from http://www.census.gov/prod/cen2010/briefs/c2010br-09.pdf

4 Livney, M. G., Clark, C. M., Karlawish, J. H., Cartmell, S., Negrón, M., Nuñez, J., … & Arnold, S. E. (2011). Ethnoracial differences in the clinical characteristics of Alzheimer's disease at initial presentation at an urban Alzheimer's disease center. *The American Journal of Geriatric Psychiatry, 19*(5), 430–439.

5 2015 Alzheimer's disease facts and figures. (2015). *Alzheimer's & Dementia: The Journal of the Alzheimer's Association, 11*(3), 332.

6 Sun, F., Hilgeman, M. M., Durkin, D. W., Allen, R. S., & Burgio, L. D. (2009). Perceived income inadequacy as a predictor of psychological distress in Alzheimer's caregivers. *Psychology and Aging, 24*(1), 177.

7 Guskiewicz, K. M., Marshall, S. W., Bailes, J., McCrea, M., Cantu, R. C., Randolph, C., & Jordan, B. D. (2005). Association between recurrent concussion and late-life cognitive impairment in retired professional football players. *Neurosurgery, 57*(4), 719–726.

8 Lövheim, H., Gilthorpe, J., Adolfsson, R., Nilsson, L. G., & Elgh, F. (2015). Reactivated herpes simplex infection increases the risk of Alzheimer's disease. *Alzheimer's & Dementia, 11*(6), 593–599.

9 Pearce, N. (2012). Helping families through dementia care-related conflicts. *Social Work Today, 12*(3), p. 18. Retrieved from: http://www.socialworktoday.com/archive/051412p18.shtml.

10 Lieberman, M. A., & Fisher, L. (1999). The effects of family conflict resolution and decision making on the provision of help for an elder with Alzheimer's disease. *The Gerontologist, 39*(2), 159–166.

11 Steadman, P. L., Tremont, G., & Davis, J. D. (2007). Premorbid relationship satisfaction and caregiver burden in dementia caregivers. *Journal of Geriatric Psychiatry and Neurology, 20*(2), 115–119.

12 Podgorski, C. (2014). Dementia and difficult family conversations: Tips and tools [PDF document]. Alzheimers.org. Retreived from: http://www.alz.org/centralnewyork/documents/dc14_navdiff-disc.pdf.

13 Brotons, M., & Marti, P. (2003). Music therapy with Alzheimer's patients and their family caregivers: A pilot project. *Journal of Music Therapy, 40*(2), 138–150.

14 Dooley, N. R., & Hinojosa, J. (2004). Improving quality of life for persons with Alzheimer's disease and their family caregivers: Brief occupational therapy intervention. *American Journal of Occupational Therapy, 58*(5), 561–569.

15 Schulz, R., Burgio, L., Burns, R., Eisdorfer, C., Gallagher-Thompson, D., Gitlin, L. N., & Mahoney, D. F. (2003). Resources for enhancing Alzheimer's caregiver health (REACH): Overview, site-specific outcomes, and future directions. *The Gerontologist, 43*(4), 514–520.

16 Alzheimer's Association. (n.d.). Retrieved January 30, 2017, from http://www.alz.org/advocacy/federal-priorities.asp#napa

Figure Sources

1 Figure 6.1: Source: https://commons.wikimedia.org/wiki/File:Alzheimers_brain.jpg.

2 Figure 6.2: Copyright © The Prime Minister's Office (CC BY-SA 2.0) at https://www.flickr.com/photos/number10gov/7017124741/sizes/l/in/set-72157629306277768/.

3 Figure 6.3: Copyright © Neuropathologyblog (CC BY-SA 3.0) at https://commons.wikimedia.org/wiki/File:Autopsy_brain.jpg.

4 Figure 6.4: Source: https://commons.wikimedia.org/wiki/File:Characteristics_of_AD.jpg.

5 Figure 6.5: Source: https://pixabay.com/p-441408/?no_redirect.

6 Figure 6.6: From: "Grandpa: Do You Know Who I Am?," https://i.ytimg.com/vi/1G0yHKBPrY8/maxresdefault.jpg. Copyright © 2009 by PBS: Public Broadcasting Service.

CHAPTER SEVEN

Cancer

Coauthors:
**Genevieve Dash, M.S., Sue K. Adams, Ph.D.,
Sarah Feldstein Ewing, Ph.D.**

@AmericanCancer

Receiving a cancer diagnosis is an emotionally and physically exhausting experience. Patients and loved ones experience a wide range of emotional reactions. The physical effects of cancer on the body and the side effects associated with cancer treatments take a toll on both physical and psychological health, and learning how to navigate others' reactions to the diagnosis can either cause distress or bring people closer together. As you read this chapter, be forewarned that the information in this chapter is a bit technical. We suggest that you think about a loved one or friend who has been diagnosed with cancer and use what you know about that person's experience as a way to anchor the information to your own life. By the end of this chapter, you will be familiar with the causes of cancer, what the symptoms and progression of cancer look like, how cancer is diagnosed and treated, and the emotional and social implications of the disease for the individual and their family. You will also be introduced to the complex relationships between cancer and genetics, environmental factors, and social influences.

What Is Cancer?
Cancer is a major public health concern, both in the United States and around the world. Cancer is a leading cause of death in the United States, second only to heart disease. The *National Cancer Institute (NCI)* estimates that in this year alone, almost 1.7 million new cases of cancer will be diagnosed and almost 600,000 people will die from cancer in the United States.[1] Cancer is also the leading cause of death worldwide, and the *World Health Organization (WHO)* estimates the number of

new cancer cases is expected to rise to 22 million across the globe over the next 20 years.[2] In addition to the impact that cancer has on individuals and families, the cost of care for the disease is extraordinary: Costs reached $125 billion in the U.S. in 2010 and are expected to increase to $156 billion by 2020.[3] If you do not already know someone who has been diagnosed with cancer, you will.

There are over 100 types of cancer, which vary in their place of origin, progression, and ability to be treated. Most generally, *cancer* refers to a collection of diseases that cause the body's cells to divide uncontrollably and spread into surrounding tissues, often causing lumps called *tumors*. Normally, cells function by dividing to replace old and dying cells as needed. When cancer is present, new cells begin to form when and where they should not. They continue to divide and duplicate, causing a buildup of excess cells that form tumors and make it challenging, or impossible, for the body to function normally. Some tumors are *benign*, or noncancerous, and others are *malignant*, or cancerous. Benign tumors do not spread but can grow to be very large. Malignant tumors can grow back after being removed and spread to other tissues when some of the tumor's cells break off and move through the body via the blood or *lymphatic system*. The lymphatic system is a network of tissues and organs that gets rid of toxins and is important to immune system function. It is part of the circulatory system that is spread throughout the entire body, making it an easy way for tumor cells to travel to different parts of the body.

When cancer develops, old or damaged cells are not replaced. They continue to survive in the body because cancer cells are able to ignore *apoptosis*, or the process of programmed cell death that the body uses to get rid of unnecessary cells. Cancer cells grow at an abnormally accelerated rate as compared to healthy cells, and they begin to crowd out healthy cells. Cancer cells are very smart and very tricky. They are able to influence their *microenvironment*, or the normal cells, molecules and blood vessels that surround the tumor. Through this control tumors are supplied with oxygen, nutrients, and waste removal processes. Cancer cells are able to dodge the body's immune system so that the immune system does not remove dead and dying cells, and cancer can survive in the body. Tumors are also able to use the body's immune system to prevent it from killing cancer cells. While lumps and tumors are the most obvious sign of cancer, some types of cancer, such as leukemia (cancer of the blood), do not form solid tumors.

Types of Cancers

Cancers are typically named for the place in the body in which the disease originates but may also be named for the formative cell or type of tissue in which the cancer forms. Cancers found in the part of the body in which they formed are termed *primary cancers*. Cancers are termed *metastatic* if they spread outside of the primary part of the body in which the cancer formed; the process of cancer spreading is called *metastasis*. Whether or not the cancer spreads, or *metastasizes*, it is still named for the place in which the cancer originated. For illustration, a cancer that originated in the lungs (primary cancer) can metastasize and travel to the brain (which is the secondary site).

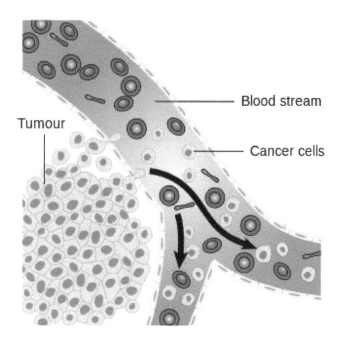

FIGURE 7.1   Cancer cells metastasizing to a different part of the body via the blood stream

There are many types of cancer, and they can start anywhere in the body. This section will briefly review the five major categories and some of the specific types of cancers that fall into them. These five main types of cancer are *carcinomas, sarcomas, melanomas, lymphomas, leukemias, and myelomas*, which differ in the type of tissue from which they originate. These are broad terms to categorize types of cancer, and more specific cancers (e.g., breast, lung) fall in to these categories; these more specific types are, obviously, named based on the part of the body in which the cancer originates and are the typical terminology used when describing cancers. There are many other types of cancer that are not reviewed below. For a more comprehensive list of cancer types and their etiology, progression, and treatment, please visit the NCI website (www.cancer.gov).[4]

- Carcinomas: This is the most common type of cancer, accounting for over 90% of cancers. Carcinomas primarily impact individuals age 50 or older. They are formed by *epithelial cells*, or the cells that cover the internal and external surfaces of the body, such as skin, breast, colon, prostate, stomach, lungs, bladder, kidney, and uterus.
- Melanomas: This type of cancer begins in cells that make the pigment that gives skin its color. Most melanomas form on the skin, but they can also form on other pigmented tissues, such as in the eye. Melanoma is the least common but deadliest and most aggressive form of skin cancer. It can spread quickly to other parts of the body if it is not quickly diagnosed. Individuals with fair skin are at particularly high risk for this form of cancer. Preventing melanoma is an important reason to wear sunscreen, as sun exposure is a major risk factor.

- Sarcomas: Sarcomas are cancers that form in bones and soft tissues such as muscle, fat, blood vessels, lymph vessels, tendons, and ligaments. Some examples of sarcomas are bone, muscle, fat, nerve, cartilage, and blood cancers, with bone cancer being the most common. These types of cancers only account for about 1% of all cancer cases and can impact people of any age.
- Lymphoma: Lymphoma is a cancer that forms in the cells of the lymph system. Lymphoma occurs when abnormal *lymphocytes*, or the white blood cells in the immune system, build up in lymph nodes and lymph vessels. Common forms of lymphoma are Hodgkin's Lymphoma (which usually occurs in children and is very curable) and Non-Hodgkin's Lymphoma (which more commonly occurs in adults and is very aggressive).
- Leukemia: Leukemia, which is a cancer of the blood, begins in on the blood-forming tissue of the bone marrow. Instead of forming tumors, large numbers of abnormal white blood cells build up in the blood and bone marrow.

Health Disparities

A number of factors, including insurance coverage and living near health care centers, influence the likelihood of receiving regular health care and screenings. The NCI defines "cancer health disparities" as "adverse differences in cancer incidence (new cases), cancer prevalence (all existing cases), cancer death (mortality), cancer survivorship, and burden of cancer or related health conditions that exist among specific population groups in the United States."[5] The NCI implemented the "Surveillance, Epidemiology, and End Results (SEER)" program to investigate cancer prevalence and survival rates among the United States population.[6] This program gathers data from diverse groups to create a more accurate picture of the cancer health disparities occurring in the U.S., covering individuals of various racial, ethnic, and socioeconomic backgrounds. The data presented in this chapter are from this program, using data collected in the United States from 1975–2013.[7]

Socioeconomic Status and Environment

Health disparities primarily impact individuals of low socioeconomic status (SES), a factor that is complexly tied to income, educational attainment, and many other variables that work together to impact health-related outcomes. SES predicts quality of life factors, including insurance coverage, access to health care and preventative screenings, education, certain occupations, and healthy living conditions, beyond race or ethnicity. All of these factors are tied to cancer risk. SES also appears to play a role in behavioral risks of cancer, including smoking, alcohol consumption, and diet and exercise, with individuals of low SES being more likely to engage in adverse behaviors that increase cancer risk.

Race and Gender

Cancer mortality is higher among men than women, and African Americans experience the highest rate of mortality due to cancer. Cancer mortality among African Americans is significantly higher than whites; the death rate is 25% higher for African Americans than for white Americans when accounting for all cancers combined. Overall, cancer mortality is highest among African American men and lowest among Pacific Islander women.[8]

Prostate cancer is more common among African American men, as is death associated with the disease. It appears that the disease is more aggressive and progresses more quickly in African American men. According to the NCI, the incidence of prostate cancer is 60% higher among African American men than it is among American men of European descent.[9] Similarly, the prostate cancer mortality rate for African American men is 44.2%, while it is 19.1% for whites.[10] Colorectal cancer is also more common among African Americans, as is death due to the disease. Research by the NCI identified 20 genes that are mutated in the presence of colorectal cancer and found that a majority of these are most common in African Americans. The mortality rates for colorectal cancer for African American men were also higher compared to other racial and ethnic groups.[11] Clearly, there is a major discrepancy in the appearance and progression of this disease across groups.

White women are most frequently diagnosed with breast cancer. However, African-American women are disproportionately impacted by breast cancer, particularly in that individuals of this population have a much poorer prognosis with the disease and are more likely to die from it. Triple-negative breast cancer, an aggressive subtype of the disease, is more common in this population but does not fully account for the lower survival rates. Preliminary research shows that a different genetic mutation may be a causal factor in breast cancer among African-American women. While incidences of breast cancer are less frequent in African-American women compared to white women, the mortality rates are higher in African-American women as compared to whites. This is the highest mortality rate for breast cancer across all racial and ethnic groups. Additionally, rates of cervical cancer and death associated with it are higher among Hispanic and African-American women, with incidence rates of 9.4 and 8.9 and mortality rates of 2.9 and 3.6, respectively.[12]

This data shows us that incidence rates can vary greatly across various racial and gender groups. It also sheds light on some of the more complex issues at play with respect to cancer prognosis and mortality: we can see that even though whites are more likely to be diagnosed with many cancers, African Americans are more likely to die from them. This type of information only begins to skim the surface of the complex issues at play that contribute to major disparities in health outcomes across race and gender, including health education, access to health care, beliefs about health and lifestyle factors.

Healthy People 2020

Healthy People 2020 has set goals to reduce the number of new cancer cases in addition to reducing the illness, disability, and death caused by the disease. This agenda focuses on monitoring trends, incidence, mortality, and survival rates of cancer as a means of addressing the progress made in eradicating it. Healthy People 2020's objectives are to 1) reduce the cancer death rate, 2) increase the proportion of cancer survivors, 3) increase the rates of cancer screening, and 4) increase public knowledge about cancer.[13] This is a crucial accomplishment, as one third of all cancer cases are preventable, and many specific cancers are preventable through reduction of risk factors.

Risk Factors and Causes of Cancer

Risk factors for cancer increase a person's risk for developing the disease but do not necessarily cause the disease. However, there is significant overlap between risk factors and causes of cancer. Below, we will discuss a few of the most common risk factors and causes of cancer.

Age

Age appears to be the most important risk factor for cancer. The *median age* of cancer diagnoses is 66. This means that half of people diagnosed with cancer are under age 66, and half of people diagnosed with cancer are over age 66.[14] Cancer can occur at any age, but getting older seems to be the risk factor most highly related to cancer as a general trend. Given the way cancer develops, this makes logical sense: the longer a person is alive, the more opportunities there are for a gene to mutate or to be exposed to environmental factors that can lead to cancer-causing mutations. In addition, some specific cancers are more common in particular age groups. For example, bone cancer is most frequently diagnosed in individuals under age 20, with 25% of diagnosis occurring in this age group. Similarly, 10% of leukemia diagnosis occurs in individuals under age 20, and *neuroblastoma*, or cancers that form on nerve tissue, are more common in children and adolescents than they are in adults.[15]

Environmental Factors

Environmental factors contribute to cancer risk. These include exposure to radiation, such as UV rays from the sun that can cause damage to DNA. Skin cancer is by far the most common form of cancer, with about 5.4 million diagnosed each year. Other environmental exposures can be in air, water, food, and other everyday materials. Some of these include asbestos, formaldehyde, soot, and wood dust. You might be surprised how often you come into contact with these materials in your everyday life. Asbestos is used in construction, formaldehyde is an ingredient in many brands of nail polish, and soot and wood dust can be found in many homes.

Immunosuppression

Immunosuppression, or reduction of immune system activity, can increase cancer risk. Immunosuppression can be caused by medications or infections such as HIV and makes the immune system less effective in detecting and destroying cancer cells. Other infections can also increase risk for cancer or even cause it. These include human papillomavirus (HPV), hepatitis B (HBV), and hepatitis C (HCV). Vaccinations, protected sex, and not sharing needles can help prevent infection.

Genes

When we hear about a "genetic disease," we usually think of an illness that "runs in the family." However, the term "genetic disease" can also mean that the disease is caused by changes to the genes that control cell functioning. Both are the case for cancer. While cancer risk can be inherited, cancer is a genetic disease in that it is caused by changes to genes within an individual. These changes can be inherited or caused by environmental factors. Cancer is a genetic disease that is caused by genes inherited from parents, mutations and errors as cells divide, and/or changes to genes that occur due to environmental factors. Inherited gene mutations account for a minority of cancer cases, making up only 5–10% of identified cancer cases.[16] *Hereditary cancer syndromes* are disorders that predispose certain individuals to developing certain cancers. This is the "runs-in-the-family" aspect of cancer. However, inheriting the mutation does not necessarily mean that cancer will occur. Genetic tests, such as the BRCA 1 and 2 tests for breast cancer, also have been developed to detect the presence of mutations that can cause cancer.

Obesity

Obesity has been associated with esophageal, pancreatic, thyroid, colorectal, breast, endometrial, gallbladder, and kidney cancers.[17] Obesity can increase cancer risk for a number of reasons. First, fat tissue produces estrogen, high levels of which have been linked to certain cancers. Higher levels of estrogen in the body due to hormone therapy or due to exposure for a long time (e.g., early menstruation, late pregnancy, late menopause, never giving birth) can be a cancer risk. In fact, having given birth and breastfeeding for at least six months are protective factors against estrogen-related cancer. Second, obesity causes high levels of *insulin* (the same hormone implicated in diabetes). Insulin can promote tumor development, as well as an abundance of hormones (e.g., *leptin*) that can promote the process of cell division and production. Third, obesity has also been linked to chronic inflammation throughout the body. In a healthy person, damaged tissue releases chemicals that initiate the inflammatory process, during which white blood cells cause cells to grow and divide to repair the injury. In a case of chronic inflammation, this process begins when there is not an injury to repair and does not end. This causes damage to DNA that can lead to cancer. As a result, weight loss can potentially reduce the cancer risk associated with obesity.

Nutrition and Diet

While no specific foods have been directly linked to cancer, an unhealthy diet could be considered a *secondary cause* due to its role in causing obesity, which in turn can lead to cancer. In addition to alcohol, artificial sweeteners and charred meats (such as barbecue) have been identified as potentially risky. Conversely, some foods, including garlic and tea, have been identified as possibly protective against cancer, although little evidence exists to support this claim. Diet is also implicated secondarily through the risk factor of obesity, which has been associated with esophageal, colorectal, breast, endometrium, and kidney cancers.[18]

Lifestyle Factors

Smoking cigarettes and using tobacco are some of the most well-known and notorious causes of cancer. Tobacco is the leading cause of cancer incidence and death. Lung cancer is by far the most common cancer type aside from skin cancer. Smoking can also cause cancer of the larynx, mouth, esophagus, throat, bladder, kidney, liver, stomach, pancreas, colon, rectum, and cervix. Even smokeless tobacco, such as chewing tobacco, can cause mouth, esophageal, and pancreatic cancer. Although intensive public health efforts have been implemented to reduce smoking rates, and smoking rates in the United States have significantly decreased, smoking remains one of the most prominent causes of cancer. Drinking alcohol can also lead to cancer, and risk is compounded for people who both smoke and drink. Alcohol use increases risk of cancer in the mouth, throat, larynx, esophagus, liver, and breast. Risk is associated with amount of drinking, meaning that, unsurprisingly, people who drink more are more likely to get cancer.

Environment

The most common environmental cause of cancer is UV rays from sunlight exposure. Other environmental carcinogens include secondhand smoke and exposure to substances such as *radon*, a radioactive gas given off by rock and soil that can leach into one's home through the foundation and can cause lung cancer after long-term exposure. Anyone living in a rocky area should consider occasional radon testing.

Radiation involves the use of radon and is used in X-rays, CT scans, and PET scans. These are methods used in treating cancer and are discussed later in the chapter. Radiation treatments can cause cell damage that leads to *second cancer*, or cancer that is caused by cancer treatment, although the benefits of using these tests that involve radiation typically outweigh the risk involved. Despite the notions of many a conspiracy theorist, radiation from cell phones has not been found to cause cancer.

Symptoms and Diagnosis of Cancer

Cancer can be difficult to detect. While some cancers present themselves more overtly, such as skin cancer, others are harder to identify. This is why *screening* is such an important preventative measure. Screenings look for cancer before symptoms appear as a means of detecting cancer before it progresses to an advanced stage. Some risks of screenings include false positives, false negatives, some health risks (such as with radiation), and the fact that simply finding cancer does not mean that treatment will be helpful. However, screening is typically conducted as a general rule of prevention. For example, the *Centers for Disease Control and Prevention (CDC)*[19] suggests that women receive mammograms and pap smears, and that men receive prostate exams even when there are no symptoms of cancer. Other screening methods include physical exams to look for lumps, history interviews to gather information on health habits and past illnesses, lab tests to examine tissue, blood, and urine, imaging procedures to check for tumors, and genetic tests to look for gene mutations. For some, these screening tests come back negative, and for others, symptoms are identified. This section will discuss some of the general signs and symptoms of cancer.

Signs and Symptoms

As has been discussed throughout the chapter, tumors are the hallmark sign of cancer. Cancer causes malignant tumors that can grow and spread throughout the body and even grow back after being removed. Thus, the most obvious symptom would be a lump underneath the skin. In addition to this physical change that cancer causes, there are a number of other biological and cognitive signs and symptoms of cancer. In some cancers, such as brain cancer, even a small tumor can cause impactful symptoms, such as seizures or a significant change in someone's personality. In other cancers, such as pancreatic cancer, symptoms do not emerge until a tumor is large enough to negatively impact surrounding organs.

Some general signs of cancer may include unexplained weight loss, fever, fatigue, pain, and skin changes, although these signs are often related to other unrelated ailments. However, particular signs and symptoms are specific to different cancer types. According to the NCI and CDC,[20] the following are some examples of signs and symptoms specific to particular cancers.

- *Skin cancer*: skin changes such as a new mole, a change in an existing mole, changes in skin pigmentation, or a sore that does not heal. The CDC provides an easy way to remember the signs of skin cancer: "A-B-C-D-E." "A" is for "asymmetrical," meaning that the mole or spot is irregular. "B" is for "border," meaning that the border of the mole is irregular. "C" is for "color," meaning that the color is uneven or inconsistent. "D" is for "diameter," meaning that the mole or spot is larger than a pea. "E" is for "evolving," meaning that the mole or spot has changed over time.
- *Oral cancer:* sores in the mouth that do not heal.
- *Breast cancer*: a new lump in the breast or underarm area, swelling of the breast, irritation of breast skin and/or nipple, inversion of the nipple,

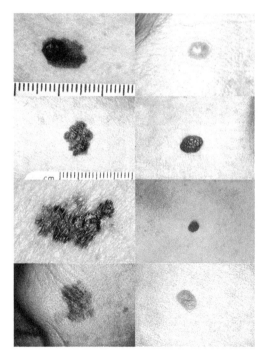

FIGURE 7.2 **Various photos of skin cancer: Be aware that skin cancer presents in different ways**

breasts and nipples changing in size or shape, bloody discharge expelled from the nipples, and changes in the texture of breast skin.

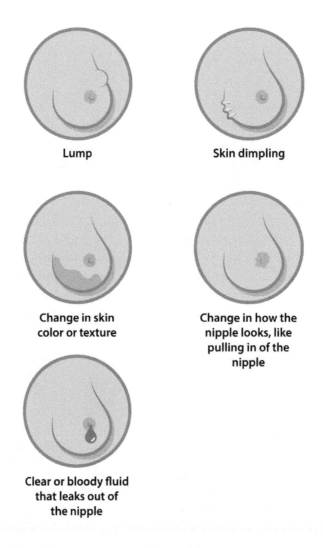

Lump

Skin dimpling

Change in skin
color or texture

Change in how the
nipple looks, like
pulling in of the
nipple

Clear or bloody fluid
that leaks out of
the nipple

FIGURE 7.3   The symptoms of breast cancer

- *Colon cancer*: stomach pain, persistent cramps, unexplained weight loss, constipation, diarrhea, blood in the stool, or other bowel changes.
- *Bladder, prostate,* and *kidney cancer*: pain during urination and blood in the urine. Signs and symptoms of prostate cancer also include difficulty urinating, frequency of urination, weak flow of urine, painful ejaculation, and persistent back, hip, or pelvic pain.
- *Lung cancer*: chest pain, shortness of breath and wheezing, persistent coughing, and coughing up blood.
- *Vulvar cancer*: itching, burning and bleeding on the vulva, changes in the color of the vulvar skin, skin changes with the appearance of rashes or warts, persistent sores, lumps, or ulcers, and pelvic pain, particularly during sex.

- *Uterine, ovarian, vaginal,* and *cervical cancer:* abnormal vaginal discharge and bleeding. *Uterine, ovarian,* and *vaginal* cancers can also cause pelvic pain. Other symptoms of *ovarian cancer* include back pain, bloating, feeling full quickly, frequent urination, and a change in bowel habits. *Cervical cancer* does not have many other signs and symptoms. The absence of signs and symptoms highlights how important screenings are, as cancer can become advanced without signs and symptoms to warn the sufferer of the disease.

This is by no means an exhaustive list of all cancers and their signs and symptoms. The fact that many of these symptoms can be caused by other diseases highlights the importance of knowing one's body, performing regular screenings, and communicating with health care providers about unusual symptoms.

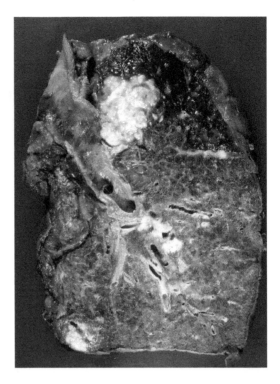

FIGURE 7.4   Lung Cancer (Squamous Cell Carcinoma)

Stages

Some cancers progress more quickly than others. The stages of cancer refer to the progression of the disease, including information on the size of a tumor and how far it has spread. There are multiple staging systems, but most include information about where the tumor is located, the cell type, the tumor size, whether the cancer has spread to another part of the body, and the *tumor grade*, or how abnormal the cancer cells look and how likely the tumor is predicted to spread. The stage of cancer also gives information on severity, chances of survival, best treatment approaches, and clinical trial treatment options. The higher the stage, the more advanced the cancer is; in the lower stages, the cancer has not spread significantly, while the higher stages indicate that the disease has spread more prominently throughout the body. At stage 0, abnormal cells are present but have not spread. While this is not considered cancer at this stage, it may become cancer. At stages I-III, cancer is present, and the higher number indicates a larger tumor and more pervasive spreading of cancer throughout the body. At stage IV, cancer has spread to distant parts of the body. In describing a cancer diagnosis, the stage is typically included; for example, someone might tell a patient that she has "stage two breast cancer."[21]

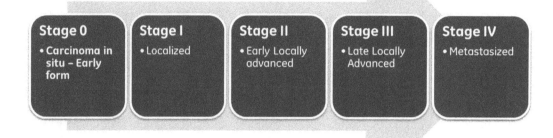

Stage 0	Stage I	Stage II	Stage III	Stage IV
• Carcinoma in situ – Early form	• Localized	• Early Locally advanced	• Late Locally Advanced	• Metastasized

FIGURE 7.5   Stages of Cancer (0-IV): Early detection and treatment is best

Prognosis

A *prognosis* is an estimate of how a disease will progress. Because a prognosis is estimated based on statistics about people with the same type of cancer, it is not always accurate and is based on an educated guess. A patient's prognosis depends on many factors. The type, stage, and location of the cancer play a major role, as do individual characteristics of the person with cancer. Age and health are important, as are lifestyle factors such as diet and exercise. Additionally, response to treatment is important in determining prognosis. Some people respond to treatment better than others, and those with more treatment-resistant conditions have a poorer prognosis.

Cancer can also be described as being *cured* or in *remission*. When someone is considered cured, there is no evidence of cancer after treatment, and the cancer has been completely eradicated. This means that no trace of cancer is in the body, and the cancer will not return. When cancer is in remission, the signs and symptoms of cancer are reduced or eliminated partially or completely, but cancer cells are still in the body. Cancer can be in either *full* or *partial* remission. In partial remission the signs and symptoms are significantly reduced, and in complete remissions the person has no signs or symptoms at all. It can be quite difficult to distinguish whether someone is cured or in remission.

Diagnostic Methods

Because many tissue changes and unusual tumor growths are benign or noncancerous, it is important to verify that these bodily changes are indeed cancer. Tissues within the body experience normal changes which are not necessarily cancerous. For example, have you ever had a wart or skin tag? These are forms of excessive skin growth that are not cancerous. There are a number of methods to determine if cancer is present in the body.

A noninvasive method of testing for cancer is through *lab tests*. Many types of laboratory tests are used for diagnostic purposes. Different tests are used in diagnosing particular cancers, and laboratory tests are often used in conjunction with imaging procedures as a means of making the most accurate diagnosis possible. For example, complete blood count (CBC) tests measure the number of different types of blood cells, including platelets and red and white blood cells, as well as *hemoglobin*, or the protein that carries oxygen. This type of test is often used in diagnosing leukemia. Sputum cytology (spit or saliva) detects the presence of abnormal cells in mucus and is used in the diagnosis of lung cancer. Urinalysis detects the presence of various substances, such as blood cells and proteins, in the urine and is used in diagnosing kidney cancer.

Surgery can also be used to diagnose and stage cancer. Tissue samples are collected surgically in a procedure called a *biopsy*. In this approach, a needle, or a thin, lighted tube called an endoscope, or surgery is used to collect a tissue sample to be tested. Then, a *pathologist*, or someone who looks for the presence of a disease, determines whether or not cancer is present. Surgery can also be used to find out how much cancer has spread by examining areas around the cancer.

Imaging procedures are also used to determine if cancer is present in the body. *Ultrasounds*, the same method doctors use to examine a fetus inside the mother's body, use a magnet to create computerized images of internal organs. *X-rays*, a method that is often used to examine bones for fractures and breaks, uses a low dose of radiation to create images of the inside of the body. In *computerized tomography* (CT) scans, multiple X-ray images are used to create a more detailed picture of internal organs. This can help to detect tumors growing inside the body. *Nuclear scans* create pictures of bones and organs by using a radioactive tracer that a scanner measures and turns into an image. *Positron emission tomography* (PET) scans create a three-dimensional image of the body by using a tracer that disperses throughout the body and collects in the tissue and organs. PET scans can detect changes happening in the organs, providing information on how organs are functioning.

Treatments

Various types of cancers are treated differently. The treatment approach depends on many factors, including the type, stage, and location of cancer. Often, multiple types of treatment are used in conjunction in an attempt to eradicate the cancer cells and tumors. There are many treatment approaches, and new and innovative types of cancer treatment are constantly being researched.

Medical Approaches

Surgery is used to remove cancerous, and sometimes benign, tumors and lumps. In *curative surgery*, the procedure is used to remove all cancer inside the body.[22] Surgery is also used to *debulk* cancer, meaning that it removes only some of the tumors present.[23] This type of surgery is used when tumors are too close to vital organs and tissues, so removing them would be too dangerous or damaging. This surgical approach is typically used in conjunction with other treatments. *Palliative surgery* may also be used in patients with advanced cancer in an effort to make them more comfortable or ease pain caused by tumors.[24] Surgery is classically accomplished by making incisions in the skin, muscle, and other parts of the body, although newer and less invasive surgical techniques are being developed. These approaches include (but are not limited to) laser surgery, in which tumors are essentially burned away, and cryosurgery, in which liquid nitrogen is used to freeze and eradicate abnormal cells. A number of side effects come with surgery, including blood clots, tissue damage, pain, and infection.

Chemotherapy administers medicine, either intravenously or in pill form, that kills cancer cells and/or slows their growth. It is most effective for late-stage cancer, in part because too many tumors may be present throughout the body for surgery to be viable. Chemotherapy can have many negative side effects, which include fatigue, vomiting, hair loss, and nerve problems.[25] Chemotherapy can be used alone or in conjunction with others types of treatment.

Radiation is similar to an X-ray, and, as its name suggests, uses radiation to kill cancer cells by damaging their DNA. However, radiation also kills normal cells, which causes side effects, including fatigue, memory loss, skin irritation, and infertility.[26] Thus, doctors need to be precise in where they aim the radiation.

Nutrition Therapy

Nutrition therapy integrates nutrition into the process of cancer treatment and involves monitoring a patient's nutritional intake. This is important because individuals with cancer may lose the desire to eat. According to the NCI[27], this is not uncommon, and almost all patients experience significant weight loss by the time their cancer is in the advanced stage. Certain cancer treatments can also change the taste and smell of food, making eating less appealing. When people with cancer do not consume enough food or their body does not absorb enough nutrients, they may become *malnourished*. Malnourishment can cause weakness, fatigue, and immune system deficiencies. Proper nutrition can help minimize the negative effects of co-occurring conditions such as diabetes and heart disease and keeps the body in better shape to fight cancer. Nutrition therapy is particularly important for cancer patients because their nutritional needs can greatly differ from the usual nutritional guidelines. Because tumors can change how the body absorbs nutrients, an individual with cancer may be consuming enough calories, but his or her body is unable to access the nutrients in the food he or she is consuming. Thus, specialized diets and nutrition therapy can be crucial to keeping a cancer patient's body in optimal shape for fighting the disease.

Cancer Across the Lifespan

When I teach about cancer in the classroom, one of the first questions that I ask my students is "What is the first word that comes to your mind when you hear the word cancer?" If you are like 80% of students, you answered that question with the word *death*. Our associations with cancer very significantly impacts how we react to and cope with the diagnosis of cancer in either our loved ones or ourselves. Adults often let their minds go to the darkest place before pulling themselves up to fight the battle of their lifetime. However, for children who have not developed the association between cancer and mortality, their ability to cope, function, and demonstrate extreme resilience in spite of the disease is remarkable. Although cancer most obviously affects the patient's family and friends, it is important to view the diagnosis through an ecological lens and appreciate that the diagnosis will affect all areas of life.

Childhood

Cancers that develop in children are often different than those that develop in adults, as they are less commonly linked to behavioral, environmental, and lifestyle factors. According to the NCI, cancer remains one of the most common causes of death among children, with 32.1 cancer diagnoses per 100,000 children aged 0–14 years. Even though childhood cancer rates have decreased by 70% in the past 40 years, the disease remains a significant health issue for young children. An estimated 5% of childhood cancers are caused by inherited genetic mutations, but the remaining 95% of cases are largely not understood. The most common cancers among children aged 0–14 years are acute lymphocytic leukemia, brain and other central nervous system tumors, and neuroblastoma (which is cancer in immature nerve cells). These three types of cancer account for more than half of new childhood cancer cases.[28]

Children with cancer can face very different physical effects than adults. Because children's bodies are going through a rapid phase of development, their bodies are actually better able to receive more intensive treatment, so they are often given higher doses of radiation over a shorter period of time. However, some of the side effects of chemotherapy can cause more side effects for children and can cause developmental damage, leading to impairment of growth or second cancer. Children can even experience *late effects*, or side effects of chemotherapy that occur years after receiving treatment. This adds the burden of needing lifelong aftercare for survivors of childhood cancer.

On a more positive note, children are more likely to have a wide social network of support, including family, friends, schoolmates, and teachers. Because there are many people closely involved in a child's life, they will have a wide network of support for both themselves and their family members who are coping with the difficulties of a cancer diagnosis. However, caregivers should remain mindful to the fact that children may benefit from a "cancer-free" zone, where they focus on the tasks of normal childhood, such as learning, play, and socializing without having to be reminded about their illness.

Adolescence and Young Adulthood

Cancer is more common among adolescents and young adults age 15–39 years than in younger children, with approximately 70,000 annual cancer diagnoses in adolescents and young adults in the United States.[29] The most commonly diagnosed cancers in adolescence include Hodgkin's lymphoma, melanoma, testicular cancer, thyroid cancer, and sarcoma.

Adolescents often seek to develop autonomy and independence from their parents. However, because they are still minors, their parents are legally responsible for making all medical decisions. This can cause difficulty in treating adolescents who may be old enough to understand their circumstances but too young to invoke the right to receive treatment. This conflict emphasizes the importance of clear communication between the adolescent and his/her parents about medical decisions. Similarly, a particular challenge with cancer in young adults is being somewhat stuck between pediatric and adult health care providers. Most doctors specialize in treating either young children or older adults, so adolescents and young adults may feel isolated and out of place. This issue can also make coordinating care difficult, as young adults are also more likely to be without health care than individuals in other age groups. For this reason, and because young adults tend to be in generally good health and are less likely to attend regular doctor visits or receive screenings, cancer in young adults is often detected at a more advanced stage as compared to other age groups.

Lastly, adolescence is a particularly difficult time for children to cope with the cancer diagnosis of a parent. Adolescents are at a developmental stage where they can comprehend the gravity of the diagnosis. They are also torn between balancing the demands of helping to care for an ill parent while also wanting to spend more time with their friends. Gender differences also exist in how adolescents cope with a cancer diagnosis. Males typically engage in active problem-focused coping strategies, such as trying to solve the problem, avoiding the problem, distractions, and sticking to routines to keep things "normal." Females tend to use emotion-coping strategies, such as talking about their problem, experiencing sadness or fear, and looking to social support for help.[30] Adolescents may also worry about the chances of inheriting the cancer in the future.

Older Adulthood

Given that a longer lifespan increases the chance of exposure to carcinogens and other environmental risks, it follows that incidence of cancer increases through older age. As the average lifespan increases, and the United States population gets progressively older, the incidence of cancer is likely to increase and disproportionately impact older adult populations. Older adults may also be perceived differently by health care providers and therefore receive different treatment. They may receive less aggressive treatment, as they are seen as unable to tolerate a full regimen or because some doctors may not believe it is "worth it" to implement a full treatment regimen to someone of advanced age.

Adult Caregivers

Caregivers can be partners/spouses, family members, close friends, or paid employees. Most often, the person providing care for a person with cancer is an unpaid family member. The role of a caregiver includes accomplishing daily tasks, transportation to treatment, administering medication, managing side effects, communicating with other family members and friends, and assessing the progression of the disease and the effectiveness of treatment. Family members are often untrained in caregiving skills and can become overwhelmed by the duties and tasks associated with the many responsibilities of caretaking.

Taking care of a person suffering from cancer can be extremely stressful and emotionally and physically draining. Caregiving can be particularly challenging for family members taking care of a person they love while watching the person get increasingly sick from cancer or its treatment. Caregivers can succumb to extreme stress, negatively impacting their psychological and physical well-being. Caregivers report stress levels exceeding population norms and high levels of depression.[31] This emotional response to caretaking can compromise the quality of care provided and fracture the relationship between the caregiver and the person for whom they are caring. It is important for caregivers to implement self-care routines to reduce the amount of stress in caring for an individual with cancer.

Caregivers and patients may also experience a phenomenon called *anticipatory grief*. Anticipatory grief is experienced when patients and loved ones are expecting any type of functional loss or death as a result of the cancer diagnosis. These losses can include the prospect of death but also include the loss of functioning, independence, roles in the family, and/or hope for the future. As a result, the patient or loved one may have intensified emotional responses such as separation anxiety, isolation, and resentment, which may cause the patient or loved ones to avoid the situation altogether. (As you will learn in the anxiety chapter, avoidance is the most powerful and natural response to uncomfortable situations). However, it is important for the patient and the family to process the reality of the losses, complete any unfinished physical or emotional business with the dying person, begin to adapt to life without their loved one, and plan for the future.[32]

Family Dynamic and Role Changes

A cancer diagnosis for one individual can have implications for immediate and extended family members. Persons diagnosed with cancer may notice that family and friends begin treating them differently, and their role within the family structure may change as their physical, mental, and emotional capacities change. An immediately noticeable change within the family structure is scheduling around treatment. Cancer treatment is incredibly time consuming, both in time spent at the hospital and in the time coping with and recovering from its effects. Because treatment can be so incapacitating, individuals with cancer, their families, and their friends will likely need to adjust their schedules around treatment. This can impact work schedules and need for childcare, again highlighting the financial burden of this disease that increases the challenges for people of low SES.

Role Changes

When a family member is diagnosed with cancer, his or her role within the family may change, making it necessary for others in the household to adjust their place in the family structure. As an individual with cancer goes through treatment or becomes increasingly afflicted, he or she may be less capable of accomplishing the same tasks that he or she was able to complete before. The person may need help paying bills, cooking meals, doing household chores, shopping, mowing the lawn, caring for children or caring for himself or herself. This can lead to a spouse taking on more household duties or changing status to the head of the household (if not already), or doing chores not previously required. Similarly, children may become more parentified as they are called upon to pick up duties and chores previously accomplished by a parent. Furthermore, in households where one child is diagnosed with cancer, the family will also have to navigate how to ensure that other siblings are nurtured and receive adequate attention throughout the course of the illness. Similar to other illnesses, it is common for siblings to experience feelings of rejection, isolation, and a lack of attention. Most parents do not consciously ignore their other children, but the demands of cancer treatment require parents to spend a significant amount of time attending treatments, delivering medications, and talking with health care providers and insurance companies, as well as keeping a watchful eye on the child's symptoms and well-being. Parents should be reminded to actively nurture siblings throughout the course of the disease.

Finances

Financial concerns are also commonly reported stressors among cancer patients. Because an individual with cancer may not be able to continue working, either due to treatment or the progression of the disease, money can become a major stressor for the individual and the family. Cancer can be a major financial burden in and of itself, an issue that is compounded by the fact that many people are unable to work while they are in treatment or because they are too sick. Furthermore, without work, a person suffering from cancer may lose health insurance. These issues present their own problems and can also cause extreme stress and conflict within the family structure.

Impact of Cancer on Individual, Family, and Community Well Being
Psychological Impact of Cancer

Many feelings and emotions can come with a cancer diagnosis. These include overwhelming feelings, such as feeling out of control and helpless, experiencing stress from a disrupted routine, and frustration from not understanding an inundation of new medical terms. Denial is also common in that many people have trouble believing or accepting that they have been diagnosed with cancer. Many people experience anger, such as wondering "why me," and feeling anger at loved ones, medical professionals, and God. Fear, stress, depression, and anxiety are also common due to confrontation with pain, sickness, figuring out how to take care of one's family, dealing with employment and paying bills, having to come to terms with death, and experiencing a sense of loss. Other emotions often experienced by individuals diagnosed with cancer include guilt, such as blaming oneself for upsetting their family and feeling like a burden, loneliness, feeling as though friends are distant, being too sick to socialize, and feeling as though others do not understand, and gratitude, as though cancer was a wakeup call to pay attention to what is truly important in life. Reframing cancer from something you "die from" to something you need to "live with" can be a helpful strategy for coping with the many negative emotions associated with a cancer diagnosis. Eventually, many people come to feel hope after they experience acceptance, which can be achieved through activities such as planning for their family's future, living life to the fullest, spending time outside in nature, and self-reflection.

Suicide

Risk of suicide is also a particular concern in individuals who are terminally ill. Nearly 50% of terminally ill cancer patients have thoughts of suicide[33], although these thoughts are usually fleeting. Suicidal thoughts are often associated with a temporary loss of control or heightened anxiety about the future. These thoughts or actions may also be a cry for help to alleviate the pain and psychological distress associated with late-stage cancer. Many cancer patients may engage in behaviors that will allow them to have a method of suicide if needed, such as pill hoarding or securing a handgun. It is important to remember that very few cancer patients actually end their own lives; rather, these behaviors are a way of holding onto to the last thing that they can control—their life.

Social Impact of Cancer

Cancer impacts much more than the afflicted individual. The person's family, friends, and colleagues can also feel the impact of a cancer diagnosis. The individual's self-esteem and how the person perceive himself or herself in relation to others is also likely to be affected. Those who lose weight or their hair to cancer treatment may feel as though their loved ones are treating them differently or even experience changing interactions with strangers and feel as though they are looked at differently when they walk down the street. The social impact of cancer is far-reaching and pervasive. The social impacts of cancer can also be on a scale larger than specific interpersonal relationships. Hara and Blum (2009) make the observation that the social expectation of an individual with cancer to "beat" the disease and be a "survivor" can cause pressure and stress to "get over" their experience once the disease is cured or in remission.[34] Moving on from cancer is a challenging prospect, considering the impact that the disease has on long-term health prospects, finances, and employment, and the expectation for things to "return to normal" can be challenging and unrealistic. Living with a "new normal" is a more realistic way to think about the situation. Survivors may experience long-term or permanent effects of cancer and cancer treatment, their life trajectory may be altered, and the impact of dealing with cancer and preventing its return can be farther reaching than anticipated.

Sexuality

Cancer can greatly impact personal relationships, particularly in the sphere of sex and sexuality. Fifty eight percent of cancer survivors report "sexual changes," and 25% report "dating problems."[35] Impaired physical functioning and changes in personal appearance adversely impact self-esteem and interpersonal intimacy. The NCI reports that cancer survivors may have to live with hair loss, skin changes, weight changes, lost limbs, and infertility.[36] Other components of dealing with cancer, such as carrying a colostomy bag, can lead to feelings of shame and embarrassment. It is common to experience a decreased sex drive due to cancer and its treatment, as well as the depression and anxiety that can accompany such a diagnosis. Physical limitations due to cancer that prohibit sexual activity as it was experienced previously can also play a role in sexual problems. The NCI suggests that talking about these issues with the therapist and/

or partner, finding ways to be intimate outside of sex, and trying new ways of feeling physical can be beneficial.

Employment

Hara and Blum (2009) discuss the stigma of being a cancer survivor in American society, in situations such as navigating the workplace and dealing with insurance.[37] Survivors may not receive appropriate accommodations from their workplace (e.g., scheduling around treatment), may fear job loss due to missed work, and may be passed over for promotions. Cancer survivors may also experience inflexibility in their career choices, as they may feel as though they have to stay in a particular job due to the risk of jeopardizing health-insurance benefits. Medical treatment can lead to the threat of unemployment, debt, and difficulty obtaining life and disability insurance. One study indicated that 25% of cancer survivors under age 65 have health insurance deferred or did not obtain follow-up care due to prohibitive costs, and that the same was true for 70% of those without insurance.[38] Clearly, the ongoing, long-term social issues of a cancer survivor are far-reaching and have the potential to be greatly inhibiting.

Community Efforts to Help Reduce Impact and Cope with Cancer

Some highly recognizable cancer charities include the American Cancer Society, the Lance Armstrong Foundation (LiveStrong.org), and Susan G. Komen for the Cure. The latter hosts highly attended national events such as Walk for the Cure. The breast cancer community is an example of a community that has mobilized significant fundraising and research activities to better the lives of women around the country diagnosed with breast cancer, investing over $2.6 billion in the fight against breast cancer.[39] Other types of cancers, however, do not receive the same level of publicity and outreach. It is important to note that those who are diagnosed with rare types of cancer may feel isolated and alienated from the larger cancer community and may not have the privilege of advocacy, research, and treatment development compared to more common cancers.

Hospice and Palliative Care

Many cancer patients and their families have experienced the true blessing which is hospice and palliative care. As terminally ill cancer patients near the end of life, they qualify to receive *hospice* care. Hospice care is a form of care provided to keep patients medically comfortable once it has been deemed by their physicians that they have less than six months to live, and they will no longer be engaging in aggressive medical therapies. Hospice can be delivered at a hospice facility or in the home. Once a patient's pain is alleviated, he or she can focus on living the rest of his or her life to the fullest, as well as on the emotional and practical issues of dying. Many patients also receive *palliative care* either at the end of life or throughout their illness, which helps to keep patients physically comfortable throughout the illness. Palliative care is provided for patients who may still be undergoing active treatment and want comfort and symptom relief during their disease. Both of these programs fill an important gap in helping people to navigate their illnesses and/or end their lives with dignity and comfort.

Conclusion

By now, you should have a fundamental understanding of what cancer is, how it develops, and how it is treated. Cancer is complex and far-reaching, and extensive research into the cause of and treatment options for the disease is ongoing. Cancer mortality rates have been steadily declining, but the disease remains a primary cause of death in the United States and around the world. In the U.S., cancer disproportionately affects individuals from low socioeconomic status, and by this point in the book you should have a clear picture of the factors that contribute to these health disparities. Clearly, cancer is a complex issue with a vast network of variables that play into the process of the disease, as well as how individuals, families, and communities cope with the disease.

Case Study

Alexander is an eight-year-old Cambodian boy who was diagnosed with lymphoma in 2007. Alexander's mother was able to care for him until he was four years old, at which time he went to live with his biological father and two older, female siblings. He had weekly visits with his father's family prior to his move. His father and siblings lived in the family's rented, multifamily home with Alexander's paternal grandparents, who moved to the United States 15 years ago and spoke limited English. Alexander could not speak Cambodian. When Alexander was seven years old, his father was incarcerated due to multiple charges of physical and sexual assault on women, and he also assaulted Alexander's older sisters. Alexander's grandparents remained convinced of their son's innocence. They attempted to advocate for their son; however, their language barrier often interfered with their ability to convey important information. Alexander's grandparents could not afford an attorney due to limited economic resources.

Soon after Alexander was diagnosed with lymphoma, his mother resumed contact with the family and communicated interest in being part of Alexander's life (i.e., regaining custody). Due to Alexander's complex medical regimen, there were concerns about her ability to effectively care for Alexander. Therefore, the court ordered that visits should be in a public place and scheduled initial visits to occur at the hospital during Alexander's medical visits. His mother showed up for the first visit. Although Alexander was happy to see her, he was also cautious given the fact that he did not know her well. In the next five months, she did not show up for another scheduled visit. His grandmother was the primary health caregiver, accompanying Alexander to every hospital visit. She was extremely dedicated to Alexander's medical care. In fact, Alexander was admitted into the Intensive Care Unit for three days due to a serious infection that scabbed his lips, mouth, and esophagus, and his grandmother stayed with him around the clock. She was becoming increasingly overwhelmed, but her primary motivation was Alexander's well-being.

Alexander was identified as a child who may benefit from psychotherapy given his internalization of his feelings regarding his family situation and illness. Therapy occurred in the cancer clinic while Alexander received chemotherapy. Alexander took three or four sessions to warm up to the therapis, but soon revealed himself as an affable, inquisitive, and sensitive eight-year-old boy. He often asked the therapist to accompany him to spinal tap surgeries, because he stated that his grandmother became too nervous. He later stated that he was embarrassed by his grandmother because she did not speak English well and did not know the culture. His embarrassment also affected his social life, and he chose not to have friends over due to similar acculturation issues. Academically, Alexander's teachers reported that although he was a quiet child, he was a good student and had a few friends in the classroom. Alexander, however, has not been able to attend school for the past two months due to illness and has received tutoring.

During the second-to-last psychotherapy session (which was when Alexander was hospitalized in the Intensive Care Unit for the infection) and before the therapist left the institution, Alexander disclosed that his father had hit him with a closed fist and left a mark. He also disclosed that his paternal grandparents had punished him on occasion by locking him in the dark basement and locking him out of the house for hours at a time. These methods of discipline, however, did not result in any type of physical injury. Alexander was very concerned about his disclosure of these past events as he did not want his grandparents to "get angry" and "get in trouble by social services." He was told that if social services suspected abuse, they would remove him from the home. Alexander's providers reported the disclosure to social services, as required by state law. The therapist also spoke with Alexander's grandmother and emphasized the importance of not punishing Alexander for this disclosure. His grandmother understood. Alexander was very angry at the therapist, but during the last psychotherapy session told her that he forgave her and would miss her.

Notes

1 National Cancer Institute (n.d.). Retrieved from http://cancer.gov.

2 Stewart, B. and Wild, C.P. (eds.), International Agency for Research on Cancer, WHO. (2014) *World cancer report 2014* [Online]. Public Health Well. Available from: http://www.thehealthwell.info/node/725845 [Accessed 6 February, 2017].

3 Mariotto, A.B., Yabroff, K.R., Shao, Y., Feuer, E. J., & Brown, M. L. (2011). Projections of the cost of cancer care in the United States: 2010–2020. *Journal of the National Cancer Institute, 103*(2).

4 National Cancer Institute (n.d.). Retrieved from http://cancer.gov.

5 Howlader, N., Noone, A. M., Krapcho, M., et al. (eds). SEER cancer statistics review, 1975–2011. National Cancer Institute. Bethesda, MD. http://seer.cancer.gov/csr/1975_2011/, based on November 2013 SEER data submission, posted to the SEER web site, April 2014.

6 Surveillance, epidemiology, and end results (SEER) program, SEER*stat database: Incidence—SEER 17 regs limited-use, Nov 2006 sub (2000–2004)—linked to county attributes—total U.S., 1969–2004. National Cancer Institute, DCCPS, Surveillance Research Program, Cancer Statistics Branch, released April 2007, based on the November 2006 submission. http://www.seer.cancer.gov

7   Howlader, N., Noone, A.M., Krapcho, M., Miller, D., Bishop, K., Altekruse, S. F., Kosary, C. L., Yu, M., Ruhl, J., Tatalovich, Z., Mariotto, A., Lewis, D. R., Chen, H. S., Feuer, E. J., Cronin, K. A. (eds). SEER cancer statistics review, 1975–2013, National Cancer Institute. Bethesda, MD, http://seer.cancer.gov/csr/1975_2013/, based on November 2015 SEER data submission, posted to the SEER web site, April 2016.

8   Cancer rates by race/ethnicity and sex (2016). Cancer Prevention and Control, Centers for Disease Control and Prevention. Retrieved from https://www.cdc.gov/cancer/dcpc/data/race.htm.

9   Howlader, N., Noone, A. M., Krapcho, M., et al. (eds). SEER cancer statistics review, 1975–2011, National Cancer Institute. http://seer.cancer.gov/csr/1975_2011/, based on November 2013 SEER data submission, posted to the SEER web site, April 2014.

10 Cancer stat facts: Prostate cancer. (2013). National Cancer Institute, Surveillance, Epidemiology, and End Results Program. Retrieved January 18, 2017, from https://seer.cancer.gov/statfacts/html/prost.html

11 Surveillance, epidemiology, and end results (SEER) program, SEER*stat database: Incidence—SEER 17 regs limited-use, Nov 2006 sub (2000–2004)—linked to county attributes—total U.S., 1969–2004. National Cancer Institute, DCCPS, Surveillance Research Program, Cancer Statistics Branch, released April 2007, based on the November 2006 submission. http://www.seer.cancer.gov

12 Whitman, S., Orsi, J., & Hurlbert, M. (2012). The racial disparity in breast cancer mortality in the 25 largest cities in the United States. *Cancer Epidemiology, 36*(2). doi:10.1016/j.canep.2011.10.012

13 Cancer. (n.d.). Healthy People 2020. Retreived from https://www.healthypeople.gov/2020/topics-objectives/topic/cancer.

14 Berger, N. A., Savvides, P., Koroukian, S. M., et al. (2006). Cancer in the elderly. *Transactions of the American Clinical and Climatological Association, 117,*147–156.

15 Ward, E., DeSantis, C., Robbins, A., Kohler, B. and Jemal, A. (2014). Childhood and adolescent cancer statistics, 2014. *CAA Cancer Journal for Clinicians, 64*: 83–103. doi:10.3322/caac.21219

16 Genetics. (2007). Cancer Research & Genetics UK. Retrieved January 18, 2017, from http://www.cancerresearchgenetics.co.uk/genetics.html

17 Wolin, K. Y., Carson, K., Colditz, G.A. (2010). Obesity and cancer. *Oncologist. 15*(6):556–565.

18 Roberts, D.L., Dive, C., & Renehan, A. G. (2010). Biological mechanisms linking obesity and cancer risk: New perspectives. *Annual Review of Medicine, 61,* 301–316.

19 Center for Disease Control and Prevention (2015). Retreived from www.cdc.gov

20 Center for Disease Control and Prevention (2015). Retreived from www.cdc.gov

21 Niederhuber, J. E. (2014). Surgical interventions in cancer. In: Abeloff, M. D., Armitage, J. O., Niederhuber, J. E,, Kastan, M. B., McKenna, W. G., eds. *Abeloff's Clinical Oncology.* 5th ed. Philadelphia, PA: Elsevier Churchill Livingstone, 372–380.

22 Hosoya, Y., Lefor, A. T. (2011). Surgical oncology: Laparoscopic surgery. In: DeVita, V. T,, Lawrence, T. S., Rosenberg, S. A., eds. *Cancer Principles & Practice of Oncology.* 9th Ed. Philadelphia, PA: Lippincott Williams & Wilkins, 277–288.

23 Hosoya, Y., Lefor, A. T. (2011). Surgical oncology: Laparoscopic surgery. In: DeVita, V. T,, Lawrence, T. S., Rosenberg, S. A., eds. *Cancer Principles & Practice of Oncology.* 9th Ed. Philadelphia, PA: Lippincott Williams & Wilkins, 277–288.

24 Hosoya, Y., Lefor, A. T. (2011). Surgical oncology: Laparoscopic surgery. In: DeVita, V. T,, Lawrence, T. S., Rosenberg, S. A., eds. *Cancer Principles & Practice of Oncology.* 9th Ed. Philadelphia, PA: Lippincott Williams & Wilkins, 277–288.

25 Oeffinger, K. C., Mertens, A. C., Sklar, C. A., Kawashima, T., Hudson, M. M., Meadows, A. T., … & Schwartz, C. L. (2006). Chronic health conditions in adult survivors of childhood cancer. *New England Journal of Medicine, 355*(15), 1572–1582.

26 Oeffinger, K. C., Mertens, A. C., Sklar, C. A., Kawashima, T., Hudson, M. M., Meadows, A. T., … & Schwartz, C. L. (2006). Chronic health conditions in adult survivors of childhood cancer. *New England Journal of Medicine, 355*(15), 1572–1582.

27 Nutrition in cancer care. (2016, January 8). Cancer.gov. Retrieved January 18, 2017, from https://www.cancer.gov/about-cancer/treatment/side-effects/appetite-loss/nutrition-hp-pdq

28 Cancer in children and adolescents. (2014, May 12). Cancer.gov. Retrieved January 30, 2017, from https://www.cancer.gov/types/childhood-cancers/child-adolescent-cancers-fact-sheet

29 Parsons, H. M., Harlan, L. C., Schmidt, S., Keegan, T. H. M., Lynch, C. F., Kent, E. E., Xiao-Cheng, W., Schwartz, S. M., Chu, R.L., Keel, G., Smith, A. W. (2015). Who treats adolescents and young adults with cancer? A report from the AYA HOPE Study. *Journal of Adolescent and Young Adult Oncology, 4*(3), 141–150. http://doi.org/10.1089/jayao.2014.0041

30 Lazarus, R. S., & Folkman, S. (1984). *Stress, appraisal, and coping.* New York: Springer.

31 Kessler, E. R., Moss, A., Eckhardt, S. G., et al. (2014). Distress among caregivers of phase I trial participants: A cross-sectional study. *Supportive Care in Cancer: Official Journal of the Multinational Association of Supportive Care in Cancer. 22*(12):3331–3340. doi:10.1007/s00520–014-2380–3.

32 Hottensen, D. (2010). Anticipatory grief in patients with cancer. *Clinical Journal of Oncology Nursing, 14*(1).

33 Rosenstein, D. L. (2011). Depression and end-of-life care for patients with cancer. *Dialogues in Clinical Neuroscience, 13*(1), 101–108.

34 Hara, R. & Blum, D. (2009). Social well-being and cancer survivorship. National Center for Biotechnology Information, U.S. National Library of Medicine. Retrieved January 17, 2017, from https://www.ncbi.nlm.nih.gov/pubmed/19856588

35 Wolff, S. N., Nichols, C., Ulman, D., Miller, A., Kho, S., Lofye, D., … & Armstrong, L. (2005, June). Survivorship: An unmet need of the patient with cancer-implications of a survey of the Lance Armstrong Foundation (LAF). In *ASCO Annual Meeting Proceedings* (Vol. 23, No. 16_suppl, p. 6032).

36 Self image and sexuality. (2017, January 23). National Cancer Institute. Retrieved January 30, 2017, from https://www.cancer.gov/about-cancer/coping/self-image

37 Hara, R. & Blum, D. (2009). Social well-being and cancer survivorship. National Center for Biotechnology Information, U.S. National Library of Medicine. Retrieved January 17, 2017, from https://www.ncbi.nlm.nih.gov/pubmed/19856588

38 Bradley, C. J., & Bednarek, H. L. (2002). Employment patterns of long-term cancer survivors. *Psychooncology, 11*(3), 188–198.

39 About us. (2017). Susan G. Komen. Retrieved from http://ww5.komen.org/AboutUs/AboutUs.html.

Figure Sources

1 Figure 7.1: Copyright © Cancer Research UK uploader (CC BY-SA 4.0) at https://commons.wikimedia.org/wiki/File:Diagram_showing_cancer_cells_spreading_into_the_blood_stream_CRUK_448.svg.

2 Figure 7.2: Source: https://upload.wikimedia.org/wikipedia/commons/thumb/4/43/Melanoma_vs_normal_mole_ABCD_rule_NCI_Visuals_Online.jpg/768px-Melanoma_vs_normal_mole_ABCD_rule_NCI_Visuals_Online.jpg.

3 Figure 7.3: Copyright © Raphseck (CC BY-SA 4.0) at https://commons.wikimedia.org/wiki/Category:Breast_cancer_stages#/media/File:Breast_cancer_illustration_en.svg.

4 Figure 7.4: Copyright © Yale Rosen (CC BY-SA 2.0) at https://www.flickr.com/photos/30950973@N03/3922611335.

5 Figure 7.5: Copyright © Simplyanon (CC BY-SA 3.0) at https://upload.wikimedia.org/wikipedia/commons/0/06/Cancer_stages.png.

CHAPTER EIGHT

Sleep Health

Coauthors:
Sue K. Adams, Ph.D., Rachel Feragne, B.S.

@sleepfoundation

As human beings, we spend 1/3 of our lives sleeping, which equates to 229,961 hours of sleep during the average lifetime. For a process that we engage in for so much of our lives, we actually know quite little about how and why we sleep. Although it is clear that sleep deprivation impacts a person's ability to function, it may be less obvious that poor sleep has major implications for communities and public health. It is estimated that 50–70 million Americans suffer from sleep disorders.[1] The exact economic cost, however, of sleep problems is hard to determine, although it is easily calculated to be in the hundreds of billions of dollars. The economic costs are both direct and indirect, and are both short- and long-term. Examples of direct economic costs include medical and mental health doctor's visits, hospital services, prescriptions, and over-the-counter medications. Indirect economic costs include illness-related morbidity and mortality, absenteeism from work, disability, decreased productivity, and work place and vehicular accidents.[2] The National Highway Traffic Safety Administration estimates that approximately 100,000 motor vehicle accidents happen each year, resulting in around 1,500 deaths.[3] Did you know that the Chernobyl accident, the Exxon Valdez oil spill, and the Challenger space shuttle accident are all thought to have been partially caused by sleepiness?

The purpose of this chapter is to introduce you to what we do know about sleep, including the function of sleep, how sleep deprivation impacts individuals, families, and communities, and the most common sleep disorders in the United States.

What Is Sleep?

Definition of Sleep

After a long hard day of work, school, or play, many people look forward to bedtime. Sleep is a rather comforting time; our head hits the pillow and we wrap ourselves in our sheets waiting to drift off into dreamland. Although many of us fall asleep easily, sleep is in fact a very complex process. By definition, sleep is "a natural periodic state of rest for the mind and body, in which the eyes usually close and consciousness is completely or partially lost, so that there is a decrease in bodily movement and responsiveness to external stimuli."[4] Sleep has a few primary functions. First, it is a time when the tissues and cells in our bodies repair themselves from damage that occurred during the day. Second, sleep helps our brain to make sense of the information that we learned during the day and move it into long-term memory. Lastly, it has also been proposed that sleep is a survival mechanism because when we sleep we are less likely to be outside in the dark and eaten by nocturnal predators.

Sleep is regulated by two systems: sleep/wake homeostasis and the circadian biological clock. After being awake for a substantial amount of time, our sleep/wake homeostasis informs our body that the need for sleep is growing, resulting in feelings of fatigue, tiredness, having low energy and decreased alertness. Sleep/wake homeostasis creates a drive for sleep and waking up, producing a balance of the two.[5] The circadian biological clock, also known as our *circadian rhythm*, regulates the timing of sleep and waking throughout the day, as well as other processes like hormone secretion and body temperature. Our sleep circadian rhythm is based on a roughly 24-hour cycle and is mainly affected by light and darkness in our environment. Our circadian rhythm increases and decreases at different times of the day. For example, adults tend to have the strongest sleep drive from 2–4 a.m. and from 1–3 p.m. (the reason why you may have trouble keeping your eyes open during afternoon classes).

As we sleep, our brain cycles through five distinct phases: stages 1, 2, 3, 4, and REM (rapid eye movement) sleep. These stages progress in order from stage 1 to REM sleep. Stages 1–4 fall in the NREM (non-rapid eye movement) sleep category. We tend to experience NREM about 75% of the time when in bed. It takes approximately 90 to 110 minutes to complete a full sleep cycle, and every time as we transition from REM sleep to stage 1, we briefly wake up. This may be the time when you roll over or pull up the covers. During the early periods of the night, the first sleep cycles contain shorter REM periods and longer deep sleep periods (stages 3 and 4). Later on in the night REM sleep periods increase while deep sleep periods decrease. The amount of REM sleep we receive depends on our stage of development. Infants for example tend to spend 50% of their sleep in REM sleep while adults spend about 20% in REM sleep.[6] Below is a brief description of what happens in each phase of sleep.[7]

Stage 1

During stage 1, known as the light theta wave stage, we begin to drift off to sleep; however, any small sound or disturbance could easily wake us up. This is the time when a person is literally between being awake and asleep. People may experience sudden muscle contractions

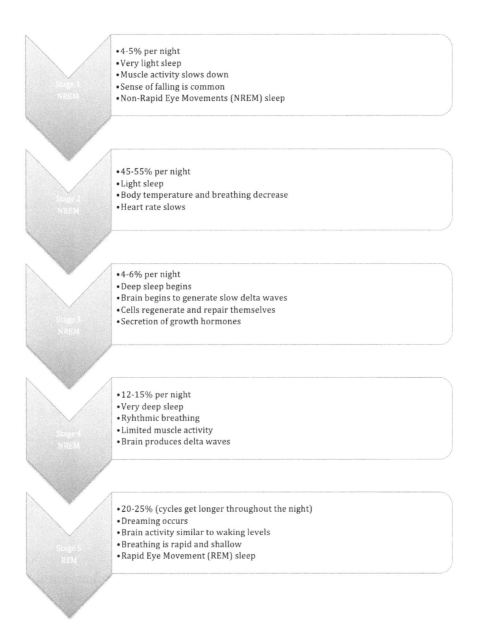

FIGURE 8.1 **The Sleep Cycle**

known as *hypnic myoclonia* usually proceeded by a sensation of feeling like you are falling. Stage 1 occupies approximately 2–5% of sleep per night.

Stage 2
Stage 2, or the true light theta wave stage, is the onset of sleep. In this stage eye movements halt, breathing and heart rate are regular, and body temperature drops. Disengagement

from the stimuli around us also occurs. We spend approximately 45–60% of sleep per night in stage 2.

Stage 3
Deeper sleep transpires in stage 3, known as the early deep slow wave stage, as our brain waves slow down and *delta waves* begin to appear. These slow waves are interspersed with small, faster waves. Stage 3 of sleep occurs in the first four hours of sleep.

Stage 4
By stage 4, also called the deep slow wave delta stage, the brain is producing delta waves almost entirely. Stages 3 and 4 are also known as the *deep sleep* phase. In both stages 3 and 4, there is no eye movement or muscle activity, breathing becomes slow, blood pressure drops, blood supply to the muscles increases, tissue growth and tissue repair occur, hormones are released, and energy is restored. Since all of these bodily functions are occurring while we sleep, we are said to be experiencing restorative sleep.

REM Sleep
The last sleep stage, REM (Rapid Eye Movement) sleep, occurs about 20–50% every night and varies due to age and stage of development. The onset of REM sleep occurs about 90 minutes after we fall asleep. During REM sleep breathing becomes faster and irregular, eyes jerk rapidly in all directions (hence the term rapid eye movement), limb muscles become paralyzed for a temporary amount of time so that a person does not act out their dreams, heart rate increases, and blood pressure escalates. While we are unaware of the bodily changes taking place during REM, waking up and remembering dreams is a sure indicator that you were in REM. Everyone dreams at night, but you only remember your dreams if you wake up in REM.

Health Disparities
Although a number of health disparities exist in sleep, the two most impactful are both age disparities. Sleep disordered breathing (SDB), which includes sleep disorders such as obstructive sleep apnea and snoring, are disproportionately affecting children and older adults in the United States. African American children are twice as likely as white children to develop SDB.[8] This is not due to increases in obesity but more likely due to chronic inflammation in the airways caused by exposure to air pollutants and cigarette smoke. SDB also affects up to 40% of older adults as they age.[9] If left untreated, SDB is associated with school problems, metabolic disorders, and future heart disease, such as stroke.

Healthy People 2020
Now that we have explored why we sleep, let's return to our discussion of the importance of sleep. As a result of the effects that sleep deprivation has on individuals, communities, and

the economy, Sleep Health was added as an objective to Healthy People 2020. The goal is to "increase public knowledge of how adequate sleep and treatment of sleep disorders improve health, productivity, wellness, quality of life, and safety on roads and in the workplace."[10] More specifically, Healthy People 2020 aims to 1) increase the number of people who are evaluated for obstructive sleep apnea (which you will learn about later), 2) reduce rates of car accidents due to drowsy driving, 3) to increase the number of adolescents who receive adequate sleep, and 4) increase the number of adults who receive adequate sleep. Healthy People 2020 aims to reach its objectives using both individual and community-based public health interventions. For instance, the National Center on Sleep Disorders Research and the National Highway Traffic Safety Administration have worked together to identify three priority issues for an educational campaign: 1) education for young males about sleepiness and driving, 2) promotion of the use of rumble strips on highways, and 3) education for shift workers about drowsy driving after shifts.[11]

Sleep Across Development

The National Sleep Foundation sets out the recommended hours of sleep each age group should receive on a daily basis. Infants, for example, need 12–15 hours of sleep per night while adults need 7–9 hours for optimal functioning. Each stage of development encompasses different challenges, strengths, and opportunities that must be faced. Also, sleep cycles change as people advance through these stages of development. We will now look into each developmental age group, focusing on specific sleep patterns and challenges that may affect sleep.

Infancy (birth-1 year)

The National Sleep Foundation states that newborns between 0–3 months old need 14–17 hours of sleep per day. It may also be appropriate for newborns to sleep 11–13 hours per day; however, anything less than 11 hours is strongly advised against. The NSF recommends infants who are 4–11 months old receive 12–15 hours of sleep per day. These numbers are averages, and some infants sleep more or less depending on their individual needs, although sleeping less than 10 hours per day is not recommended.[12]

Sleep is essential for babies' growth and development. It is the primary activity of the brain during a child's development. Circadian rhythms for infants tend to be extremely irregular the first couple months of life. This is why infants tend to sleep every three hours and do not begin to develop consistent nighttime sleeping rhythms until about six weeks old. By three to six months of age most infants have a developed sleep-wake cycle. Around 50% of infants sleep through the night by four months of age, with "sleeping through the night" being defined as six continuous hours of sleep. By nine months about 70–80% of infants are sleeping through the night.[13] Infant sleep slowly regulates over the first year until they are sleeping similar hours as their parents (which is great news for sleep-deprived parents). Now we will discuss two important topics for infants and sleep: sudden infant death syndrome (SIDS) and co-sleeping.

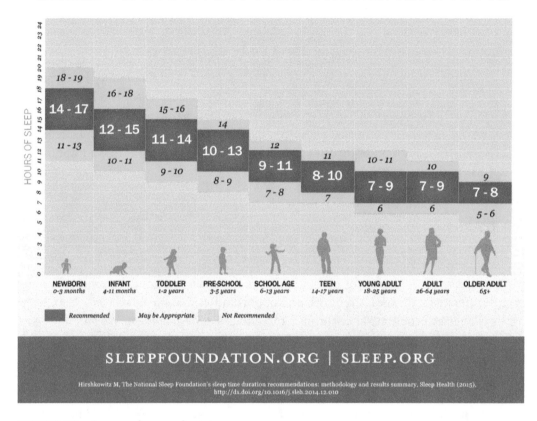

National Sleep Foundation

SLEEP DURATION RECOMMENDATIONS

SLEEPFOUNDATION.ORG | SLEEP.ORG

Hirshkowitz M, The National Sleep Foundation's sleep time duration recommendations: methodology and results summary, Sleep Health (2015). http://dx.doi.org/10.1016/j.sleh.2014.12.010

FIGURE 8.2 **Average sleep needs across age groups**

Sudden Infant Death Syndrome (SIDS)

SIDS is the unforeseen death of a child under the age of one where an autopsy cannot show any explainable cause of death. Very tragically, these babies die in their sleep, and SIDS is the leading cause of death of infants between one month and one year in the United States. Possible causes of SIDS include physical factors and sleep environment factors. *Physical factors* include brain abnormalities, low birth weight, and respiratory infections. One theory is that a brain abnormality in the baby's hippocampus and brainstem impairs the brain's ability to control breathing and heart rate patterns during sleep, and the babies never wake up. Babies may be particularly prone to experiencing this phenomenon when they are sleeping on their stomachs, as sleeping on the stomach promotes a very deep sleep. Sleep *environmental factors* include infants sleeping on a soft surface and face down and/or sleeping with parents, both of which can lead to smothering and suffocation during sleep. Risk factors of SIDS also include being a boy, being born premature, babies 0–3 months in age, babies of black and American Indian backgrounds, and those who have had siblings or cousins who have died from SIDS.[14]

In response to an increase in SIDS rates in the U.S., in 1992 the American Academy of Pediatrics began the *Back to Sleep* campaign. The Back to Sleep Campaign promotes putting babies to sleep on their backs, rather than on their sides or bellies. Since its inception, rates of SIDS have significantly decreased, although in recent years the rates have plateaued.[15] Although Back to Sleep has been an incredibly effective campaign, some parents may not follow the recommendation due to certain misconceptions. For instance, parents may fear that placing a baby to sleep on its back will cause potential choking, which is unlikely. Parents may also be given advice from older generations that belly sleeping is the most comforting type of sleep for babies. In any case, other prevention techniques have been shown to protect children from SIDS such as breastfeeding, giving infants a pacifier, not using any soft bedding or blankets in the crib, not overheating the infant by bundling with too many clothes or blankets, and having babies sleep in their own cribs rather than in a bed with adults.[16]

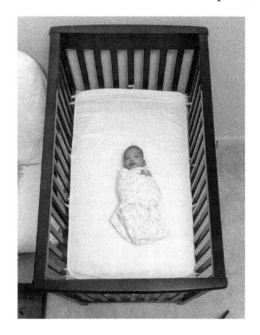

FIGURE 8.3   Safe sleep conditions for infants

Co-sleeping

Sleeping with a child in the parent's bed is referred to as co-sleeping. Sleeping with an infant in the bed versus having the infant sleep alone in a crib has been a long-standing debate and continues to be a controversial issue. Co-sleeping has both pros and cons. Pros of co-sleeping include: nighttime nursing is more convenient, mother's sleep cycle becomes in sync with the infant, increased nighttime sleep for infants, and promoting a sense of bonding and attachment with the infant. Many parents find it fulfilling to sleep with their baby for these reasons. Cons of co-sleeping potentially include: less sleep for the baby and for parents, increased risk of SIDS, and the promotion of dependence on parents.[17,18] Also, cultural and economic factors influence co-sleeping. Parents who live in small homes, apartments, or live with family or friends due to poverty may co-sleep out of necessity because they do not have the space for separate rooms.[19]

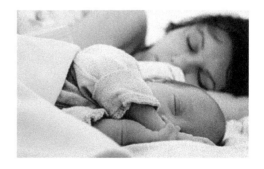

FIGURE 8.4   A mother and child co-sleeping

Co-sleeping is also the cultural norm in many parts of the world. The topic of co-sleeping will continue to be a controversial issue, and ultimately it is up to parents to decide what is best for their child and their family.

Sleep Training

Sleep training is another controversial issue in many parenting circles. If a child will not sleep alone, but parents want him or her to start sleeping alone in his room, two main sleep training techniques can be used. The first was created by Richard Ferber and is called *cry it out*.[20] In this method, the child is left to cry himself/herself to sleep. This method takes a lot of self-control on the parent's part because the natural response to a crying child is to comfort. However, cry it out is very effective, and the child will usually be able to put himself to sleep without crying after a few days. The second method is *gradual sleep extinction*.[21] In this method, the parents will go into the crying child's room after progressively longer lengths of time (e.g., after one minute, then after five minutes, then after 10 minutes). This method is also effective, and often more tolerable for parents, but takes longer to accomplish than cry it out. With either strategy, children have the ability to self-soothe after about six months of age. Therefore, these strategies should never be used before six months old. It takes a lot of work up front, but having a child who will sleep through the night feels amazing!

Toddlers (1–3 years) and Preschoolers (3–5 years)

Toddlers between the ages of one and two need approximately 11–14 hours of sleep, including naps.[22] Naps may occur more than once per day and can last one to three hours depending on when parents choose to wake their toddler. Once toddlers reach 18 months of age, naptimes tend to decrease to one nap per day. Although the sleep guidelines are clear, many toddlers do not receive the appropriate amount of sleep needed to restore their energy. Common sleep problems that toddlers experience include resisting going to bed, nighttime awakenings, nighttime fears and nightmares. In fact, it is more common than not for toddlers to experience nighttime awakening, which is useful information for parents so that they do not have unrealistic expectations that toddlers sleep straight through the night. Let's take some time to discuss a few of the reasons for why toddlers have difficulty sleeping.

Resisting Going to Bed

Toddlers may resist going to sleep for many reasons. Toddlers' brains are developing at a fast rate. They are constantly experiencing and learning new things, and, therefore, their motor, cognitive, and social abilities are on overdrive. Toddlers may resist sleep because they fear they are missing exciting and new opportunities. They may be attempting to exert control over the situation, especially since they are in the "terrible twos" or are "threenagers." They may resist sleep due to separation anxiety from parents, and sleeping alone in a dark room often does not help any separation woes. Lastly, toddlers may build up a fear of bedtime using their imagination, for example thinking that a scary character from a story or television show is lurking under the bed.

Nighttime Awakenings

Waking up during the night is very common among toddlers, and a number of reasons contribute to nighttime awakenings. For example, early in toddlerhood they may wake up out of habit, since nighttime feedings were part of their normal routine in infancy. Toddlers may also wake up during the night if they napped too close to bedtime, as late naps can affect the sleep quality and quantity toddlers receive. Nighttime awakenings may also occur from having nighttime fears and waking up from nightmares.

Nighttime Fears and Nightmares

Nightmares are frightening dreams that create feelings of fear, distress, and anxiety. Having these fearful thoughts and dreams can make children fear bedtime. Nightmares are common among toddlers due to their vivid, ever-growing imagination, their newfound independence to be able to explore new environments, and the developmental ability to verbalize the content of their dreams.

To improve the sleep habits of toddlers, parents should stick to a regular wake-up and bedtime schedule. Going to bed at a certain time will condition toddlers to become tired around the same time every night. Although it is counterintuitive, putting a child to bed too late can lead to a worse nights' sleep. Further, if children are fearful of the dark and being alone, nightlights or a hallway light can be helpful. Giving toddlers an object to sleep with, such as a teddy bear, can help reduce their fears of sleeping alone. Regarding nightmares, parents should provide verbal or physical reassurance if the child is crying but keep the interaction to a minimum. It can be difficult to talk a toddler out of the idea that their fears are real, so work with their imaginations to minimize their distress by spraying "nightmare or monster spray" before bedtime. Finally, bedtime routines are essential. Creating a relaxing bedtime routine with approximately five to six soothing activities, such as bathing, reading a story before bed and cuddling, is a great way to prime the child that sleep is coming!

Preschoolers, aged 3–5 years, typically sleep 10–13 hours per night,[23] Although most still require naps, some preschoolers will stop napping. Like toddlers, preschoolers tend to suffer from the same types of sleep problems. Since preschoolers are continuously developing and learning new things, and their imaginations are growing, this leads preschoolers to commonly experience nighttime fears and nightmares. Preschoolers are very capable of sharing their fears, and often sleep in regular beds, so they are more likely to get up in the middle of the night seeking their parents for comfort when they have scary dreams.

School-Age Children (6–12 years)

The National Sleep Foundation recommends that school-age children need approximately 9–11 hours of sleep per night.[24] As children pass from preschool age to school-age, sleep habits become more stable. In general, school-aged children are better at following bedtime routines, waking up and going to sleep around the same time every night. Children in this stage of development, however, are met with increasing external demands from school, extracurricular activities, peers, and family. School obligations (i.e., homework, the school day, and bus rides) take up a large portion of children's free time. When the school day is over, many children have a fair amount of homework, as schools are working to complete all mandated curriculum in a timely manner. Stress related to increased homework demands can lead to delayed sleep. Children may be involved in extracurricular activities, such as sports or music classes, or play dates all of which may take place after school. Juggling this with the general demands of the family, preparing and eating dinner, having a bath or shower, downtime to relax, and parental demands such as employment and household chores can be overwhelming for even the most organized of families. In a world where there seem to be too few hours in a day, children's sleep quality and quantity often suffer.

Attention Deficit/Hyperactivity Disorder (ADHD) and Sleep

Now we are going to take some time to discuss another important factor that impairs sleep in children, Attention Deficit/Hyperactivity Disorder (ADHD). ADHD is a disorder resulting from the misfiring of a number of important brain centers that control behavior, attention, and activity. ADHD makes it harder for certain behaviors to be controlled. While it is common for all children to have behavior problems at times, children with ADHD have frequent and severe behavior problems that interfere with living a normal life. Three common behavior symptoms children with ADHD exhibit include inattention, impulsivity, and hyperactivity.[25] Inattention is defined as having a hard time paying attention, being disorganized, being easily distracted, and daydreaming excessively. Children with ADHD have a hard time paying attention during the school day, especially when going to class six hours every day. Impulsivity is defined as acting and speaking without thinking. Children who are impulsive tend to be impatient and interrupt others while speaking. Hyperactivity is when children are constantly moving and have difficulty staying in the same spot for long periods of time. Sitting in a classroom for long periods of time can be very difficult for children with ADHD. Like school, sleep is an area in which children with ADHD also tend to struggle.

Approximately 25–50% of children and adolescents with ADHD report sleep problems.[26] Interestingly, research suggests that the brain center that controls attention and behavior also controls the regulation of the sleep-wake cycle. It makes sense why ADHD and sleep problems are so closely related. Hyperactivity in children results in having restless sleep, having a hard time falling asleep, and having a difficult time staying asleep. Children on ADHD medications may also experience a *rebound effect* close to bedtime, which is when the medication wears off and the ADHD symptoms return in full force. Clearly, this will interfere with sleep. Also, when children are sleep deprived, they do not look "sleepy" but rather get very inattentive, impulsive, and fidgety. Some children who are diagnosed with ADHD may not have organic ADHD but rather ADHD-like symptoms caused by poor sleep.

Wetting the Bed

Bedwetting, also known as nocturnal enuresis, occurs when children wet their bed during sleep. Approximately seven million children in the United States wet their bed on a regular basis.[27] For children learning to potty-train and up to age seven, occasional bedwetting is seen as a normative behavior, as a person's muscles, nerves, brain, and spinal cord are learning how to be in sync with one another. If bedwetting continues past age seven, the child may have an underlying medical condition or possible trauma, and the child's pediatrician should be notified.

Adolescents (13–17)

Adolescence is characterized by multiple transitions in life, and sleep is no different. Although most adolescents continue to require nine to 9½ hours of sleep per night, multiple demands cause them to get only between seven to 7½ hours per night.[28] Females also report more sleep deprivation than males. This leads to a significant accumulation of sleep debt, which is the accumulation of the amount of sleep missed over the course of a week. No wonder why adolescents usually sleep late on the weekends—they have to make up approximately 25% of sleep debt to feel fully rested!

Reasons why adolescence are chronically sleep deprived include puberty and life demands. Puberty shifts the circadian rhythm by about two hours.[29] Therefore, teens want to go to bed two hours later and wake up two hours later, and this is a natural biological rhythm that will not be outgrown until the transition to adulthood. Our society, however, does not function to accommodate adolescent sleep needs. School start time gets earlier as children age, with most high schools beginning earlier than middle school. In districts where start time is delayed by a half hour or so, they have seen increases in alertness, academic performance, and mood.[30] In addition, adolescents have increased life demands such as more and harder academic work, extracurricular activities, employment, and technology use. As parents loosen the reigns and allow teens more autonomy over their sleep schedules, it is easy to see the combination of these factors contribute to sleepy teens.

Young Adults and College Students (18–25)

As young adults transition into adult sleep patterns, they continue to require approximately eight to nine hours of sleep per night in order to function at their best.[31] Whether they are enrolled in college or are working full-time, young adults continue to experience the burden of lifestyle demands, and college students report twice as many sleep problems as the general population.[32] Specifically, college students report that increased academic demands, not wanting to be the first to go to bed and miss something important, nighttime being the primary time to socialize with current and old friends, and the stresses of living in dormitories all impact sleep.[33] Interestingly, some researchers have found that sleep deprivation is linked to lower GPA in college,[34] so making sleep a priority can increase grades.

Young adults are also susceptible to the effects of technology use late at night. Using a cell phone or watching television before bed may seem like a normal and mundane task; however, the brain is being stimulated by the device's blue light to think that it is daytime, therefore suppressing the secretion of the sleep hormone, melatonin. Waking up to texts after falling asleep dysregulates the sleep cycle, and if the text is emotional, the person will likely have trouble getting back to sleep. Studies have shown that using technology immediately before bed will decrease overall sleep time and if used compulsively (i.e., before bedtime, during the night), could lead to significant sleep disruption.[35] Please, turn off your phones. Very rarely will you miss something super important.

Adulthood

On average, adults require eight hours of sleep. Here is an interesting fact: Human sleep is biphasic, which means that we are pre-programmed to sleep four hours, wake up for a brief time, and then go back to sleep for another four hours. American adults are sleep deprived, with 25% of U.S. adults reporting insufficient sleep at least 15 out of every 30 days.[36] Racial disparities exist, with Hispanic or Latino adults getting the most sleep (71%) compared to black and white Americans, and black Americans are more likely than others to experience "short sleep duration."[37] There are also significant public health concerns, with 7% of men between the ages of 25 and 34 likely to fall asleep while driving.[38]

A gender health disparity exists between men and women, with women experiencing more sleep problems than men. Certain factors may contribute to this finding, including higher rates of anxiety that can make it hard for women to fall asleep and biological processes at different life stages. Pregnant woman are particularly vulnerable, with 30% reporting that they rarely received a good night's sleep, 84% reporting insomnia, and 40% reporting an increase in sleep-disordered breathing. As a pregnancy progresses, it leads to discomfort while lying down and an increase in mucus secretions in the sinus cavities (hence, the snoring). Finally, menopausal women report less sleep throughout the night, as well as an increase in sleep-disordered breathing.[39] Specifically, one study found that 67% of women who are menstruating report more insomnia during their cycle, and 33% reported more disturbed sleep. Taken together, some women have a difficult time getting a good night's sleep.

Older Adults

As adults age, many things change including their sleep. Adults over the age of 65 spend significantly less time in stages 3 and 4 of sleep. Since stages 3 and 4 are where memory consolidation occurs, these changes in sleep patterns could be a factor in cognitive impairment. Their REM cycles are also shorter and less frequent, and their sleep is often interrupted by periods of wakefulness. Biological factors such as increased aches and pains and more frequent trips to the bathroom caused by certain medications may cause these nighttime awakenings. Older adults also have shifts in their circadian rhythms, which can cause them to fall asleep early in the evening and wake up early in the morning, We also see that 20–40% of older adults experience sleep-disordered breathing as they age, and sleep-disordered breathing is linked with increased risk of stroke and death. The good news is that 76% of adults over the age of 65 report getting sufficient sleep, which is a higher percentage than adults under 65 who report sufficient sleep.[40] [41] Despite the fact that they may be sleeping less throughout the night, as older adults approach retirement age, they benefit from a more leisurely lifestyle that includes time to nap during the day.

How Long to Nap

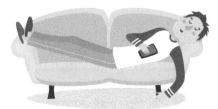

10-20 minutes	30 minutes	60 minutes
The power nap is ideal for a boost in energy. This length lets you stay in the light stages of sleep, making it easier to wake up.	Sleeping this long may cause sleep inertia, which is a groggy feeling upon waking that can last up to 30 minutes.	Napping for this length of time can result in remembering facts, faces and names, but can cause sleep inertia.

90 minutes

This is a full cycle of sleep (including all NREM and REM), and can result in improved emotional, procedural memory and creativity. Sleep inertia is usually avoided since the person cycled through a full sleep cycle.

FIGURE 8.5   Guidelines for how long adults should nap

Impact of Sleep on Individual Health, Communities, and Public Health

Biological Implications

Adequate sleep is a key component of living a healthy lifestyle and maintaining both physical and mental health. Physically, when a person does not get enough sleep, he or she is more likely to experience decreased immune functioning (which partially explains why college students often get sick during or after finals). People can experience deregulated metabolism, which could result in health issues such as weight gain, as well as insulin resistance, increased cortisol levels, inflammation throughout the body, and heart disease.[42] Lack of sleep increases the risk of obesity; people who sleep fewer hours have been shown to crave calorie-dense food, especially carbohydrates. This phenomenon may occur due to hormone imbalances. Sleep helps maintain a healthy balance of hormones that make you feel hungry (ghrelin) and full (lepton). When the body does not get enough sleep, then ghrelin levels go up, and lepton levels go down. As a result, people feel hungrier when they are not well rested. Sleep also affects how the body reacts to insulin hormones, which control blood glucose levels. Lack of sleep leads to higher levels of blood sugar, which increases one's risk for diabetes.[43] We also see that people who are sleep deprived may be more likely to make poorer behavioral choices, such as increased alcohol and drug use, engaging in risky sexual behavior, and overuse of prescribed and/or non-prescribed stimulant medication to counteract drowsiness.[44] Excessive daytime sleepiness can also make people vulnerable to injury and death while driving, as daytime drowsiness can lead to lapses in attention and delayed response times.[45]

Psychological Implications

Psychologically, sleep deprivation affects cognition (that is, how people think), as well as their mood. Poor sleep is related to reduced short-term memory, long-term memory, and concentration, decreased learning abilities, and poor productivity at school and work. Poor sleep is also associated with increased depression, anxiety, trouble managing stress, family and peer conflicts, and impulsivity.[46] To sum it up, sleep deprivation affects the entire body and mind—from top to bottom, inside out, and a person cannot function at peak performance without proper sleep!

Moving Toward Psychological Self-Awareness: Dreaming
Why We Dream

Typically, humans spend two to three hours dreaming each night, therefore having hundreds of thousands of dreams during a lifetime. Dreams, occurring in the REM sleep stage, are images, thoughts, sounds, voices, and sensations experienced when sleeping. Dreams can include people we know, people we have never met, places we have been, places we have never been, activities we have done, activities we have never engaged in, and so on. What is the ultimate function and purpose of dreaming? To this day scientists have not figured out the exact reasons why we dream during sleep, but they do have some theories.

Sigmund Freud, founder of psychoanalysis, analyzed dreams for many years in order to understand aspects of people's personality. Freud believed dreams are a window into humans' unconscious thoughts and desires. Freud believed nothing occurs at random, rather every thought, action, and image people experience is motivated by the unconscious mind to some degree. Many times dreams bring out these wishes and thoughts from the unconscious mind without the person's knowledge. Therefore, Freud felt that dreams are an important factor into understanding the unconscious mind where true desires, thoughts, and needs are held.

While many accept Freud's dream theory, some criticize his outlook. Alfred Adler, an Austrian psychiatrist, believed dreams reflect one's current lifestyle and offer possible solutions to problems. Adler saw dreams as problem-solving devices to be incorporated into one's waking life. Unlike Freud, Adler did not believe individuals' thoughts, desires, and behaviors are stored in the unconscious mind. While Freud believed that the conscious mind and the unconscious mind work against each other (the unconscious mind is always trying to come out while the conscious mind tries to stop it from emerging), Adler believed they function the same whether we are asleep or awake.[47] Since Adler's view focuses on dreams being a problem-solving tool, he theorized a direct correlation between dreams and the number of problems a person has. In other words, the more dreams a person has, the more problems that person has. The fewer dreams a person has, the fewer problems he or she has. While both Freud and Alder proposed varying theories about dreams and their functions, there is no definitive explanation of why people dream. Dreams can be good or bad, happy or sad, and exciting or frightening, and always fascinating! What do you think your dreams are telling you?

Medical and Behavioral Health Interventions

Sleep disorders are changes in a person's sleeping patterns or habits that in turn negatively affect health and well-being. An estimated 60 million people in the United States are currently suffering from a sleep disorder. Out of those 60 million, 40 million are suffering from a chronic sleep disorder and 20 million from an occasional sleep disorder.[48] While sleep disorders vary in length and persistence, each disorder can be placed into one of three categories: lack of sleep, disturbed sleep, and excessive sleep. Since there is an abundance of sleep disorders, this section will focus on the most common sleep disorders that affect Americans, including insomnia, restless legs syndrome, obtrusive sleep apnea (OSA), and night terrors.

Insomnia

Symptoms

More than three million people in the U.S. per year suffer from insomnia,[49] and typically people who suffer from insomnia are adults. By definition, insomnia is persistent difficulty with falling asleep and staying asleep. To be diagnosed with chronic insomnia, a person must have symptoms for three nights per week for four weeks in a row. Otherwise, they would have what is called acute insomnia. People with insomnia tend to have too much of a wake drive and too little of a sleep drive. Only one cycle can be functioning at a time; therefore, if your wake cycle is strong, there is little if any chance you will fall asleep.

Predisposing, Precipitating, and Perpetuating Factors

Factors that contribute to insomnia are divided into three categories: predisposing factors, precipitating factors, and perpetuating factors.[50] *Predisposing factors* are genetic and other factors that increase a person's likelihood to respond to internal and external stressors. For instance, a person's personality, sleep-wake cycle, age, past experience of trauma, or lack of coping mechanisms may make it more likely for a person to be sensitive to developing insomnia. *Precipitating factors* are short-term stressors that override a person's sleep-wake cycle. For example, factors such as stressful situations, a noisy environment, certain medical conditions such as autism, and mental health conditions such as anxiety and depression would make it more likely for a person to develop insomnia. Lastly, *perpetuating factors* are factors that reinforce poor sleep. These include things like doing work in or spending a lot of time in bed (because it reinforces the *sleep association* that bed is for work and not sleep), worrying about lack of sleep, unrealistic sleep expectations, stimulant drug use, technology, and inconsistent bedtime and wake times.

Treatments

The interventions for insomnia include behavioral and medical strategies. To address the behavioral causes of insomnia, it would first be recommended that people engage in stimulus control. Stimulus control involves limiting or controlling the things that are done in the bedroom to decrease the sleep association between bed and wakefulness. For instance, a person would be instructed that he or she cannot eat, read, rest, etc. in bed. The person could be instructed to move the clocks out of the bedroom so that he or she does not "clock watch." Cognitive Behavioral Therapy is a very effective treatment for insomnia and teaches people to challenge unhealthy beliefs about sleep. Also, relaxation strategies can be helpful in calming the body before bed. Medically, a number of prescription (e.g., Ambien®) and non-prescription drugs (e.g., Tylenol PM®) exist to treat insomnia. In fact, medications to treat insomnia are a billion-dollar industry. The problem with using medications without behavioral strategies, however, is that people never learn to change their behaviors. When they stop the medications, their sleep problems will likely return.

Restless Leg Syndrome

Symptoms

Imagine you are lying in your favorite comfy chair watching TV or reading a novel. Your body is slowly releasing any tension you are holding, becoming relaxed and at ease, except for your legs. Restless leg syndrome (RLS) is defined as a strong, *irresistible* urge to move one's legs. Sensations such as tingling, numbness, and even pain can accompany this sleep disorder. Symptoms of RLS tend to begin in the evening hours and continue throughout the night. In order to feel relief, people tend to move, rub, and stretch their legs. These tactics are short-lived as the leg uneasiness often returns.

RLS is more common among women than men. Although RLS affects individuals of all ages, people 45–65 years of age are the most typical patients. People under the age of 45 who develop RLS are considered early-onset cases and experience symptoms at a slower rate. Older individuals over 65 with RLS tend to have leg sensations that occur almost every night. More than 50% of people with RLS are diagnosed with primary RLS, meaning their sleep disorder is not associated with any other medical issue(s) they may or may not have.[51]

Risk Factors

Regarding family history, the chances of developing RLS increases ten-fold if an immediate family member has RLS. Therefore, genetics is a strong risk and causal factor in this sleep disorder. Medical disorders, such as Parkinson's disease, kidney failure, diabetes, and anemia can also increase the likelihood of developing RLS symptoms. Pregnancy is also a factor that can lead to having temporary RLS, specifically after 20 weeks of gestation. In most cases RLS is a temporary sleeping disorder that can be resolved through diverse treatments.

Treatments

One of the best ways to reduce symptoms of RLS is to have a regular exercise routine. Walking, riding a bike, massaging the legs, light stretching and taking hot baths are just a few of the ways RLS symptoms can be reduced. Lowering caffeine and alcohol intake has also shown to be effective at reducing RLS. RLS is certainly a disorder that should be discussed with a health care provider. Although some medications have been known to cause RLS, many medications can treat RLS, and sometimes an iron supplement to counteract anemia is all that is needed to reverse the symptoms of RLS.

Obstructive Sleep Apnea (OSA)

Symptoms

Obstructive Sleep Apnea (OSA) is a type of sleep-disordered breathing characterized by consistent episodes of not breathing throughout the night, or apneas. Apneic episodes, meaning "without wind," occur when the throat muscles relax, narrowing and eventually blocking the airway.[52] When the brain realizes that the person has not breathed in oxygen for a period of time, it triggers a loud snore, gasp, or choking sound to stimulate the airway to open. The problem is that every time a person experiences an apneic episode the sleep cycle resets, causing a very **unrestful** night of sleep.

OSA symptoms affect 25 million people, approximately 4% of adult men and 2% of adult women in the United States.[53] While it seems men suffer from OSA more than women, this gender gap closes in old age when women become more susceptible. More adults tend to have OSA than children, although it is possible for children to have this sleeping disorder especially if they are overweight. Symptoms of OSA include LOUD snoring (like a freight train passing by your window loud), waking up throughout the night, gasping, choking, excessive movements and sweating during the night, sore throat, dry mouth, and headaches in the morning. Most people with OSA also experience daytime sleepiness despite spending a significant time in bed sleeping. Although OSA is related to heart disease, people do not die from the apneic episodes.

Risk Factors

A number of factors put a person at risk for developing OSA. Having a large neck circumference, a history of snoring, being overweight, drinking alcohol, hypertension, smoking, and having issues with one's airway passage can predispose someone to OSA. Retrognathia, which is a small recessed jaw, can also push the tongue back into the airway, resulting in OSA.

Treatments

There are many treatment options for OSA patients. In order to treat OSA, the severity of the condition must first be taken into account. Treatment can include two types: behavioral treatments and/or medical treatments. Behavioral treatments consist of weight loss to help re-open the airway passages in the neck, avoiding depressant drugs and alcohol that can relax the muscles, using nasal strips to prevent congestion and snoring, and adjusting one's sleeping position so

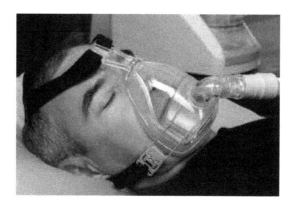

FIGURE 8.6 **A CPAP machine that cover both the nose and mouth**

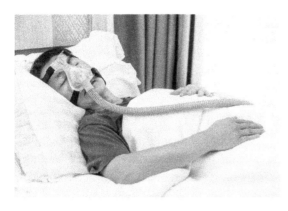

FIGURE 8.7 **Man wearing CPAP machine that** covers the nose only

that a person is sleeping on his or her side, rather than on the back which allows fat tissue to put pressure on the throat. Medical treatments include having surgery to remove tonsils and adenoids which block the airway, using oral devices that stop the tongue from falling to the back of the throat, and Continuous Positive Airway Resistance (CPAP). CPAP is a mask that is worn over the mouth and/or nose and delivers a constant stream of air through the airway, forcing it to remain open throughout the night. Although this is considered the gold standard treatment for OSA and when used correctly is very effective (and many times life-changing), CPAP can be hard to tolerate and bulky, making it hard to find a comfortable position for sleep.[54]

Parasomnias: Night Terrors, Sleepwalking, and Sleeptalking
Symptoms
Parasomnias are a group of sleep disorders that occur when a person is falling asleep or in between sleep stages, and involves abnormal movements, behaviors, emotions, perceptions, and dreams. If you have ever experienced the feeling that you were awake but could not move, otherwise known as sleep paralysis, you have had a parasomniac event. Seeing or hearing something that is not actually there is also an example of a parasomnia.

One specific type of parasomnia, called a Night or Sleep Terror is relatively common in children, affecting up to 6% of children between the ages of one to eight years old.[55] Unlike nightmares, which occur during REM sleep when a person is dreaming, night terrors occur in NREM sleep during the transition from Stage 3 to Stage 4 sleep. A night terror can be characterized by frequent and recurring episodes of intense fear and crying during sleep, with NO recollection of the event. Night terrors vary greatly in their duration, ranging anywhere from a few minutes to up to 30 minutes. Night terrors can also include other behaviors, such as sleepwalking and sleep talking. Children tend to be difficult to comfort or even inconsolable when experiencing a night terror because they are still asleep. In some extreme cases, children may walk out of the house or become clumsy in their movements, putting themselves in harm's way. The good news is that night terrors are usually harmless to the child, especially since they have no recollection of it happening. The bad news is that the rest of the family will likely be woken up from the crying and thrashing that happens during the night terror and will likely be very alarmed by what is happening one door over.

Risk Factors
Although night terrors affect both boys and girls, boys are more likely to experience them on a regular basis.[56] Genetics also plays a role in parasomnias, so if a parent has a history

of night terrors, the children may also have night terrors. While there is no known cause for night terrors and sleepwalking, they may result from stressful life events, illness, sleep deprivation, and certain medications. This sleeping problem tends to be outgrown once children reach adolescence.

Treatments

When children are having a night terror or sleepwalking, it is best to lead them back to their room and not wake them. Parents should reassure their child with words, although the child likely will not hear them because he or she is still technically asleep. Parents should also calmly bring the child back to his bed. Waking up a child can lead to confusion and disorientation—just imagine if you last remembered falling asleep in your bed, and someone woke you up in the basement. Creepy, right? Because parasomnias are often triggered by sleep deprivation, parents should ensure that children are getting enough sleep every night. Also, because night terrors occur at approximately the same time each night (approximately two to three hours after sleep onset), parents can do a "scheduled awakening." Scheduled awakenings involve gently waking the child up 15–30 minutes before the night terror will likely occur, which resets the sleep cycle and prevents the night terror from happening.[57] Lastly, some tips to keep children safe during sleepwalking events are locking all windows and doors at night, installing a security system in the house or a small alarm on the child's bedroom door, locking up potentially dangerous objects such as knives, etc., not allowing the child to sleep in a bunk bed, and installing safety gates in front of all stairs and doorways.

Conclusion

Sleep is a vital process for humans to achieve their best performance throughout the day. Without adequate sleep, our bodies are very quickly affected, and we experience a number of negative effects including decreased immune system protection, impaired mood, and cognitive issues. As people's lives become more complicated, children, adolescents, and adults are experiencing dramatic increases in sleep disorders. The encouraging news is that sleep health is a national priority, and a number of promising behavioral and medical interventions can help improve sleep.

Case Study

The following is an example of a clinical case report of a pediatric patient in a sleep clinic. As you read the case study, identify the risk factors and symptoms of the sleep disorders that you read about in the chapter. Also identify strategies that might be effective for treating the sleep disorder.

History of Presenting Illness

Nathaniel is a seven-year-old white boy whose parents sought consultation with the sleep clinic after an episode of sleepwalking. The information reported below was obtained from direct interviews with Nathaniel and his parents and from a review of the following records: sleep clinic intake forms, child behavior checklist, restless sleep questionnaire, and children's sleep habits questionnaire. Nathaniel's parents are seeking additional recommendations to ensure Nathaniel's safety during any future sleepwalking episodes, as well as recommendations on preventing future episodes.

Developmental/Medical History

Nathaniel lives at home with his father, mother, and older sister. Nathaniel's father completed high school and is employed as an alarm technician. His mother also completed college and is employed as a project manager. Nathaniel met all developmental milestones as expected. He reportedly does well in school, has many friends, exercises regularly and does not consume caffeine. He has never been hospitalized and does not have a history of medical or emotional problems. Nathaniel has an allergy to mold. Nathaniel's family history is positive for mental health problems. His father and paternal grandfather have been reportedly diagnosed with Depression and his maternal grandfather has been diagnosed with Substance Abuse Disorder (Alcohol), with a Rule Out of Obstructive Sleep Apnea.

Clinical Intake

Nathaniel's parents reported that Nathaniel's only episode of sleepwalking occurred on March 4. He was found by a neighbor, who is a police officer, at 11:30 p.m. approximately one half mile away from their home. According to Nathaniel's parents, their neighbor described his behavior as "out of it" and "in a fog." His eyes were open, and he was talking, but his speech was not sensible. As he began to regain awareness, he became very frightened, but he was able to tell the police officer where he lived, at which time the officer brought him home.

His parents reported that in the nights prior to the episode Nathaniel had minor changes in his sleep routine. For two nights prior, he had been sleeping without his nightlight. Nathaniel expressed some fears about sleeping in the dark, but his parents were not overly concerned. Nathaniel's parents also reported that he has been snoring more loudly at night. Nathaniel has a good bedtime routine, consisting of taking a shower, reading, and playing with Legos. On an average night, he falls asleep on his own, in his own bed, within 15 minutes.

Approximately once every two months, Nathaniel awakens in the middle of the night from nightmares. The content of the nightmares often includes black furry monsters or animals, such as ostriches and coyotes, chasing him. Nathaniel is able to recall these dreams the next morning. His parents reported that they live in the woods, and during the night they can hear coyotes from the house, which may be contributing to Nathaniel's nightmares. In order to fall back asleep Nathaniel will play some music or seek out his parents for comfort. No sleep terrors were reported.

Nathaniel's family history is positive for parasomnias. His father had a history of sleep-walking and sleeptalking dating back to his own childhood. His paternal aunt also experienced one known episode of sleepwalking. His father and grandfather are also loud snorers and experience daytime fatigue but have never been assessed for the presence of a sleep disorder. Nathaniel also presents with risk factors and symptoms for obstructive sleep apnea, including family history of OSA, retrognathia, and snoring.

Nathaniel's current sleep patterns are as follows:
Bed time: 9:00 p.m.
Sleep onset latency: 15 minutes
Wake after sleep onset: awakens for five minutes before midnight to use the bathroom
Early morning awakenings: n/a
Waking time: 6:45 a.m. (weekdays); 7:15 a.m. (weekends)
Napping: n/a
Total sleep time: 10½ hours

Notes

1 Colton, H. R., & Altevogt, B. M., eds. (2006). Sleep disorders and sleep deprivation: An unmet public health problem. Washington, DC: National Academies Press.

2 Hossain, J. L. & Shapiro, C. M. (2002). The prevalence, cost implications, and management of sleep disorders: An overview. *Sleep and Breathing, 6*(2), 85–102.

3 Drowsy driving: facts and stats. (2016). National Sleep Foundation, Washington, DC. Retrieved from http://drowsydriving.org/about/facts-and-stats/

4 Stedman, T. L. (2005). *Stedman's medical dictionary for the health professions and nursing.* Philadelphia, PA: Lippincott Williams & Wilkins.

5 Sleep drive and your body clock. (2016). National Sleep Foundation. Retrieved from https://sleepfoundation.org/sleep-topics/sleep-drive-and-your-body-clock

6 Stages of sleep. (2018, January 22). Tuck. Retrieved from http://www.sleepdex.org/stages.htm

7 What happens when you sleep? (2016). National Sleep Foundation. Retrieved from https://sleepfoundation.org/how-sleep-works/what-happens-when-you-sleep

8 Spilsbury, J. C., Storfer-Isser, A., Kirchner, H. L., et al. (2006). Neighborhood disadvantage as a risk factor for pediatric obstructive sleep apnea. *Journal of Pediatrics.149*(3): 342–7.

9 Redline, S., Yenokyan, G., Gottlieb, D. J., et al. (2010). Obstructive sleep apnea hypopnea and incident stroke: The sleep heart health study. *American Journal of Respiratory and Critical Care Medicine, 182*(2), 269–77.

10 Sleep health. (n.d.). Healthy People 2020. Retrieved January 30, 2017, from https://www.healthypeople.gov/2020/topics-objectives/topic/sleep-health

11 Drowsy driving and automobile crashes. (1998). National Heart, Lung, and Blood Institute; National Center on Sleep Disorders Research. Retrieved from https://www.nhlbi.nih.gov/files/docs/resources/sleep/drsy_drv.pdf

12 Sudden infant death syndrome and sleep. (2016). National Sleep Foundation. Retrieved from https://sleepfoundation.org/sleep-disorders-problems/sudden-infant-death-syndrome-and-sleep

13 Sudden infant death syndrome and sleep. (2016). National Sleep Foundation. Retrieved from https://sleepfoundation.org/sleep-disorders-problems/sudden-infant-death-syndrome-and-sleep

14 Sudden infant death syndrome (SIDS) risk factors. (2016, October 28). Mayo Clinic. Retrieved January 16, 2017, from http://www.mayoclinic.org/diseases-conditions/sudden-infant-death-syndrome/basics/risk-factors/con-20020269

15 Research on back sleeping and SIDS. (n.d.). Eunice Kennedy Shriver National Institute of Child Health and Human Development. Retrieved January 16, 2017, from https://www.nichd.nih.gov/sts/campaign/science/Pages/backsleeping.aspx

16 SIDS and other sleep-related infant deaths: Expansion of recommendations for a safe infant sleeping environment. (2011, November). *Pediatrics*. http://pediatrics.aappublications.org/content/pediatrics/early/2011/10/12/peds.2011-2284.full.pdf

17 Co-sleeping pros and cons. (2015). Health Research Funding. Retrieved from http://healthresearchfunding.org/co-sleeping-pros-cons/

18 Safe cosleeping guidelines. (2016). University of Notre Dame, Mother-Baby Behavioral Sleep Laboratory. Retrieved from http://cosleeping.nd.edu/safe-co-sleeping-guidelines/

19 Co-sleeping pros and cons. (2015). Health Research Funding. Retrieved from http://healthresearchfunding.org/co-sleeping-pros-cons/

20 Stress, cortisol, and getting your baby to sleep. (2013). ChildrensMD. Retrieved from http://childrensmd.org/browse-by-age-group/newborn-infants/stress-cortisol-and-getting-your-baby-to-sleep/

21 Stress, cortisol, and getting your baby to sleep. (2013). ChildrensMD. Retrieved from http://childrensmd.org/browse-by-age-group/newborn-infants/stress-cortisol-and-getting-your-baby-to-sleep/

22 Children and sleep. (2016). National Sleep Foundation. Retrieved from https://sleepfoundation.org/sleep-topics/children-and-sleep

23 Children and sleep. (2016). National Sleep Foundation. Retrieved from https://sleepfoundation.org/sleep-topics/children-and-sleep

24 Children and sleep. (2016). National Sleep Foundation. Retrieved from https://sleepfoundation.org/sleep-topics/children-and-sleep

25 CHADD: The national resource on ADHD. (2015). CHADD: The National Resource on ADHD. Retrieved January 16, 2017, from http://www.help4adhd.org/

26 Owens, J. A. (2009). A clinical overview of sleep and Attention Deficit Hyperactivity Disorder in children and adolescents. *Journal of the Canadian Academy of Child and Adolescent Psychiatry*, *18*(2), 92–102.

27 Bedwetting. (2016). National Sleep Foundation. Retrieved from https://sleepfoundation.org/sleep-disorders-problems/bedwetting-and-sleep

28 Wolfson, A. R., & Carskadon, M. A. (1998). Sleep schedules and daytime functioning in adolescents. *Child Development*, *69*(4), 875–887.

29 Sleep and teens. (n.d.). UCLA Health. Retrieved from http://sleepcenter.ucla.edu/sleep-and-teens

30 Start time recommendations, etc. (2016, December 11). Schoolstarttime.org. Retrieved January 16, 2017, from https://schoolstarttime.org/2011/08/28/time-specific-start-time-recommendations/

31 How much sleep do we really need? (2016). National Sleep Foundation. Retrieved from https://sleepfoundation.org/how-sleep-works/how-much-sleep-do-we-really-need

32 Buboltz, Jr., W. C., Brown, F., & Soper, B. (2001). Sleep habits and patterns of college students: a preliminary study. *Journal of American College Health*, *50*(3), 131–135.

33 Adams, S. K., & Kisler, T. S. (2013). Sleep quality as a mediator between technology-related sleep quality, depression, and anxiety. *Cyberpsychology, Behavior & Social Networking*, *16*(1), 25–30. doi:10.1089/cyber.2012.0157

34 Buboltz, Jr., W. C., Brown, F., & Soper, B. (2001). Sleep habits and patterns of college students: a preliminary study. *Journal of American College Health*, *50*(3), 131–135.

35 Grandner, M. A., Gallagher, R. A. L., & Gooneratne, N. S. (2013). The use of technology at night: Impact on sleep and health. *Journal of Clinical Sleep Medicine*, *9*(12),1301–1302.

36 Perceived insufficient rest or sleep among adults: United States, 2008. (2009, October 30). *MMWR*. *58*(42), 1175–9.

37 CDC declares sleep disorders a public health epidemic. (2014, December 13). Advanced Sleep Medicine Services, Inc. Retrieved January 30, 2017, from http://www.sleepdr.com/blog/cdc-declares-sleep-disorders-a-public-epidemic

38 CDC declares sleep disorders a public health epidemic. (2014, December 13). Advanced Sleep Medicine Services, Inc. Retrieved January 30, 2017, from http://www.sleepdr.com/blog/cdc-declares-sleep-disorders-a-public-epidemic

39 Colton, H. R., & Altevogt, B. M., eds. (2006). Sleep disorders and sleep deprivation: An unmet public health problem. Washington, DC: National Academies Press.

40 Redline, S., Yenokyan, G., Gottlieb, D. J., et al. (2010). Obstructive sleep apnea hypopnea and incident stroke: The sleep heart health study. *American Journal of Respiratory and Critical Care Medicine.182*(2), 269–77.

41 Punjabi, N. M., Caffo, B. S., Goodwin, J. L., et al. (2009, August 6) Sleep-disordered breathing and mortality: A prospective cohort study. *PLOS Medicine*. (8), e1000132.

42 Knutson, K. L., Spiegel, K., Penev, P., & Van Cauter, E. (2007). The metabolic consequences of sleep deprivation. *Sleep Medicine Reviews*, *11*(3), 163–178.

43 Overweight and obesity. (2012, July 13). National Heart, Lung, and Blood Institute, NIH. Retrieved January 30, 2017, from http://www.nhlbi.nih.gov/health/health-topics/topics/obe/causes

44 Harrison, Y., & Horne, J. A. (2000). The impact of sleep deprivation on decision making: A review. *Journal of Experimental Psychology: Applied*, *6*(3), 236.

45 Drowsy driving: Facts and stats. (2016). National Sleep Foundation. Retrieved from http://drowsydriving.org/about/facts-and-stats/

46 Alhola, P., & Polo-Kantola, P. (2007). Sleep deprivation: Impact on cognitive performance. *Neuropsychiatric Disease and Treatment*, *3*(5), 553–567.

47 Jung, C. G., Adler, G., Fordham, M., & Read, H. (2014). *Symbols of transformation* (Vol. 5). London: Routledge.

48 Sleep disorders. (2016). Anxiety and Depression Association of America (ADAA). Retrieved from https://www.adaa.org/understanding-anxiety/related-illnesses/sleep-disorders

49 What is insomnia? (2016). National Sleep Foundation. Retrieved from https://sleepfoundation.org/insomnia/content/what-is-insomnia

50 Insomnia. (2015). CRC Health. Retrieved from http://www.crchealth.com/treatment/ pain-relief-sleep-disorder-treatment/sleep-disorders/

51 Restless legs syndrome (RLS). (2012). Tuck. Retrieved January 16, 2017, from http://www .sleepdex.org/rls.htm

52 Reversible airflow obstruction: Topics by Science.gov. (n.d.). Science.gov. Retrieved January 16, 2017, from https://www.science.gov/topicpages/r/reversible airflow obstruction.html

53 Obstructive sleep apnea: Overview. (2015, July 30). PubMed Health, U.S. National Library of Medicine. Retrieved January 30, 2017, from https://www.ncbi.nlm.nih.gov/pubmedhealth/ PMH0072458/

54 CPAP: treating sleep apnea. (2016). National Sleep Foundation. Retrieved from https:// sleepfoundation.org/sleep-disorders-problems/continuous-positive-airway

55 Night terrors. (2017). KidsHealth from Nemours. Retrieved from http://kidshealth.org/en/ parents/terrors.html

56 Sleep terror disorder. (n.d.). Encyclopedia of Mental Disorders. Retrieved January 16, 2017, from http://www.minddisorders.com/Py-Z/Sleep-terror-disorder.html

57 Richards, D. W., (1996–2006). Night terrors resource center. Retrieved from http://www .nightterrors.org/

Figure Sources

1 Figure 8.2: National Sleep Foundation, https://sleepfoundation.org/sites/default/files/STREP-changes_1.png. Copyright © 2015 by National Sleep Foundation. Reprinted with permission.

2 Figure 8.3: Source: https://www.flickr.com/photos/nichd/18311550489.

3 Figure 8.4: Copyright © sima dimitric (CC BY-SA 2.0) at https://www.flickr.com/photos/ simajr/5462142145.

4 Figure 8.5: Copyright © 2017 Depositphotos/MSSA.

5 Figure 8.6: Copyright © PruebasBMA (CC BY-SA 3.0) at https://commons.wikimedia.org/wiki/ File:CPAP.png.

6 Figure 8.7: Copyright © 2017 Depositphotos/cpoungpeth.

CHAPTER NINE

Mental Health

Coauthors:
Caroline Segal, M.A., Sue K. Adams, Ph.D.

@NAMICommunicate

Mental Health Disorders: An Overview

Everybody goes through stress and hardship in life. Sometimes these experiences can motivate people to reflect, adapt, persevere, and grow, and sometimes they can knock them to the ground. Mental health has to do with how we respond to life events, how we interact with others, and how we function in our everyday lives. Our mental state influences how we think, feel, and behave. When mental health is poor, accomplishing a simple task can feel like an insurmountable challenge—like trying to walk a mile with heavy chains around our ankles. Poor mental health can slow us down physically and psychologically, making it difficult to focus on daily tasks, to make decisions, to have a conversation, sometimes even just to get out of bed.

It can be difficult to draw the line between struggling and suffering. At what point does poor mental health become a diagnosable mental illness? How do you tell the difference between sadness and depression? Nervousness and anxiety? Restlessness and ADHD? Every mental health disorder has its own list of symptoms to help identify that line. The entire list of all mental illnesses currently recognized by the American Psychiatric Association is published in a manual entitled the *Diagnostic and Statistical Manual of Mental Disorders - 5* (or the DSM-5), which is currently in its fifth edition.

A general rule of thumb, however, is that mental health becomes a concern when the symptoms start to get in the way of a person's ability to function normally. For example, sadness can be adaptive; it can help a person slow down, reflect, and make sense of things. Sadness can even bring people together, like when a group of people comes together to grieve the loss of a shared loved one. That kind of sadness is normal, even helpful, and not necessarily grounds for concern. However, if sadness becomes impairing—if someone stops going to class and his or her grades drop, or someone develops poor diet and exercise habits and increases the risk of diabetes or heart problems—those are important signals of something serious.

In a lot of ways, mental health is similar to physical health, and, in fact, they influence each other quite a bit. Just like physical health, maintaining mental health takes work. In the same way one might try to eat healthy, exercise, and wash his or her hands to preserve physical health, one can take actions to improve mental health as well (actually, a lot of the same ones). In addition to good nutrition, regular physical activity, and hygiene habits, one can improve mental health by setting realistic goals, taking breaks from stressful activities, and surrounding oneself with people who are positive and encouraging. A person can pay attention to any negative self-talk he or she might engage in and try talking to himself or herself the way he or she would talk to a friend. Getting enough sleep plays a huge role in mental health, and even drinking a lot of water can do wonders to help a person feel good.

This chapter will provide an overview of mental health issues, population trends, and intervention efforts in America. In the following chapter, you will learn about the symptoms, causes, and treatment of the two most common mental health disorders: anxiety and depression.

Mental Health Statistics

In a given year, nearly one in every five adults living in the United States experiences mental illness, and one half of chronic mental illness begins by the age of 14.[1] That equates to an estimated 18.1% (43.6 million) of U.S. adults suffering from any mental illness and 4.2% (9.8 million) suffering from a seriously debilitating mental illness.[2] Mental health issues are the world's leading cause of disability.[3] In the United States, major depressive disorder ranks fifth in terms of disability-adjusted life years (DALYs), which is the sum of years lost to both disability and premature death. Anxiety comes in at 13th, and schizophrenia, a rare but extremely debilitating condition, takes its spot at #27.[4] The cost to society of mental health disorders is colossal. Severe mental illness alone costs the United States nearly $200 billion in lost earnings every year.[5] Throw in the cost of disability payments and health care, and we have clearly got ourselves a serious public health issue.

Health Disparities

Similar to physical health disorders that you have already learned about, mental health disorders disproportionately affect people from low-income, minority backgrounds. Unlike physical health disorders, however, significant stigma still exists in mental health. Unfortunately, a lot remains unknown about mental health disparities. As you read the following sections, challenge yourself to think about why those health disparities might exist, as well as what missing information would help us understand those disparities better. Think about cultural differences between groups and how that might impact somebody's expression

TABLE 9.1   Mental Health Facts in America

FACT: 43.8 million adults experience mental illnes in a given year

1 in 5 adults in America experience a mental illness.

Nearly 1 in 25 (10 million) adults in America live with a serious mental illness.

One-half of all chronic mental illness begins by the age of 14; three-quarters by the age of 24.

Prevalence of Mental Illness by Diagnosis

1.1% 1 in 100 (2.4 million) American adults live with schizophrenia.

2.6% (6.1 million) of American adults live with bipolar disorder.

6.9% (16 million) of American adults live with major depression.

18.1% (42 million) of American adults live with anxiety disorders.

Consequences

10.2m Approximately 10.2 million adults have co-occurring mental health and addiction disorders.

26% Approximately 26% of homeless adults staying in shelters live with serious mental illness.

24% Approximately 24% of state prisoners have "a recent history of a mental health condition".

Impact

1st Depression is the leading cause of disability worldwide, and is a major contributor to the global burden of disease.

-$193b Serious mental illness costs America $193.2 billion in lost earning every year.

90% of those who die by suicide have an underlying mental illness. Suicide is the 10th leading cause of death in the U.S.

Treatment in America

60% Nearly 60% of adults with a mental illness didn't receive mental health services in the previous year.

50% Nearly 50% of youth aged 8-15didn't receive mental health services in the previous year.

African American & Hispanic Americans used mental health services at about 1/2 the rate of whites in the past year and Asian Americans at about 1/3 the rate.

Ways to Get Help

Talk with your doctor

Connect with other individuals and families

Learn more about mental illness

Visit NAMI.org

TABLE 9.1   Mental Health Fact Sheet In America (NAMI)

of distress, views of mental health professionals, barriers to accessing services, and the utilization of services that do exist.

Race and Ethnicity

Recent data show that adults in the United States who identify as multiracial are at the highest risk for mental health issues (24.9% report experience with mental illness). This group is followed closely by American Indians and Alaska Natives (22.7%) and then white adults (19%). At the low end of the spectrum, Asian Americans report the lowest rates of mental illness (13.4%), followed by Hispanic populations (15.3%) and black adults (16.8%).[6]

It is important, however, to interpret these statistics with caution. Even with numbers this specific, it is unknown how many people from each group have an unidentified mental illness. We also have to consider how each of these groups defines mental illness. Many Asian American cultures, for example, view mental illness as a source of shame and a poor reflection of the community.[7] Therefore, it is hard to say whether Asian Americans truly experience lower rates of mental illness than other racial and ethnic groups or whether those in distress are less likely to identify themselves.

Certain ethnic minority groups also experience what we call "culture-bound syndromes," which are expressions of mental illness specific to a cultural group. For example, *ataque de nervios* is a condition commonly seen in Hispanic populations, with symptoms including screaming, crying, trembling, and aggression, usually in response to stress. Culture-bound syndromes are not currently recognized by U.S. mental health care; we do not assess for them, and insurance does not cover treatment for them. Therefore, we cannot possibly identify the true scope of mental illness in minority populations, but just because our health care system does not see it does not mean it is not there.

To better understand racial and ethnic disparities, we can also look at data on service use. The groups that most commonly seek treatment for mental health issues are multiracial populations, white adults, and American Indian and Alaska natives. In fact, these groups utilize services about twice as often as black and Hispanic adults, and three to four times more often than Asian adults.[8] There are many reasons for why these trends exist. For example, studies show that racial minorities have more barriers to care. They are more likely to be low income and thus less likely to have health insurance coverage.[9] For immigrant groups, language may be a barrier, as most providers in the U.S. are English-speaking. Some groups, such as Native Americans, are more likely to live in rural or isolated areas where care may not be available.[10]

It also important to consider what services look like. Many people from cultural minority groups drop out of treatment early. This is in part due to stigma, as well as the unfortunate reality that many therapists from majority backgrounds have a poor understanding of the issues pertaining to racial and ethnic minorities. Another common barrier to continuing services is mistrust of health care providers. This sentiment is particularly strong among African-American populations, who have historically been mistreated by health care providers.[11]

Lastly, it is important to consider alternative ways people deal with distress. Ethnic and racial minorities are more likely to seek help from friends and family than from formal service providers. Among cultures where religion is strongly interwoven into the community fabric, people also turn to spiritual leaders for guidance. Additionally, many cultural groups turn to traditional medicine practices. For example, acupuncture and massage are common practices in Chinese traditional medicine, and teas, oils, and spiritual rituals are often used in Latin American folk healing. Therefore, the numbers we have on rates of mental illness and service use paint part of a picture of what is happening across racial and ethnic groups, but the unseen details make the picture complete.

Gender

Men and women generally experience mental illness at equal rates, but gender prevalence differs between specific disorders. For example, women are significantly more likely than men to have depression and anxiety. Women are also more likely to experience posttraumatic stress disorder (PTSD), which is a condition marked by significant mental, emotional, and physiological distress in response to a trauma. Men, on the other hand, are more likely than women to have substance use disorders or impulse-control disorders (like ADHD or disorders having to do with aggression and rebelliousness).[12] With regard to suicide, an interesting pattern emerges: women are three times more likely to *attempt* suicide than men, but men are four times more likely to *complete* suicide than women.[13]

Men and women also appear to deal with mental health issues in different ways. Women tend to seek treatment for mental health issues more often than men. In particular, women are more likely to work with therapists, social workers, and medical professionals to treat mental illness; men are slightly more likely than women to try self-help groups (for example, Alcoholics Anonymous).[14]

Transgender and Gender Nonconforming

There has been increasing attention in recent years to the mental health experiences of transgender and gender-nonconforming individuals, who are people whose gender identity does not completely match their sex assigned at birth. Until very recently, identifying as transgender or gender nonconforming (or TGNC) was considered a mental illness in and of itself. This label was stigmatizing and invalidating, and it only served to increase prejudice and discrimination against TGNC people. Although the American Psychiatric Association has changed its stance on gender nonconformity, the mental health field has a long way to go toward better understanding and serving the TGNC community.

As of now, what we know is this: transgender and gender-nonconforming people face substantial discrimination in schools, in the workplace, in health care, in the legal system, and even in their own neighborhoods. They are at higher risk for violence, poverty, and homelessness. The stigma associated with a TGNC identity, rather than the identity itself, leads to increased risk of mental illness. Two out of five transgender and gender-nonconforming people attempt suicide, which is *25 times as many* as the general population. The

TABLE 9.2   Mental Health Facts — Multicultural

FACT: Mental health affects everyone regardless of culture, race, ethnicity, gender or sexual orientation.

1 in every 5 adults in America experience a mental illness.

Nearly 1 in 25 (10 million) adults in America live with a serious mental illness.

One-half of all chronic mental illness begins by the age of 14; three-quarters by the age of 24.

Prevalence of Mental Illness by Diagnosis

16.3% Hispanic adults living with a mental health condition.

19.3% White adults living with a mental health condition.

18.6% Black adults living with a mental health condition.

13.9% Asian adults living with a mental health condition.

28.3% American Indian/Alaska Native (AI/AN) adults living with a mental health condition.

LGBTQ Community

2x LGBTQ individuals are 2 or more times more likely as straight individuals to have a mental health condition.

11% of transgender individuals reported being denied care by mental health clinics due to bias or discrimination.

2-3X Lesbian, gay, bisexual, transgender and questioning (LGBTQ) youth are 2 to 3 times more likely to attempt suicide than straight youth.

Use of Mental Health Services among Adults (2008-2012)

	Male	Female
White	11.3%	21.5%
Black	6.6%	10.3%
AI/AN	16.3%	15.5%
Asian	4.4%	5.3%
Hispanic	5.5%	9.2%

Critical Issues Faced by Multicultural Communities

Less access to treatment · Culturally insensitive health care system · Less likely to receive treatment

Racism, bias, homophobia · Poorer quality of care · Language barriers · Lower rates of health insurance

TABLE 9.2   Mental Health Multicultural Fact Sheet (NAMI)

vast majority of TGNC people seek therapy at some point in their lives, but as it stands, too few therapists understand the issues and dangers many TGNC people face.[15]

Socioeconomic Status

A consistent and strong relationship has been shown between socioeconomic status and rates of mental illness: the lower one's socioeconomic status, as determined by income, education, and occupation, the higher the risk of mental illness. An important question to ask is: *Why?* Does mental illness change socioeconomic status (SES), or does socioeconomic status impact mental health?

The answer is most likely a little bit of both. In terms of mental illness' impact on SES, remember that mental illness is a leading cause of disability, meaning it impacts income and work status. Mental illness also leads to school dropout, meaning it impacts education level. However, more research has looked at the effect of SES on mental health. Economic stress, specifically, seems to play a large role in this relationship. Consider people who are unemployed, who live in poverty, who reside in shelters or have to sleep on the street. Consider the risk of violence and other potentially traumatic experiences in low-income neighborhoods. The population on the whole faces a significant amount of stress and relatively few resources to manage that stress, especially since many people in low-SES neighborhoods are uninsured.

Consider one last contributing factor to the relationship between mental illness and SES. Mental hospitals were established as long-term care facilities for people with severe mental illness who could not otherwise function in society. For centuries, treatment of patients in those hospitals was anything but humane; patients were chained, beaten, or altogether ignored—hard to even call it "treatment." Things came to a head toward the end of the 20th century, which marked the "deinstitutionalization" movement. The idea behind deinstitutionalization was to close down mental institutions that were maltreating patients and to reintegrate those patients into society. Unfortunately, the transition plan was not executed particularly successfully. Most of those patients had nowhere to go—no families, friends, or communities to receive them. As a result, many patients went to the streets (one third of the homeless population is comprised of people with severe mental illness) or ended up in jails and prisons (constituting one in six inmates). In fact, seven times as many severely mentally ill individuals are homeless or in prison than are currently receiving treatment in psychiatric hospitals.[16]

Geography

Lastly, rates of mental illness vary across each state, but the reasons why are poorly understood. Prevalence of mental illness is highest in Oregon, Utah, and West Virginia (about 21–22%) and lowest in New Jersey, North Dakota, and Maryland (about 16–17%).[17] We have a lot more to learn about what connects these sets of states in order to understand why residents of some states fare better than residents of others. What is a little clearer is how geography influences availability of mental *health care.* States in the northeast have substantially greater treatment opportunities than states in the south. In fact, there are four times as many providers per person in Massachusetts, Maine, and Vermont, compared to West Virginia, Texas, and Alabama.[18] In general, people in rural areas have the most difficulty accessing mental health care. Some have to drive up to two hours one way just to get to a therapist's office, and most people cannot manage to do that on a regular basis.

A possible solution to this problem is the advent of a practice called *teletherapy*. Teletherapy is the idea of providing mental health care over the phone or through video chats. It is gaining popularity as an alternative to traditional therapy because it reduces transportation time and cost, but a number of ethical questions remain. What happens if somebody has a mental health emergency, and the therapist cannot physically ensure that he or she gets to a hospital or other safe space? Does receiving therapy through a screen, with potential connectivity issues, detract from the therapeutic relationship? Also, licensure is granted state by state—can a therapist treat someone who lives in Minnesota if he or she is licensed in California? Teletherapy is a promising direction for the field, but the debate over these ethical issues is unlikely to end soon.

Healthy People 2020

Healthy People 2020 has identified mental health objectives that fall into two general categories: mental health status improvement and treatment expansion. Mental health status improvement focuses on reducing suicide rates in adults and adolescents, reducing eating disorders in adolescents, and reducing major depression episodes in adolescents and adults. Treatment expansion focuses on eight areas to help promote access to treatment; increase referrals for mental health services for children, adolescents, adults and the homeless; increase screenings for depression by health care providers; and increase the number of people with mental health disorders who are employed. The goal is to improve these targets by 10% by the year 2020.

Mental Health Across Development

Life stage plays an important role in the expression of mental illness. As a person makes his or her way through the life cycle, he or she is faced with different developmental challenges, life circumstances, and capacity for coping skills. Many disorders are chronic, meaning people struggle with them their whole lives, but notable patterns appear across age ranges.

Childhood

Starting with childhood, the more common disorders tend to stem from difficulties with regulating behavior and developing autonomy. We see these difficulties more often in childhood than in other life stages because they represent the major developmental tasks for this life stage. For example, attention deficit hyperactivity disorder (ADHD) has to do with difficulties sustaining attention, managing impulses, and controlling energy levels, tasks that are difficult for most children but exceedingly more so in children with ADHD. Similarly, certain forms of anxiety are more common in childhood, such as separation

TABLE 9.3   Mental Health Facts — Children & Teens

FACT: 1 in 5 children ages 13-18 have, or will have a serious mental illness.

20% of youth ages 13-18 live with a mental health condition.

11% of youth have a mood disorder.

10% of youth have a behavior or conduct disorder.

8% of youth have an anxiety disorder.

Impact

50% of all lifetime cases of mental illness begin by age 14 and 75% by age 24.

10 yrs The average delay between onset of symptoms and intervention is 8-10 years.

50% Approximately 50% of students age 14 and older with a mental illness drop out of high school

70% of youth in state and local juvenile justice systems have a mental illness.

Suicide

3rd Suicide is the 3rd leading cause of death in youth ages 10 - 24.

90% of those who died by suicide had an underlying mental illness

Warning Signs

Feeling very sad or withdrawn for more than 2 weeks • Trying to harm or kill oneself • Repeated use of drugs or alcohol

Out-of-control, risk-taking behaviors • Extreme difficulty in concentrating or staying still • Intense worries or fear

4 Things Parents Can Do

1. Talk with your pediatrician	2. Get a referral to a mental health specialist
3. Work with the school	4. Connect with other families

TABLE 9.3   Mental Health Fact Sheet in Children and Teens (NAMI)

anxiety disorder, because children are faced with the nerve-wracking task of learning to separate from their parents (e.g. when they go to school for the first time), speak for themselves, and make their own decisions. These disorders occur throughout the lifespan, but they are most likely to start in childhood.[19]

Adolescence

When people reach the teenage years and early adulthood, their main developmental task is to search for meaning and identity—what really matters? What do they stand for? What should they do with their lives? Who should they end up with? These existential questions rarely have easy answers, and many identify feeling helpless and lost at this stage of the game. Consequently, anxiety remains a common struggle, and rates of depression increase. Suicidal thoughts, in particular, are highest in this life stage (7.4% of adults ages 18–25).[20] Social belonging also takes on new meaning starting in adolescence. Body image becomes a more prominent concern after the onset of puberty, with a corresponding rise in eating disorders between childhood and adolescence, and substance use rises significantly, with substance use disorders most often developing during adolescence and early adulthood.[21] Schizophrenia, a rare disorder characterized by hallucinations, delusions, and/or loss of touch with reality, also spikes in onset between adolescence and early adulthood. The reason why is not well understood, but it is thought that important changes in brain development at this time might have something to do with it. It is also important to note that half of people in the U.S. with mental health disorders first experience their illness by the time they turn 14 (¾ by the time they turn 24),[22] and the earlier the onset of a mental health disorder, the more likely it is to be chronic. As a result, childhood through early adulthood represents important age periods for prevention and early intervention efforts.

College Students

College students are at particularly high risk for mental health issues. They face constant deadlines and academic pressure. They might be trying to fit in with a new social scene. Perhaps they are away from home for the first time and feeling homesick. They are entering a new chapter of life as they transition into adulthood. There is a lot going on, and all these forms of stress can add up and take a toll on overall wellbeing. Eighty percent of students report feeling overwhelmed by their responsibilities, and half of students suffer academically as a result.[23] Students with poor mental health are at greater risk of poor adjustment, dropping out of school, and committing suicide.

Altogether, one in four college students suffers from mental illness.[24] That is even higher than the national average, which shows that one in five adults in the U.S. lives with a mental health disorder.[25] Depression and anxiety are the most common mental health issues that college students experience, as well as high rates of bipolar disorder, posttraumatic stress disorder, eating disorders, and schizophrenia, among others.

Many schools offer counseling services to struggling students, often for free or at a low cost. Academic accommodations are also often available, such as extra time and extra help, but students need to take the initiative to seek out these services, which can be daunting. It is helpful for students to become familiar with the school's policies so that they know where to go for help if needed. They should find out where therapy is offered, what kind of therapy is offered (and for how long—schools really differ on this one), and how to make an appointment. They should pay attention to what services are offered by the Dean's Office or the school's Office of Disabilities—they can usually help students work with professors to get their needs met—and what advocacy groups are represented on campus. Most importantly, learning to recognize symptoms, identify risk factors, and take care of mental health can make a huge difference for college students.

Adulthood

Once into adulthood, new challenges arise: People struggle to establish a professional identity, often dealing with the risk of lay-offs, pressure to get promoted, and more of those existential questions about what career path to take. Relationships in this stage are also associated with significant stress—both marriage and divorce rank among the top 10 most stressful life events.[26]

Let us not forget that the miracle of birth is not always joyous. Women who are pregnant or recently gave birth are at high risk for mental health issues, most commonly depression and anxiety, and with all of the physical and neurological shifts of pregnancy, psychosis (which is a very serious disconnection from reality) becomes an increased risk, too. All parents, regardless of whether they personally experienced pregnancy, are faced with the responsibility of keeping another human alive—and not just alive, but happy, healthy, and thriving. Finances, schedules, and increased household responsibilities get tied in with attachment, parent-child conflicts, and the development of parenting values to create ongoing stress. Although most parents say that parenting is a rewarding experience, it is important to recognize that the stress that it creates can take a serious toll. Taken together, anxiety, depression, and substance use disorders remain common among adults.

Older Adulthood

A sometimes forgotten population, but one that is at extremely high risk for mental health issues, is older adults. Older adults deal with many life changes, including retirement, death of friends and family, and changes in health and stamina. As people age, they may lose their ability to live independently, and it can be devastating to no longer be able to do the things they used to do every day, like prepare meals, go for long walks, or even tasks as simple as getting dressed. Many are surprised to learn that older adults are the most likely age group to commit suicide (nearly 20% of people 85 or older).[27] Unfortunately, depression among the elderly often goes unnoticed, sometimes because people are living alone and do not have much contact with others, but even in nursing homes, staff rarely identify depression before it is too late.[28] Another mental health condition common among the elderly is dementia. Dementia affects memory, thought process, and everyday behaviors, making it very hard to live independently.

Impact of Mental Health Disorders on Wellbeing

Biological Impact

Mental health and physical health are highly linked. People with physical health conditions, such as chronic pain, brain injuries, terminal illnesses, etc., are at greater risk for mental health issues such as depression. Similarly, experiencing a mental health issue puts a person at greater risk for developing a physical malady. There are a couple of possible explanations for this. First of all, suffering from a mental health disorder can make it hard for people to take care of themselves. Diet and exercise may fall to the wayside, people often miss doctor's appointments, and even hygiene can suffer. Secondly, mental health issues take a direct toll on the body's health and wellness.

Psychoneuroimmunology studies the connection between the mind, the brain, and the immune system. Have you ever noticed that people tend to get sick around finals? Experiencing stressful emotions reduces immune functioning, making people more susceptible to illness and disease. Victims of trauma are disproportionately likely to experience heart disease, diabetes, and cancer.[29] Depression can lead to chronic pain.[30] A whole category of mental health disorders are experienced physically, with symptoms as common as a headache or as unusual as temporary blindness, paralysis, and seizures. The good news is that psychoneuroimmunology goes both ways. Happy people tend to be healthy people. Taking care of mental health by taking breaks from work, maintaining friendships, staying active, making responsible decisions, and getting treatment for symptoms of distress can all help to keep physical health intact.

Psychological Impact

Unfortunately, mental health issues remain a heavy source of stigma. Despite the fact that nearly half of adults in the U.S. are expected to live through a mental health disorder at some point in their lives,[31] people are often reluctant to speak up when they need help for fear of what others will think of them. Nearly one in four college students feel that their university is not supportive regarding mental health issues, and many are concerned they will be penalized by their professors if they disclose.[32] Some students say that they avoid going to their institution's mental health center due to concerns about confidentiality, namely that they fear their peers might see them or that they may know some of the clinic staff from other settings.

In many cases, people with mental health issues are concerned that they will be considered crazy, dangerous, even contagious, and that friends and family will reject them. Sadly, these concerns are not always unwarranted—there does continue to be discrimination against people with mental illness in terms of hiring practices, educational opportunities, health care benefits, and even housing applications. Many people subscribe to the myth that people with mental health issues are violent, when the facts show no such association. If anything, it is the opposite; people with mental health disorders are four times more likely than the general population to be a *victim* of a violent act.[33]

In addition to the risk of stigma from others, people with mental health issues may also experience stigma from themselves. Some people who struggle with mental illness feel ashamed, think less of themselves, or doubt their ability to get better. In addition to the symptoms of their disorder, these tendencies can substantially increase psychological suffering. Due to the combined effects of stigma, discrimination, fear, and other access barriers, many people shy away from getting treatment. In recent years, nearly 60% of adults with mental illness did not receive treatment.[34] Among children, that percentage is even higher.

Social Impact

Mental health issues can impact the wellbeing of many interpersonal relationships. Consider the functioning of a family of a child with a mental health disorder. His parents may feel guilt or stigma of their own, which could put a burden on their own relationship. A single parent may feel helpless to help the child without the support of a spouse. Parents undergo the additional stress of figuring out where to go for treatment, overcoming any barriers such as insurance issues, transportation, and finding a sitter for their other kids, and managing the child's distress at home. Then you have siblings, who may struggle to understand what is going on, why the affected child gets different or extra attention from their parents, or whether they will develop a mental health issue, too. Siblings may have trouble knowing how to play with or speak to him, or they may be inclined to tease him, all of which can leave him feeling isolated.

Now let's consider friendships—the availability or absence of support from friends can make a big difference in somebody's recovery. Our close friends are who we go to when we are struggling, have a secret, or just need someone to talk to. Sometimes friends play an important role in helping somebody recognize the signs of distress and encouraging the person to seek appropriate care. Sometimes friends do not make the connection and instead see changes in behavior (whether they be the withdrawal common in depression, the risky behaviors seen in bipolar disorder, or the erraticism characteristic of schizophrenia) as annoying or insensitive. The worst thing that can happen to somebody dealing with the early stages of mental illness is to lose social support. Although the illness can place a significant burden on friends and family, it is important for them to listen, learn, and be patient as everybody navigates this hurdle together.

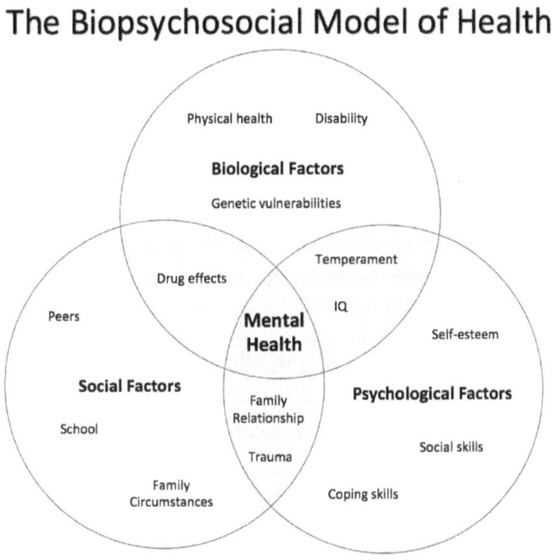

The Biopsychosocial Model of Health

FIGURE 9.1 Applying the Biopsychosocial Model of Health to Mental Health

Suicide

Suicide is the tenth-leading cause of death in the United States, and the second-leading cause of death specifically among college students.[35] People have many different motives to attempt suicide that range from a cry for help without intent to die to a genuine intention to end one's life. Not all people who attempt suicide have a diagnosed mental health issue, but the risk of suicidality drastically increases among those that do. People with depression and bipolar disorder, for example, are 20 to 30 times more likely to attempt suicide than the general population.[36,37]

What is especially scary is that people who have *recently recovered* from depression are among the highest risk for suicide. These are people who may not have had the energy to follow through on suicidal thoughts during their depression but in the recovery stage experience increased energy and motivation. Additionally, people who are recovering from depression and starting to feel better may stop attending therapy, taking medication, or reaching out for help. Especially if the depression was prompted by a significant life change, somebody may have received significant social support from loved ones during their time of need, and that support may start to dwindle as things get better.

In these moments, when concern decreases and friends look the other way, people might need help the most. If you or someone you know is experiencing suicidal thoughts or struggling with emotional distress, call the National Suicide Prevention Lifeline: 1-800-273-TALK.

Community-Wide Efforts to Improve Mental Health

While advocacy for improved mental health has been active for over a century, the last couple of decades have seen an explosion of research on program outcomes, giving us a scientific basis from which to identify at-risk populations, develop effective policies, and systematically intervene. A number of organizations in the United States, such as the National Alliance on Mental Illness (NAMI), Mental Health America (MHA), and the National Institute of Mental Health (NIMH), focus efforts on improving mental health outcomes through research, education, and advocacy. Additionally, federal efforts to improve access to mental health care, such as the Affordable Care Act, are steadily increasing. For every dollar invested in mental health, you can expect to save between $2-$10 in health care, disability, and justice system costs—in other words, mental health is a pretty darn good investment.[38]

There are multiple levels at which prevention and intervention efforts occur. The Substance Abuse and Mental Health Services Administration (SAMHSA) has outlined a "Continuum of Care" highlighting each of these levels: promotion, prevention, treatment, and recovery. Within each of these levels of care, we work to increase protective factors and/or decrease risk factors. Protective factors are qualities that reduce risk for mental illness. Some examples include social connection, good self-esteem, strong education, access to positive role models, and healthy exercise habits. Risk factors are qualities that increase risk for mental illness, such as homelessness, peer rejection, living in an unsafe neighborhood, unemployment, poor relationship with parents, etc. In the following section, we will spend a little time discussing each step of the continuum of care, how protective and risk factors are considered, and what populations are targeted.

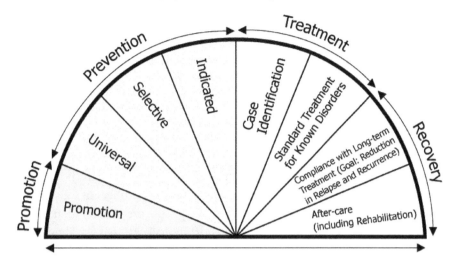

FIGURE 9.2   SAMSHA's Continuum of Care

Promotion

Mental health promotion is perhaps the broadest area of focus for mental health initiatives. It involves creating environments that support positive mental health practices for the entire population. Here we focus on increasing protective factors—what do we need our society to look like to be able to encourage healthy habits, positive coping skills, and community engagement? Promotion efforts strive to increase general wellbeing and social functioning, which not only helps to reduce rates of mental illness, but also improves physical health, productivity, and connectedness. Consider some examples: Development of parks and playgrounds promote exercise, playtime, and possibly parent-child bonding; investing in school systems promotes education, development of mastery, and building a network of support; implementing community gardens promotes good nutrition, development of life skills, and community engagement. These actions may not appear to be directly connected to "mental health," but the beauty of the promotion stage is that it benefits us in so many ways!

Prevention

When it comes to prevention efforts, we increase our focus on risk factors. The Institute of Medicine (IOM) describes three tiers of prevention efforts: universal, selective, and indicated.[39] The tiers represent different levels of risk, and as the level of risk increases, the targeted population becomes more specific.

Universal

Universal prevention programs focus on a given population, regardless of individual levels of risk. For example, some hospitals require all pregnant patients and their partners to attend parenting classes before they deliver. The goal of these classes is to ensure that new parents have a basic understanding of prenatal and infant care. They can be considered prevention programs because they help to prevent significant risk factors for medical and mental illness, including substance use during pregnancy, early deliveries, low birth weight, poor infant-parent attachment, and so on. Participants in the class are not selected based on whether they exhibit one of those risk factors already; rather, the entire population of soon-to-be-parents is involved in order to have the highest reach. Thus, these classes are considered a *universal* prevention effort.

Selective

Universal prevention programs may be sufficient for many members of the population, but inevitably a subset of the population needs more services to reach the same end goal. Selective prevention programs do just that—they focus on members of a given population who are at risk for developing mental illness. These people are usually identified through screening measures, such as questionnaires or short interviews, that ask about various risk factors. The Big Brothers Big Sisters program is an example of a selective program. It targets school-aged youth (population) who come from single-parent households (risk factor) and pairs them with an adult mentor. Studies show that participation in Big Brothers Big Sisters leads to improvements in grades, better parent-child relationships, less aggression, and less substance use.[40] These outcomes are great, so it may seem like this program should be available universally, but there is just no way to find mentors for the entire population of school-aged children, and it is likely that the program would not be as effective for kids who already have multiple adult role models in their lives. Therefore, Big Brothers Big Sisters is offered on a *selective* basis; it targets the members of the larger population that are at greater risk for poor outcomes and would thus benefit the most.

Indicated

The final tier of prevention consists of indicated programs, which go above and beyond selective programs to reach people who are not only high risk, but who are already showing definitive signs or symptoms of a possible mental illness. In this way, indicated programs focus on an even smaller set of the population than selective programs, and they function both as prevention *and* early intervention for the given problem. For example, the Incredible Years program is a therapeutic program for young children that promotes emotional wellbeing and appropriate social behaviors while also reducing aggression and disruptive behaviors.[41] The program is usually delivered in small groups to children who act out in class, have difficulty regulating their impulses, and struggle to build positive relationships—behaviors that predict future mental illness and may already be early symptoms of mental illness.

Treatment

When somebody is already experiencing full-blown symptoms of mental illness, he or she is in need of treatment. For mental health issues, treatment usually consists of some form of talk therapy, medication for psychiatric conditions, also called *psychotropic* medication, or a combination of the two. In the Anxiety and Depression chapter, you will learn more about specific forms of treatment for common mental health conditions. In the meantime, recovery after treatment is an important time that informs prognosis.

Recovery After Treatment

Many people recover from their mental illness, meaning they no longer show symptoms, but that does not mean the work ends there. People who have experienced mental illness in the past are prone to experience it again in the future, so mental health professionals view the recovery phase more like a maintenance phase; we do whatever we can to *maintain* psychological stability. People sometimes make the mistake of going back to old patterns once they feel better, but that is basically like telling somebody who has been sober for a year to celebrate with a drink. The recovery phase is a prime time to consider common triggers for distress and to make corresponding changes in the environment. For example, a person might use the recovery phase to make a game plan for how he will schedule study time during finals so that he does not get overwhelmed. If fighting with a friend or a romantic partner is a trigger, it would be important to work on communication skills.

A common misconception among people who take medication for their mental illness is that they do not need to take it when symptoms go away. Can you guess what tends to happen to these people? The symptoms come back. Unless the prescriber tells the patient otherwise, it is important to keep taking that medication. In many cases, the reason the person feels better is *because* he or she is actively taking medication, and stopping suddenly can have dangerous effects on the body. The same goes for other routines a person may have established during the treatment phase. If the person found a regular exercise routine, a change in diet, a meditation ritual, or any other habit that has helped manage symptoms in the long-term, then the task during recovery is to find a way to keep it up. Maybe the person can throw in a couple more "cheat days" than he or she had when the symptoms were at their worst, but if he or she notices unpleasant feelings coming back, it is important to take charge and implement the structure needed to prevent a relapse.

Advocacy Efforts

Mental illness remains one of the most pervasive and detrimental public-health concerns facing the United States. By educating yourself on warning signs, vulnerable populations, prevention strategies, and available resources, you can do a great service to yourself, your friends, and the greater community. There are often opportunities to be involved in campus advocacy for mental wellness through such organizations as the National Alliance on Mental Illness (NAMI), Active Minds and the Jed Foundation, as well as through your college's psychology department or counseling center.

For example, NAMI is the nation's largest grassroots mental health organization that advocates for policy changes to improve the lives of families and make mental health treatment more accessible to all. Founded in 1979 by a small group of families sitting around a kitchen table, NAMI has grown into the nation's leading voice on mental health, with its main focus being to educate the public about mental health disorders. On a policy level, NAMI advocates for an array of issues including 1) securing funding for scientific research, 2) protecting access to treatment and services, and 3) attaining equal medical benefits for mental health services as currently exist for medical conditions.[42] NAMI is a powerful advocate on behalf of Americans to encourage Congress to pass mental health reform bills that will affect millions through policy change.

Conclusion

With one in every five Americans experiencing mental illness, providing mental health screenings, appropriate referrals, and access to mental care treatment are a national priority. Mental health conditions are rarely the result of one event but rather a result of complex causes and risk factors, including genetics, environment and lifestyle factors. Our hope is that one day the stigma associated with mental health subsides, and all people afflicted with mental health disorders engage in early and consistent treatment and receive support from family, friends, community members, and policy makers to increase the likelihood of recovery.

Case Study

STIGMA AND MENTAL DISORDERS

The purpose of this exercise is to promote self-reflection, empathy for others, and knowledge about how to fight stigma. Consider what types of thoughts and beliefs you hold toward individuals with mental health disorders by answering the questions below. After you have completed the questions, expand your knowledge of where those thoughts and beliefs came from by reading about what stigma is, common misconceptions, and steps to combat stigma.

1. What are your preconceived notions of people with mental health disorders? Is there a difference between someone diagnosed with anxiety versus schizophrenia? Or depression versus narcissistic personality disorder?
2. How do you think that stigma influences your interactions with others?
3. How do you think your preconceived notions impact the way that individuals with mental health disorders perceive themselves and their self worth?
4. What types of services are offered at your university to treat students with mental health disorders? What types of stigma might be associated with using these services, if any?
5. How might you go about combating stigma at your college or university?
6. (Question number 6 is listed at the end of this section)

Stigma and Mental Disorders

What Is Stigma?

The following is from the *World Health Organization's Advocacy for Mental Health Policy and Service Guidance Package*.[43] Stigma is something about a person that causes her or him to have a deeply compromised social standing, a mark of shame or discredit. Many persons with serious mental disorders appear to be different because of their symptoms or the side-effects of their medication. Other people may notice the differences, fail to understand them, or feel uncomfortable about the persons affected and act in a negative way toward them. This exacerbates both symptoms and disability in persons with mental disorders.

Common Misconceptions About People with Mental Disorders

People with mental disorders are often thought to be

- Lazy
- Unpredictable
- Unintelligent
- Unreliable
- Worthless
- Irresponsible
- Stupid
- Untreatable
- Unsafe to be with
- Without conscience
- Violent
- Incompetent to marry and raise children
- Out of control
- Unable to work
- Always in need of supervision
- Increasingly unwell throughout life
- Possessed by demons
- In need of hospitalization
- Recipients of divine punishment

What Are the Effects of Stigma?

- Unwillingness of persons with mental disorders to seek help
- Isolation and difficulty in making friends
- Damage to self-esteem and self-confidence
- Denial of adequate housing, loans, health insurance and jobs because of mental disorders
- Adverse effect on the evolution of mental disorders and disability

- Families are more socially isolated and have increased levels of stress
- Fewer resources are provided for mental health than for other areas of health

How to Combat Stigma

a) Community education on mental disorders (prevalence, causes, symptoms, treatment, myths and prejudices)

b) Anti-stigma training for teachers and health workers

c) Psychoeducation for consumers and families on how to live with persons who have mental disorders

d) Empowerment of consumer and family organizations (as described in this module)

e) Improvement of mental health services (quality, access, deinstitutionalization, community care)

f) Legislation on the rights of persons with mental disorders

g) Education of persons working in the mass media aimed at changing stereotypes and misconceptions about mental disorders

h) Development of demonstration areas with community care and social integration for persons with mental disorders

Question #6: Now that you have gained some new ideas about how to reduce stigma, what steps could your college take to encourage the use of mental health services on campus?

Notes

1 Mental health by the numbers. (2015). National Alliance on Mental Illness. Retrieved January 30, 2017, from http://www.nami.org/Learn-More/Mental-Health-By-the-Numbers

2 Behavioral health trends in the United States: Results from the 2014 National Survey on Drug Use and Health. HHS Publication No. SMA 15-4927, NSDUH Series H-50. (2015). Center for Behavioral Health Statistics and Quality. Available from http://www.samhsa.gov/data/sites/default/files/NSDUH-FRR1-2014/NSDUH-FRR1-2014.htm

3 Whiteford, H. A., Degenhardt, L., Rehm, J., Baxter, A. J., Ferrari, A. J., Erksine, H. E., et al. (2013). Global burden of disease attributable to mental and substance use disorders: Findings from the Global Burden of Disease Study 2010. *Lancet, 283*(9904), 1575–1586.

4 The state of U.S. health, 1990–2010: Burden of diseases, injuries, and risk factors. (2013). *Journal of the American Medical Association, 310*(6), 591–608.

5 Kessler, R. C., Heeringa, S., Lakoma, M. D., Petukhova, M., Rupp, A. E., Schoenbaum, M., et al. (2008). The individual-level and societal-level effects of mental disorders on earnings in the United States: Results from the National Comorbidity Survey Replication. *American Journal of Psychiatry, 165*(6), 703–711.

6 Prevention and early intervention B4Stage4: The state of mental health in America 2016 [Report]. (2016). Mental Health America. Retrieved August 18, 2016 from http://www.mentalhealthamerica.net/sites/default/files/2016%20MH%20in%20America%20FINAL.pdf

7 Chu, J. P., & Sue, S. (2011). Asian American mental health: What we know and what we don't know. *Online Readings in Psychology and Culture, 3*(1), 1–18.

8 Mental Health America (2016). [This listing is incomplete. Could it be the same as 302?]

9 *Disparities in health care quality among racial and ethnic minority groups: Selected findings from the 2010 National Health Care Quality and Disparities Reports* (Publication # 11-0005-3-EF). (2014). U.S. Department of Health and Human Services. Rockville, MD: Agency for Health Care Research and Quality.

10 Leong, F. T. L., & Kalibatseva, Z. (2011). Cross-cultural barriers to mental health services in the United States. *Cerebrum, 5,* 1–13.

11 Snowden, L. R., & Yamada, A. (2005). Cultural differences in access to care. *Annual Review of Clinical Psychology, 1,* 143–166.

12 Lifetime prevalence of DSM-IV/WMH-CIDI disorders by sex and cohort [Table]. (Updated 2007). In *National Comorbidity Survey Replication.* Retrieved August 22, 2016 from www.hcp.med.harvard.edu/ncs/ftpdir/NCS-R_Lifetime_Prevalence_Estimates.pdf

13 Suicide statistics. (2014). American Foundation for Suicide Prevention. Retrieved August 22, 2016 from https://afsp.org/about-suicide/suicide-statistics/

14 Jans, L., & Stoddard, S. (1999). *Chartbook on women and disability in the United States* [Report]. Washington, D.C.: U.S. National Institute on Disability and Rehabilitation Research.

15 Levitt, H. M., & Ippolito, M. R. (2014). Being transgender: Navigating minority stressors and developing authentic self-presentation. *Psychology of Women Quarterly, 38*(1), 46–64.

16 Torrey, E. F., Kennard, A. D., Eslinger, D., Lamb, R., & Pavle, J. (2010). *More mentally ill persons are in jails and prisons than hospitals: A survey of the States.* Arlington, VA: Treatment Advocacy Center.

17 Mental Health America (2016) [This listing is incomplete. Could it be the same as 302?]

18 Mental Health America (2016) [This listing is incomplete. Could it be the same as 302?]

19 Kessler, R. C., Berglund, P., Demler, O., Jin, R., Merikangas, K. R., & Walters, E. E. (2005). Lifetime prevalence and age-of-onset distributions of DSM-IV disorders in the National Comorbidity Survey Replication. *Archives of General Psychiatry, 62*(6), 593–602.

20 Suicide Facts at a Glance 2015 [Fact sheet]. (2015). National Center for Injury Prevention and Control. Retrieved August 22, 2016 from www.cdc.gov/violenceprevention/pdf/suicide-data-sheet-a.PDF

21 Jones, P. B. (2013). Adult mental health disorders and their age at onset. *The British Journal of Psychiatry, 202*(s54), s5-s10.

22 Mental health facts: Children and teens [Fact sheet]. (n.d.) National Institute of Mental Health. Retrieved August 22, 2016 from www.nami.org/NAMI/media/NAMI-Media/Infographics/Children-MH-Facts-NAMI.pdf

23 Gruttadaro, D., & Crudo, D. (2012). *College students speak: A survey report on mental health.* Arlington, VA: National Alliance on Mental Illness.

24 Gruttadaro, D., & Crudo, D. (2012). *College students speak: A survey report on mental health.* Arlington, VA: National Alliance on Mental Illness.

25 *Behavioral health trends in the United States: Results from the 2014 National Survey on Drug Use and Health* (HHS Publication No. SMA 15–4927, NSDUH Series H-50). (2015). Center for Behavioral Health Statistics and Quality. Retrieved from http://www.samhsa.gov/data/

26 Holmes, T. H., & Rahe, R. H. (2000). The stress and coping inventory: An educational and research instrument. *Stress Medicine, 16,* 199–208.

27 Suicide statistics. (2014). American Foundation for Suicide Prevention. Retrieved August 22, 2016 from https://afsp.org/about-suicide/suicide-statistics/

28 Bagley, H., Cordingley, L., Burns, A., Mozley, C. G., Sutcliffe, C. Challis, D., et al. (2000). Recognition of depression by staff in nursing and residential homes. *Journal of Clinical Nursing, 9*(3), 445–450.

29 Kendall-Tackett, K. (2009). Psychological trauma and physical health: A psychoneuroimmunology approach to etiology of negative health effects and possible interventions. *Psychological Trauma: Theory, Research, Practice, and Policy, 1*(1), 35–48.

30 Trivedi, M. H. (2004). The link between depression and physical symptoms. *The Primary Care Companion to the Journal of Clinical Psychiatry, 6*(supplement 1), 12–16.

31 Reeves, W. C., Strine, T. W., Pratt, L. A., Thompson, W., Ahluwalia, I., Dhingra, S. S., et al. (2011). Mental illness surveillance among adults in the United States. *Morbidity and Mortality Weekly Report, 60*(3), 1–32.

32 Gruttadaro, D., & Crudo, D. (2012). *College students speak: A survey report on mental health.* Arlington, VA: National Alliance on Mental Illness.

33 Hughes, K., Bellis, M. A., Jones, L., Wood, S., Bates, G., Eckley, L., et al. (2012). Prevalence and risk of violence against adults with disabilities: A systematic review and meta-analysis of observational studies. *The Lancet, 379*(9826), 1621–1629.

34 *The state of mental health in America 2016* [Report]. (2016). Mental Health America. Retrieved July 15, 2016 from http://www.mentalhealthamerica.net/sites/default/files/2016%20MH%20in%20America%20FINAL.pdf

35 10 Leading causes of death by age group, United States—2014 [Chart]. (2016). National Center for Injury Prevention and Control. In *National Suicide Statistics.* Retrieved July 8, 2016, from http://www.cdc.gov/injury/images/lc-charts/leading_causes_of_death_by_age_group_2014_1050w760h.gif

36 *Depression and suicide risk* [PDF]. (2014). American Association of Suicidology.

37 Pompili, M., Gonda, X., Seafini, G., Innamorati, M., Sher, L., Amore, M., et al. (2013). Epidemiology of suicide in bipolar disorders: A systematic review of the literature. *Bipolar Disorders, 15*(5), 457–490.

38 Prevention of substance abuse and mental illness. (2016). Substance Abuse and Mental Health Services Administration. Retrieved August 25, 2016 from www.samhsa.gov/prevention

39 Springer, F., & Phillips, J. L. (2006). The IOM model: A tool for prevention planning and implementation. *Prevention Tactics, 8*(13), 1–18.

40 McGill, D. E., Mihalic, S. F., & Grotpeter, J. K. (1998). *Big Brothers, Big Sisters of America: Blueprints for violence prevention (Book 2).* Boulder, CO: Center for the Study and Prevention of Violence, Institute of Behavioral Science, University of Colorado.

41 The incredible years [Intervention Report].(2011). Institute of Educational Sciences, What Works Clearinghouse. Retrieved August 26, 2016 from https://ies.ed.gov/ncee/wwc/pdf/intervention_reports/wwc_incredibleyears_111511.pdf

42 My battle with depression. (n.d.). National Alliance on Mental Issues. Retrieved January 30, 2017, from http://www.nami.org/Get-Involved/Take-Action-on-Advocacy-Issues

43 Advocacy for mental health. (2003). World Health Organization. Retrieved January 30, 2017, from http://www.who.int/mental_health/resources/en/Advocacy.pdf

Figure Sources

1 Figure 9.1: Source: http://www.nami.org/NAMI/media/NAMI-Media/Infographics/GeneralMHFacts.pdf. Copyright © National Alliance on Mental Illness (NAMI). Reprinted with permission.

2 Figure 9.2: Source: http://www.nami.org/NAMI/media/NAMI-Media/Infographics/MulticulturalMHFacts10-23-15.pdf. Copyright © National Alliance on Mental Illness (NAMI). Reprinted with permission.

3 Figure 9.3: Source: https://www.nami.org/getattachment/Learn-More/Mental-Health-by-the-Numbers/childrenmhfacts.pdf. Copyright © National Alliance on Mental Illness (NAMI). Reprinted with permission.

4 Figure 9.5: Source: https://www.samhsa.gov/prevention.

CHAPTER TEN

Anxiety and Depressive Disorders

Coauthors:
Caroline Segal, M.S., Sue K. Adams, Ph.D.

@NIMHgov

Mental Health Disorders: Depression and Anxiety
In the last chapter, we spoke about mental health issues in a broader sense. You read about special considerations for college students; disparities in mental health issues across populations; how mental illness impacts the individual, his or her social network, and the nation as a whole; and current efforts to learn more about and improve the state of mental health in the United States. In this chapter, we will discuss two of the most pervasive mental health issues in the country, especially among college students: anxiety and depression. You will learn about the different ways these conditions present themselves, how to recognize warning signs, what causes these conditions to develop, and our current gold standards for treatment.

What Are Anxiety Disorders?
Definition
Feeling anxious from time to time is not only common, it is necessary for survival. If our ancestors never worried about safety, they would not have taken the time to build shelters, to learn which plants are poisonous, or to create weapons against predators. In today's world, it is anxiety that reminds us to look both ways before crossing the street, to go to the doctor for check-ups, and to be vigilant when walking through a bad neighborhood.

Anxiety is distinct from, but closely related to, fear. Fear is an emotional response to imminent threat—something happening in the moment, such as somebody attacking. Anxiety, on the other hand, describes the feelings a person has when anticipating future threat. Anxiety makes people plan ahead to avoid disaster, like studying before tests so or carrying an EpiPen in case of allergic reaction. In small doses, anxiety can be very helpful. However, when anxiety is *excessive, persistent, and intrusive*, it crosses the line into disorder.

Anxiety disorders typically involve unrealistic or irrational worries that do not go away. For example, it is common to worry about getting sunburned at the beach, but most people feel better when they put on sunblock. If a person has an anxiety disorder, that worry might not go away so easily. The person might reapply much more often than recommended and perseverate on the risk of getting skin cancer. He or she might avoid exposure to sunlight by putting on long sleeves and staying under an umbrella, and might feel sick if he or she notices the sun shifting his or her way. The person might even decide not to go to the beach at all because it would be safer to stay inside. While most people are reassured by the precaution of sunblock, anxiety disorders make it harder to trust one's safety and to think about something else. Altogether, nearly one in five adults and one in four children suffer from an anxiety disorder every year.[1,2] There are many different kinds of anxiety disorders, but below are brief descriptions of the most common ones.

Specific Phobia

Have you ever met somebody who is afraid of dogs or clowns or needles? A specific phobia is an intense, irrational, and persistent fear of a specific object or event. The most common kinds of specific phobias include fear of certain animals, fear of natural phenomena such as heights or thunderstorms, fear of the dark or small spaces, fear of getting sick or getting shots, and fears of loud noises or costumed characters. People with specific phobias often go to great lengths to avoid their fear, and if they cannot avoid it, they may experience significant physical and psychological distress.

Social Anxiety Disorder

It is normal to sometimes worry that people are judging you, or to be concerned about saying something stupid or embarrassing. For people with social anxiety disorder, those worries happen all the time, and they can be quite debilitating. People with social anxiety disorder have an intense fear of being judged, humiliated, or rejected by others. They struggle with social interactions, such as engaging in conversation, and often have difficulty making friends or participating in social activities. They also tend to experience significant distress when being observed, such as while giving a speech in class or performing in a play or sporting event. People with social anxiety also fear being observed in more day-to-day settings. They may avoid eating in the cafeteria or using a public bathroom for fear of potential scrutiny.

Generalized Anxiety Disorder

People with *generalized anxiety disorder* (GAD) are often described by those who know them as "worrywarts." GAD is characterized by excessive worry about a variety of things, such as grades, performances, health, family functioning, and world events. People with

GAD find it difficult to control their worrying and often spend most of their day consumed by worry thoughts. They tend to be perfectionists and to hold themselves to high, often unreachable, standards. Many experience physical side effects from excessive worrying, such as fatigue, muscle tension, and restlessness.

Panic Disorder

Have you ever gotten so nervous or worried that your heart began to race, you began to sweat, your throat closed up, it became hard to breathe, you got dizzy or maybe even blacked out, and it all happened in an instant? That experience is a *panic attack*, and many people have one at some point in their life, usually brought on by a stressful trigger, like missing a deadline or getting really bad news.

Panic disorder is the experience of having panic attacks, but ones that are *not* triggered by something specific. Rather, people with panic disorder have panic attacks that come out of the blue and for no apparent reason. They live with fear of having another panic attack because they do not have a way of knowing when it will happen. Some people are so scared of having an unexpected panic attack that they avoid leaving home altogether because they worry that if they have an attack in public, they will not be able to escape. This condition is called *agoraphobia*.

Separation Anxiety Disorder

Separation anxiety disorder is a common affliction in children, but it happens to adolescents and adults as well. Children who experience separation anxiety feel intense distress when separated from a parent or attachment figure. They have unrealistic worries or nightmares that something will happen to them or their parent that will prevent them from seeing each other again. Often this makes it hard for the child to leave home to go to school or to other children's houses, which can impair their ability to make friends. Adults with separation anxiety disorder feel the same kind of distress, but usually in the context of being separated from a romantic partner.

Causes of Anxiety Disorders

Although there are many types of anxiety disorders, they tend to share similar causal factors. Most people do not develop anxiety disorders from one single cause; rather, multiple influences work together to increase or decrease the likelihood of experiencing an anxiety disorder.

Biological Factors

Anxiety disorders have a strong genetic component. If a person has a parent or sibling with an anxiety disorder, he or she is four to six times more likely than others to develop an anxiety disorder as well.[3] Having a genetic predisposition for anxiety, however, does not mean somebody will automatically develop an anxiety disorder; rather, it means he or she is more susceptible to anxiety than others with similar life experiences.

One way we see the impact of anxiety's genetic component is through *temperament*. Temperament refers to the parts of our identity that we are born with, rather than those that are learned. It guides how we interact with and respond to our surroundings and is usually studied in babies and young children. A style of temperament that has been linked to anxiety is behavioral inhibition. Behaviorally inhibited children tend to be shy, timid, and fearful. When presented with something they've never seen before, they tend to cry, recoil, or freeze rather than investigate. Many children who are behaviorally inhibited grow up to become anxious adults.

In addition to temperament, several parts of the brain have been linked to increased anxiety. The *limbic system* is a region of the brain that is responsible for our most basic emotions, such as fear and anger. Within the limbic system lies the *amygdala*, which is responsible for integrating sensory information about emotion. The amygdala facilitates emotional "learning" and is involved in classical conditioning. The amygdala, along with its neighbor, the *hippocampus*, also helps to store memories, so you can be sure you will remember that time a dog jumped on you or how unpleasant you felt the last time you got a bad grade.

Limbic System

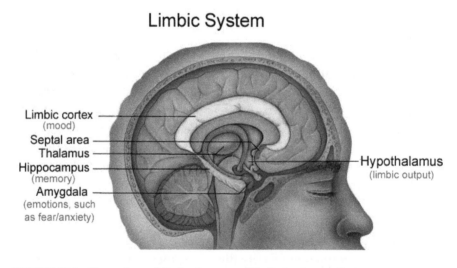

FIGURE 10.1   The regions of the brain responsible for basic emotions

Another area of the limbic system that plays a crucial role in anxiety is the *hypothalamus*. When the brain senses danger, the hypothalamus cues the body to respond by activating the *sympathetic nervous system*, which is responsible for the *fight-or-flight response*. Imagine walking through the jungle by yourself when all of a sudden, an angry lion jumps out in front of you and starts to attack. Chances are you will respond in one of two ways—either you will try to fight back, or you will try to scram as fast as you can: fight or flight. You will respond this way without thinking about it because your body is prepared to react to danger as fast as it can. It is all taken care of by the sympathetic nervous system, which commands different parts of the body to mobilize for survival. Your heart rate speeds up, your breathing accelerates, and your muscles tense. Your pupils dilate to help you see better. You begin to sweat not only to prevent you from overheating but also to make you slippery so that predators cannot catch you. The sympathetic nervous system also tells other parts of your body to stop doing their jobs for a bit so that all of your energy goes to fight-or-flight. For example, your digestion will slow, your salivary glands will take a break, and you will experience some constipation. These tasks are all carried out by two neurotransmitters, *epinephrine* and *norepinephrine*, as well as the hormone *cortisol*, better known as the "stress hormone."

Fight-or-flight is all fine and good when it is keeping you alive, but the truth is, we do not encounter many predators in modern day society; our threats include missing deadlines, being late for work, or accidentally sharing a secret. Our bodies are wired to respond this way to threat, but most of our day-to-day threats are not helped by a total physiological overhaul. This mismatch of cue and response can even make things worse—who wants to sweat profusely when giving a class presentation?

Physiologically, when the threat dissipates, the *parasympathetic nervous system* (PNS) takes over and reverses the effects of the sympathetic nervous system. Your breathing returns to normal, your muscles relax, and your heart rate regulates. Think of your PNS as a parachute (i.e., it brings you down). This feedback system is meant to protect you from exhausting your resources. With chronic anxiety, however, this feedback system can break down. People who are often anxious may have a sympathetic nervous system that is a little too eager, or a parasympathetic nervous system that sleeps on the job. Prolonged fight-or-flight comes with very unpleasant side effects, such as muscle tension, difficulty sleeping, nervous sweating, stomach problems, and constipation. In sum, your brain just wants to protect you from threat, but an anxious brain is a bit overzealous and can cause you to feel tense and alert in response to nonthreatening cues.

Psychological Factors

Our experience of anxiety is substantially influenced by how we tend to see the world. One of the most common triggers for anxiety is *perceived lack of control*. When we are not in control, we do not know what will happen, which for some people indicates that safety is not assured. Worrying is a common response to low perceived control. You may not be able to control what will happen, but you can play over all the possibilities in your mind and plan how you will react in each case. Anxious people often do this to make themselves *feel* like they have more control. The problem is that worry begets worry— once you start, it can be hard to stop. People also make the cognitive error of thinking that things worked out *because* they worried, which makes them more likely to worry about things in the future. While worrying can start as a coping mechanism to help you feel more control, it can quickly give you even less control: it can take up large amounts of time, provoke physiological stress responses, and become so habitual that you start to worry about every little thing.

How much control people feel (or crave) is often shaped by childhood experiences. Certain parenting styles are linked to greater risk for anxiety. Parents who are overprotective work hard to protect their children from danger, but they inadvertently send a message that the world is a dangerous place. When these children grow up, they might feel like they were only safe as children because they had their parents' protection, and now that they are on their own, they do not have the skills to survive. Ironically, growing up with underprotective parents can lead to the same outcome. The world is a scary place for a child, and when left alone to navigate it, the child might come to see it as chaotic and stressful. Both overprotection and underprotection can produce adults with a low perceived sense of control.

Cognitive distortions also play a major role in how people see the world. Cognitive distortions are errors in thinking that lead us to misunderstand ourselves and our surroundings. People with anxiety disorders most commonly overestimate the likelihood of a bad outcome, as well as just how bad that outcome would be. For example, someone might believe planes have a 50% chance of crashing, when the rates are actually one in five million.[4] Or someone might believe that getting a B on a single test will mean he or she will not get into college, when in reality it will probably have only a minor effect on his or her GPA. People with

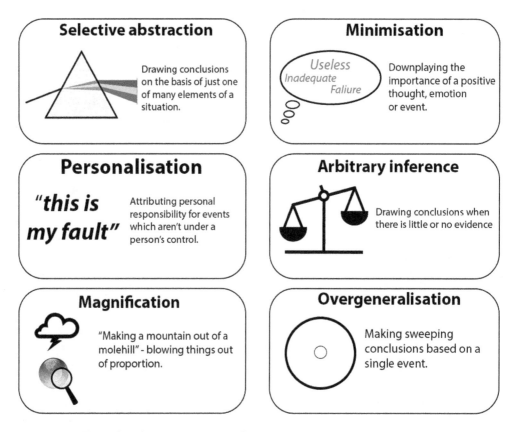

FIGURE 10.2   Examples of common cognitive distortions

anxiety disorders also tend to underestimate their ability to cope. Somebody who worries about making a mistake while giving a speech might imagine the audience reacting in horror, when more often audience members do not even notice a stumble here or there. These exaggerated expectations create a false reality in the minds of anxious people, which explains why they exhibit so much distress and prefer to run from their fears.

Two learning theories also play a role in the psychological development of anxiety. One theory is *classical conditioning*. Have you ever heard the story of the dog that began salivating whenever he heard a bell ring? This happened because Ivan Pavlov, a physiologist, rang a bell every time he gave the dog food. Soon, the dog learned to associate the sound of the bell with the promise of food, and his salivary glands responded automatically. Phobias often develop through classical conditioning, and we are usually unaware it is happening. For example, did your parents have a ritual when they fought to keep you from hearing? Maybe they closed the door to their bedroom or turned up the volume on the TV? If you came to associate those cues with your parents' fighting, which can be a very scary prospect for a child, you might develop a fear of seeing their door closed or hearing the volume increased, even though on their own, these events have nothing to do with family struggle. An unconditioned stimulus and a feared response can co-occur as little as one time for a new fear to emerge, especially if the experience is traumatic. If you get mugged in an alley, are viciously attacked by a dog, or suffer severe injuries from riding a motorcycle, those experiences can be sufficient to condition a fear of alleys, dogs, or motorcycles.

Operant conditioning also plays a role in anxiety, particularly when it comes to avoidance. Operant conditioning is the idea that we engage in behaviors more frequently if they are rewarded and less frequently if they are punished. We learn to study for tests because we are rewarded with good grades. We learn to eat less junk food because we are punished with stomachaches. When people experience anxiety, and that pesky fight-or-flight response cues unpleasant physical feelings, it does not take long to learn that removing oneself from the situation allows the parasympathetic nervous system to calm the body down. Essentially, the body rewards the person for avoiding fears by decreasing arousal. This pattern is why people who are scared of spiders avoid camping or people with social anxiety disorder keep to themselves. The problem is that avoidance is not always possible (or helpful), and the more people avoid their fears, the harder it becomes to face them.

Social Factors

A third learning theory that influences anxiety development is *social learning theory*. In short, social learning theory states that we learn from watching. This is part of the reason why anxious parents often have anxious children (there is also the genetic component). Children learn how to interact with the world by watching their parents. If their parents model anxious reactions, such as avoiding answering the phone, crying at the sight of a spider, or spewing a cascade of worried thoughts at the end of every day, children learn to do the same. It is not only parents' fault—one can learn anxious behaviors from anybody in their lives, including close friends, school teachers, and even television characters.

What Are Depression and Mood Disorders?

Definition

After anxiety, the most common category of mental health issues is *mood disorders*. Imagine moods as a spectrum, with the worst, most negative moods all the way at one end and the best, most positive moods all the way at the other. Moods that fall at either end of the spectrum are problematic, even the positive side. Most people have moods that fall somewhere in the middle. Sometimes we are up, sometimes we are down, but our highs and lows usually stick to the mild to moderate range and do not disrupt our lives in the long run. Mood disorders, on the other hand, are characterized by moods that fall at the extremes of the mood continuum and that stay there for a significant period of time. These severe and persistent moods can have detrimental effects on functioning.

There are two types of mood disorders. Depression is a *unipolar* mood disorder, meaning its symptoms tend to be towards the low end of the mood spectrum. Other mood disorders are *bipolar*, meaning symptoms fall at both the low extreme and the high extreme of the spectrum. The following sections describe the main characteristics of depression and bipolar disorders.

Depression

Depression is more than feeling sad or down; in fact, some people who suffer from depression do not experience sadness at all. Depression can present with a wide range of symptoms, so everybody's experience is unique. Some symptoms are very mood-based, such as feeling low, hopeless, guilty, or sometimes feeling nothing at all. Other symptoms are physiological, such as drastic changes in sleep or appetite. Depression can slow a person down (some people notice that they move like molasses or draw out their words) or it can speed a person up (some people report restlessness, agitation, or shakiness). It can disrupt cognitive functioning, making it hard to think straight, make decisions, or move on from an unpleasant thought or memory. It can affect one's experience of the world and make a person lose interest in activities that he or she used to love. For some people, depression leads to frequent thoughts of death. Some explain that depression feels like living underneath a pile of bricks. It may feel impossible to get out from under them, and tasks as seemingly simple as getting out of bed or taking a shower can require a huge amount of effort. Living underneath all those bricks also makes it hard to see things as they are. For example, people with depression have trouble seeing the positive; it is hard to recognize strengths, see the silver lining, or believe that good things will come. The bricks can make someone feel trapped and alone, even when he or she is in a room full of people.

One in six people suffer from depression at some point in life.[5] For some, it is triggered by a significant life event, such as divorce, losing a job, or moving to college, but for others, it can occur in the absence of a clear life change. Depression is a debilitating disorder that can make it very hard to stay productive at your job, keep up with schoolwork, and maintain healthy relationships. It is also highly *comorbid*, meaning it often co-occurs with a range of other disorders, such as anxiety, posttraumatic stress disorder, substance use, and many medical conditions. When people experience depression, they tend to withdraw from others, so if you have a friend who stops returning your calls or meeting you for lunch, he or she may not be avoiding you—it could be a sign that the person is suffering. Depression makes it hard to ask for help, so if you notice a friend pulling away and shutting people out, it might mean that he or she needs you more than ever.

Depression usually occurs in episodes, where symptoms have a beginning and an end. *Major depressive disorder* is diagnosed when an episode lasts for at least two weeks, though untreated depressive episodes often continue for three to nine months.[6] Depression can also be more chronic than episodic; *persistent depressive disorder* is a type of depression that lasts over two years without remission. Symptoms of persistent depressive disorder are usually less severe than symptoms of major depressive disorder, but sometimes that can make it harder to recognize, meaning people are more likely to suffer without treatment. Most people with either kind of depression first see symptoms before the age of 21, so college is a particularly important time to be aware of warning signs, like avoiding classes or social activities, losing interest in groups or clubs, or experiencing low self-esteem.

Bipolar Disorders

Bipolar disorder is characterized by cycles of both depression and mania, or what we call *manic episodes*. Manic episodes are in many ways in contrast with depressive episodes— instead of feeling sad or down, people experiencing mania tend to feel excessively happy; some even say they feel "high" without using any substances. People experiencing manic episodes typically feel very energized. Many report not sleeping at all or sleeping very little and still feeling ready and raring to go the next day. People in manic episodes tend to talk very rapidly, and they may jump from one idea to the next. In an interview with *Healthline,* one man with bipolar disorder explained, "I'm all over the place, dominating every conversation. I've been told I talk too fast and switch topics so quickly that it's hard for others to keep up with me. Sometimes, I can't keep up with myself."[7] Manic episodes are also characterized by increased goal-directed behavior; people tend to be very creative and ambitious during mania, and they often take on a host of new projects, such as building a house, writing a novel, starting several on-campus groups, etc.

So far, this all does not seem so bad, right? Good mood, burst of energy, and intense productivity, all with little to no sleep? Many people experiencing mania understandably enjoy these symptoms, which may discourage them from seeking treatment. Unfortunately, mania can have an ugly side. When experiencing a manic episode, people tend to exhibit impulsivity; they are more likely to spend hundreds or thousands of dollars on things they do not need (such as buying a new car on a whim), to gamble or drink excessively, or to engage in promiscuous sexual activity. Essentially, the manic brain acts before it thinks, which leads to high-risk and possibly life-threatening behavior. In more severe cases, people with mania can even exhibit psychotic symptoms, like seeing or hearing things that are not there or believing in *delusions,* which are false beliefs that people maintain even when faced with strong evidence that those beliefs are unfounded. In severe manic episodes, people commonly describe feeling "god-like" or "invincible" due to the exhilarating nature of their symptoms, which can lead them to engage in very risky behaviors, such as running into traffic or leaping from tall heights.

Like depression, bipolar disorders often first emerge during the college years, so if you or a friend start to show signs of depression, it is important to consider whether there have been any warning signs of mania as well.

Causes

Similar to anxiety, mood disorders are not caused by one single factor but rather by a confluence of biopsychosocial inputs. The following sections will discuss some of the more commonly identified causes of mood disorders.

Biological Factors

Mood disorders carry a fairly strong genetic predisposition. Someone is about three times more likely to develop a mood disorder if he or she has a parent or sibling with a mood disorder.[8] It is important to keep in mind, however, that family history alone does not determine whether someone will experience a mood disorder. It may require a significant life event or a chronic stressor to activate genetic inheritance, and even then, those genes can only increase the risk, not guarantee that one will develop the disorder.

Some of the brain regions that play a role in the development of anxiety also play a role in the development of mood disorders, which is partly why they often occur together. Remember the amygdala, the center for emotional learning? It helps people process what emotion to feel in response to different experiences. In depression, the amygdala appears to be overactive in responding to sad stimuli, which is why people who are depressed feel sadness more often. The depressed brain's amygdala also tends to drop the ball when something positive or rewarding occurs, which is why depression leads people to lose interest or enthusiasm in things they used to enjoy. In bipolar disorder, the amygdala can work too hard in both cases. It can increase your experience of sad feelings, but it can also become overly sensitive to positive stimuli, leading to surges of emotions at both extremes of the mood spectrum. Just as the amygdala works with the hippocampus to store anxious memories, so too do they collaborate to compile memories of both depressive and manic responses. These memories resurface the next time the person faces a similar stimulus as a cue to remind the person how he or she reacted before, which increases the likelihood that he or she will react that way again.

The hypothalamus is also involved in the development of mood disorders. Remember that the hypothalamus is involved in producing cortisol, the stress hormone. It may not be surprising to learn that high stress is a major risk factor for depression and bipolar disorder—both severe stress reactions to singular events, such as trauma, as well as chronic levels of stress from, say, an academically rigorous semester. The more stress a person experiences, the more cortisol is secreted, and the more cortisol secreted, the greater the risk for mood disorders. Research is beginning to show, however, that low cortisol levels are also a risk factor; low levels of cortisol may indicate dysfunction in the stress feedback system. Just like with moods themselves, the sweet spot for a healthy cortisol level is somewhere in the middle.

In addition to stress response, the hypothalamus is also involved in regulating sleep and appetite, both of which are involved in mood disorders. Irregular sleep is particularly dangerous in bipolar disorder; a manic episode can lead to decreases in sleep, but getting too little sleep can also trigger a manic episode.

Three neurotransmitters are often cited in research on mood disorders: serotonin, norepinephrine, and dopamine. *Serotonin* has been found to affect mood, appetite, digestion, sleep, sexual desire, and social functioning, all of which may be impaired in people with mood disorders. You may recall that *norepinephrine* is involved in fight or flight and is thus partly responsible for the experience of stress. *Dopamine* is involved in motivation, movement, and reward. Low levels of dopamine may explain common depressive symptoms such as lethargy and loss of interest, whereas high levels may explain common manic symptoms such as increased goal-directed activity and restlessness.

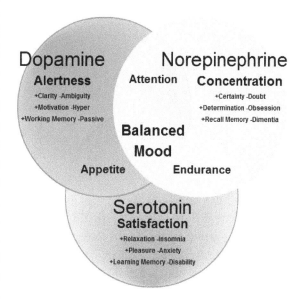

FIGURE 10.3   **The function of the neurotransmitters implicated in depression**

Psychological Factors

How we look at, think about, and understand ourselves and our surroundings is greatly influenced by our *core beliefs*, which are deep-seated principles that we hold to be true (even when they may not actually be true). We develop our core beliefs over time as we gather information about the world through life experiences. Early experiences are particularly influential, as they tend to serve as a template for what we expect in the future. For example, if your parents were neglectful and did not attend to your needs, you may come to develop a belief that you are on your own in the world and cannot depend on others. On the other hand, if your parents were responsive and caring, you may come to believe that interpersonal relationships can be very satisfying. These beliefs guide how we make sense of what happens to us throughout our lives.

People whose core beliefs tend to be negative, pessimistic, or disparaging are more likely to develop a depressive mindset. If you believe, "I am unlovable," you are more likely to blame yourself for a breakup, lose hope in relationships, and withdraw from others. If you believe, "Things never go right for me," you'll probably feel discouraged from facing challenges, putting yourself out there, maybe even leaving the comfort of your bed. Core beliefs are adaptable, but it takes a lot of hard work to change a thought process so deeply rooted in your mind.

Another facet of how we make sense of our world has to do with our *attributions*, which are the explanations we come up with for why things happen. Let's say you are sitting at a stoplight that turns green, and suddenly you get rear-ended. You might argue that it was the other driver's fault for stepping on the gas too soon, but the other driver might argue that it was *your* fault for not stepping on the gas soon enough. To what (or whom) we attribute an event is all about perspective. There are three characteristics to attributions: internal vs. external, stable vs. temporary, or global vs. specific. People who suffer from depression commonly attribute *bad* things to causes that are internal, stable, and global—very much taking the perspective that *they* caused the negative event, and it will *always* be this way. *Good* things are most often attributed to things that are external, temporary, and specific—that is, something outside the person's control caused the positive event, and it will not last.

Take, for example, somebody who just failed a test. An *internal* attribution would say that it was his fault rather than somebody else's fault (e.g., "I failed because I'm stupid"). A *stable* attribution assumes that the cause will never change ("I've always been stupid, and I'll always be stupid"). A *global* attribution would reach beyond this one event and attribute the failure to something more general ("I fail at *everything* I try to do"). Now consider someone who aced an exam. If he or she has a depressive attributional style, he or she might say, "I only did well because the professor made the test easy" (external), "It was a fluke; I probably will not do well on the next test" (unstable), or "I knew the content of this one exam, but I do not know anything that really matters" (specific). Many people who suffer from depression have developed a tendency to overemphasize the bad and explain away the good.

We spoke earlier about *cognitive distortions*, which are basically lies that the brain creates that influence how we see things. Some cognitive distortions are common among people who develop depression. For one, people who develop depression have a tendency to *discount the positive*. Basically, this means that their minds are a magnet for negative thoughts. Thoughts that make somebody feel guilty, disheartened, or bad about themselves tend to stick, and evidence that somebody has wonderful strengths, a bright future, or strong support tend to bounce back off. If someone tends to discount the positive, then negative experiences will stand out and strengthen depressive core beliefs, while he or she will be prone to ignore or write off the positive experiences.

Another common cognitive distortion in depression is *predicting the future*. The more we interact with the world, the more we come to rely on certain predictions of how things will play out. You have good reason to believe that your car will start if you turn the key in the ignition because you have probably experienced that sequence of events more than a few times. Expectations, however, are not guarantees: If your car battery dies, then turning the key *will not* start the ignition. While expecting the car to start is pretty reasonable, other predictions are not so harmless. When people fall into a pattern of pessimistic predictions, particularly ones that play into a core belief that nothing goes right for them, their risk for depression increases. Some people make predictions that they will *never* make friends, *never* graduate from school, *never* get a job, etc. When a person treats these kinds of predictions as guarantees, it discourages him or her from even trying. That discouragement can lead to hopelessness, one of the hallmark symptoms of depression.

For many people, both depressive and manic episodes can be triggered by stress. When most people hear "stress," they usually think of negative things (deadlines, family issues, health problems), but stress is not always bad. A person can also experience stress from good things, such as starting school, getting married, or visiting family for the holidays. Negative stress, or *distress*, makes us feel unpleasant, perform worse than usual, and it drains coping resources, whereas positive stress, or *eustress*, can feel exciting and motivating. However, stress is stress, and even eustress can add up and put a person at risk for a mood disorder. In depression, the number of stressful life events experienced is pretty directly correlated to the chance of having an episode.

A particularly stressful life event is a trauma. Studies show that traumatic events can actually lead to changes in the brain that look similar to what would be seen with mood disorders. Experiencing trauma substantially boosts the likelihood that one will develop depression or bipolar disorder, and the chances are higher the more trauma the person undergoes.

Social Factors

A number of social factors are specifically linked to depressive episodes, including rejection, isolation, and history of abuse. Social support plays a big role in mood disorders. Depressive episodes can be spurred on by loss of social support, such as a recent break-up, end of a close friendship, or death of a loved one. Early separation from parents is a major risk factor for depression, especially if it means experiencing a decrease in warmth, care, and attention.

While it would be unfair to blame parents for their children's mental health struggles, parents do have an unfortunate tendency to play a role. Parents can pass along cognitive distortions and depressive attributional styles to their children through modeling. Parents who exhibit poor coping skills inadvertently teach their children to behave similarly. If a parent responds to obstacles by giving up, their children may come to believe that the decks are stacked against them and their best bet in life is just to fold. If a parent models manic symptoms, such as poor self-control, impulsivity, and risky behavior, their children may pick up those tendencies as well. How parents express emotion can also be a causal factor in mood disorders. *Expressed emotion* describes how hostile, critical, and overbearing parents are towards their children. The higher the amount of expressed emotion in the household, the greater the risk.

Interventions for Anxiety and Depressive Disorders

There are two main categories of treatment for mental health issues: psychotherapy and psychopharmacology (or, more simply, medication). In many cases, the most effective treatment involves a combination of the two, but treatment decisions depend heavily on the disorder, the severity, and characteristics of the individual. A number of alternative interventions have gained popularity. Read on to learn about the most common ways we treat mental health disorders.

Psychotherapy

When many people hear the word "psychotherapy," they picture somebody lying down on a couch talking to Dr. Freud about mother issues and sexual repression. While therapy could look like this, it does not usually—at least not anymore. Several styles of psychotherapy take different approaches to working through mental health issues, but the most commonly used (and highly regarded) form of therapy is called *cognitive-behavioral therapy*, or CBT. It is an evidence-based treatment, which means a lot of sound research has validated its effectiveness. Basically, it gets proven results. Studies have shown that CBT can be an effective treatment for a wide range of mental health issues, including depression, anxiety, bipolar disorder, PTSD, substance abuse, eating disorders, and many more.[9]

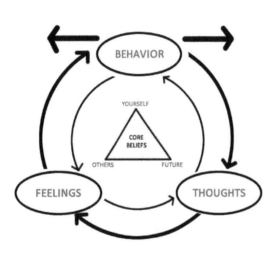

FIGURE 10.4   **Diagram of Cognitive Behavioral Therapy**

CBT explores how thoughts, feelings, and behaviors are connected. Say you were supposed to meet a friend for lunch, and she never showed up. If you think to yourself, "She probably doesn't like me and was trying to hurt me," it might lead you to feel sad, embarrassed, maybe lonely. You might leave the restaurant without calling your friend and start ignoring her attempts to reach out to you. If instead you think to yourself, "She probably had an emergency and couldn't get to the phone," your feelings might focus more on concern for your friend's wellbeing, even enhanced connectedness as you remember times you dealt with emergencies. Instead of ignoring her, you might be more inclined to call her to check in, forgive her for bailing on you, and offer to talk her through whatever is going on. In this scenario, two different thoughts about the same situation can lead to different sets of feelings and different behavioral reactions.

CBT involves a lot of collaboration between the therapist and the client, and often homework assignments are used to help the client practice new skills in everyday life. It is usually somewhat time-limited (often somewhere between eight and 20 sessions) and focused on very specific, concrete goals. Therapists use many different tools in CBT, but one involves teaching the client to challenge the thoughts he or she has that lead to negative emotions and unhelpful behaviors. CBT is often used to help people develop more realistic or helpful thoughts that they can practice using instead to improve their mood and behaviors. Another tool used in CBT, especially to treat anxiety, is called *exposure therapy*. In exposure therapy, a therapist helps a client overcome a fear by gradually exposing the person to the feared object or event in small, safe, and progressively more challenging steps. For example, somebody with a fear of spiders might start by visualizing a spider. In the next session, the person might look at a cartoon spider, then a picture of a real spider. Eventually, he or she may be asked to stand in the same room as a spider in a cage, slowly working towards the final step of holding a spider in his or her hands. If exposure therapy is rushed, the fear could be exacerbated, but when done systematically and collaboratively, the technique is overwhelmingly effective.

A more recent cognitive-behavioral tool that has steadily gained prominence in therapy is *mindfulness meditation*. Mindfulness meditation is the practice of being present and aware, staying in the moment, and leaving judgment at the door. Practicing mindfulness can help us feel more in tune with our inner and outer experiences, make us more patient and accepting, decrease stress, and increase satisfaction.

Here is a very basic mindfulness exercise to give you a taste: Pick an activity that is part of your morning routine, such as brushing your teeth. The next time you brush, bring all of your focus to the activity itself. Consider what it feels like to hold the plastic toothpaste tube in your hand, how the cap feels against your skin as you twist it open, the sound it makes as it lightly drops onto the counter. Observe the colors of the toothpaste as it slowly emerges. Can you see any dents in the paste from changes in pressure as you squeezed, or is it uniform? Consider the taste of the toothpaste as it slowly hits different parts of your tongue. Can you feel it hit each tooth? Is the temperature different from the temperature in your mouth? What is the texture like? What does your arm feel like as it moves back and forth? Pay attention to every detail of the experience, and if your mind wanders (which it will inevitably do—you will start thinking about what you have to do today, that funny thing your friend said, maybe even how silly you feel doing this exercise), do not beat yourself up for losing focus; let those thoughts come and go, and bring your attention back to brushing your teeth.

Psychopharmacology

Many medications that are used for mental health disorders are specific to each disorder, though some can be used to treat a few different conditions. For example, *selective serotonin reuptake inhibitors (SSRIs)* are a class of antidepressants that work by increasing the amount of serotonin available in the brain. Despite being called antidepressants, SSRIs are also used to treat anxiety, obsessive-compulsive disorder, and even eating disorders. SSRIs are currently the most commonly prescribed antidepressants, and you have probably heard of many leading brands, such as Prozac, Zoloft, Paxil, Celexa, and so on. Though SSRIs can be very effective, they are not without side effects, which most often include nausea, digestion issues, weight gain, restlessness, dry mouth, and decreased sex drive. SSRIs also take time to work their way through the system, so it might take a few weeks on a medication before symptoms improve.

Among anti-anxiety medications, the most common category is *benzodiazepines*. Benzo-diazepines work by increasing the effects of a neurotransmitter called *gamma-aminobutyric acid,* or *GABA*, whose job is to suppress nerve activity. Benzodiazepines are basically a sedative; they make a person feel calm, but they can make him or her feel drowsy, weak, or sometimes dizzy. Popular benzodiazepines include Valium, Ativan, Xanax, and Klonopin. These medications are usually taken as needed instead of every day (though not always), such as if someone feels an anxiety attack coming on and needs something to calm down quickly. Unfortunately, they are extremely addictive and should not be taken more often than prescribed. People with a personal or family history of addiction may also want to steer clear of these drugs, opting instead for an SSRI or a different type of anti-anxiety medication.

Alternative Therapies

A number of non-pharmacological treatment options are often used to bolster traditional therapy. Regular exercise, for example, can effectively contribute to the management of many mental health disorders. Yoga is recommended for people struggling with depression, anxiety, PTSD, ADHD, and schizophrenia. In addition, breathing exercises and meditation rituals are other basic strategies anybody can engage in to boost mental health. Even massage and acupuncture have received high marks as alternatives to medication.

Conclusion

In conclusion, anxiety and depression are highly prevalent mental health disorders that affect millions of Americans. Their causes and symptoms overlap in a number of ways, although they also have marked differences. Some very promising and effective treatment strategies can reduce the symptoms of anxiety and depression, and no one should ever suffer in silence.

Case Study

Depression

Ber is a 21-year-old, single college student in his junior year. Ber is taking six classes and works 20 hours per week in the student union. He is studying biology and lives with two roommates off-campus.

Ber reports that he has been under significant stress lately, as he has been juggling work, baseball, and a heavy course load. Two weeks ago, he failed an exam in his advanced biology class, and since then, he has been skipping classes and avoiding interactions with his professor. He states that he cannot seem to get out of bed when his alarm goes off, and that he has been sleeping from about 9 p.m. until the early afternoon. Despite getting more sleep than usual, he identifies that he still feels tired and sluggish every day.

Ber is attending school on a baseball scholarship, but he has missed more than half of his practices this month. His coach informed him that he is at risk for losing his scholarship, but Ber has been questioning whether he wants to continue playing anyway, as he no longer feels excited about the sport. His friends from the team have noted that he seems to move in slow motion these days, and they are often asking him to pick up the pace when they walk to practice together. His coach has noticed that he participates less often in drills and has gained five to 10 pounds over the past month. Ber acknowledges that he feels hungry all the time, especially when he is stressed, and that he has been snacking more often lately.

When asked how he is feeling, Ber states that he does not really know. He notes that he has not been feeling sad lately, but he also has not felt happy. Ber says that more than anything, he has been feeling numb. He says that he does not think he can improve his GPA, and he is convinced that he will not be able to get a job after college. When Ber has these thoughts, he considers dropping out of school altogether.

Anxiety

Amy is a 32-year-old, married bank teller who lives with her husband and three-year-old daughter in a small apartment building. She notes that she has always been a "worrier," but that it has not affected her life in a negative way until now. Over the past year, Amy has noticed feeling "keyed up" and irritable more days than not. She has complained of frequent stomach-aches, and about once a month she experiences an intense wave of anxiety accompanied by shortness of breath, racing heart, and dizziness. These episodes usually occur in response to a stressor, such as realizing she is late on paperwork or that she missed a doctor's appointment.

Amy has always been a cautious person, but lately she feels like she overthinks everything. Amy noticed this change after her daughter was born, when she began to worry about her parenting style, finances, her daughter's health, her marriage, etc. Amy has also been attending to the news more often lately and experiences significant distress when she hears about bad events in the world. She convinces herself that bad things will happen to her family, and she has trouble sleeping because she wakes up whenever she hears a rustle outside her window.

When asked to track how much time she spends worrying, Amy learned that worries take up more than half of her waking hours. Consequently, she has been falling behind at work, and she feels like she is missing important moments in her daughter's life because she has trouble staying present and keeping her mind from drifting. Amy's husband reports that he has been frustrated lately because he feels like he has to constantly reassure Amy that everything is okay. Amy notes that there has been a distance growing in her marriage, and that if she does not get her worrying under control, her husband and daughter will suffer.

Notes

[1] Anxiety disorders. (2015). National Alliance on Mental Illness. Retrieved from http://www.nami.org/

[2] Beesdo, K., Knappe, S., & Pine, D. S. (2009). Anxiety and anxiety disorders in children and adolescents: Developmental issues and implications for DSM-V. *Psychiatric Clinics of North America, 32*(3), 483–524.

[3] Hettema, J. M., Neale, M. C., & Kendler, K. S. (2001). A review and meta-analysis of the genetic epidemiology of anxiety disorders. *The American Journal of Psychiatry, 158*(10), 1568–1578.

[4] Haltiwanger, J. (2015). The odds of a plane crash are one in 11 million, yet you're still afraid. *Elite Daily*. Retrieved from http://www.elitedaily.com/

5 Kessler, R. C., Berglund P., Demler, O., Jin, R., Merikangas, K. R., & Walters, E. E. (2005). Lifetime prevalence and age-of-onset distributions of DSM-IV disorders in the National Comorbidity Survey Replication. *Archives of General Psychiatry, 62*(6), 593–602.

6 Maxmen, J. S., & Ward, N. G. (1995). Mood disorders. In *Essential Psychopathology and Its Treatment* (2nd ed., p. 219). New York: W. W. Norton & Company.

7 Krans, B. (2016). In their shoes: Understanding what bipolar disorder feels like. *Healthline.* Retrieved July 8, 2016, from http://www.healthline.com/health/bipolar-disorder/what-bipolar-feels-like#1

8 Goodman, S. H., & Gotlib, I. H. (1999). Risk for psychopathology in the children of depressed mothers: A developmental model for understanding mechanisms of transmission. *Psychological Review, 106*(3), 458–490.

9 Hollon, S. D., & Beck, A. T. (2013). Cognitive and cognitive-behavioral therapies. In M. J. Lambert (Ed.), *Bergin and Garfield's Handbook of Psychotherapy and Behavior Change* (6th ed., pp. 393–394). Hoboken, NJ: John Wiley & Sons.

Figure Sources

1 Figure 10.1: Copyright © BruceBlaus (CC by 3.0) at https://commons.wikimedia.org/wiki/File:Blausen_0614_LimbicSystem.png.

2 Figure 10.2: Copyright © LoudLizard (CC BY-SA 4.0) at https://upload.wikimedia.org/wikipedia/commons/d/d0/Common_Cognitive_Biases.png.

3 Figure 10.3: Copyright © Nikpapag (CC BY-SA 3.0) at https://upload.wikimedia.org/wikipedia/commons/6/63/DopamineNorepinephrineSerotoninVennDiagram.png.

4 Figure 10.4: Copyright © Urstadt (CC BY-SA 3.0) at https://en.wikipedia.org/wiki/File:Depicting_basic_tenets_of_CBT.jpg.

CHAPTER ELEVEN

Substance Use

Coauthors:
**Vanessa Somohano, M.A., Sue K. Adams, Ph.D.,
Sarah W. Feldstein Ewing, Ph.D.**

@NIDAnews

What is the first image that pops into your head when you think of the word "disease"? You might have an image of someone lying in bed with a high fever, runny nose, and aching body. Some diseases, however, are silent, can originate from within our genetic code, and remain dormant until triggered by something in our environment. Although some people have the misconception of addiction as a series of poor choices and lack of will power, many other factors are at play that make this disease much more complex than a series of decisions an individual makes. In this chapter, we will review the meaning of disease as it relates to substance addiction, specifically examining alcohol abuse, cannabis use, and opioid abuse. We will also discuss health disparities that are present in addiction populations, the impact of addiction on individuals across development and families, and intervention and treatment efforts to "fight the war on drugs."

What Is Substance Use and Substance Abuse?

According to the National Institute on Drug Abuse (NIDA),[1] addiction is a "chronic, relapsing brain disease that is characterized by compulsive seeking and use, despite harmful consequences." The Substance Abuse and Mental Health Administration[2] reports that 21.5 million people 12 years of age and older have a substance use disorder, which includes alcohol- and tobacco-use disorder. NIDA[3] estimates that addiction and abuse of alcohol, tobacco, and illicit and prescription substances costs Americans $700 billion dollars in increased health care costs, crime, and lost productivity.

Substance use is the ingestion of a particular substance. The WHO defines *substance abuse* as the harmful or hazardous use of psychoactive substances. If an individual uses or abuses a substance, it does not imply that he or she has a *Substance Use Disorder (SUD)*, which is defined as a cluster of cognitive, behavioral, and physiological symptoms indicating that an individual continues using a substance despite substance-related consequences.[4]

Often times SUD symptoms will fall under four main categories: *impaired control, social impairment, risky use,* and *pharmacological criteria.* Symptoms associated with impaired control include cravings, continued failed attempts to cease use of a substance and consuming larger amounts of a substance for longer periods of time than intended, and spending the majority of time engaged in activities revolving around using or obtaining the substance. Symptoms associated with social impairment include reduced productivity at work or school functions, interpersonal problems caused by use of a substance, and giving up important occupational or recreational activities for use of a substance. Symptoms associated with risky use include continued use despite knowledge that use is causing harmful physiological and psychological effects and using in situations that are physically hazardous, like sharing injections with others. The last grouping of symptoms under the physiological criteria category is tolerance and withdrawal. *Tolerance* is when an individual requires a greater amount of a substance to obtain a desired effect. *Withdrawal* is a set of physiological symptoms that ensues when concentrations of a substance decrease from blood or muscle tissue. Withdrawal usually occurs if a sufficient amount of a substance has been ingested over a period of time. Often times an individual will continue to use a substance to relieve withdrawal symptoms. Not all substances are known to have withdrawal symptoms, and withdrawal symptoms vary depending on the substance that is ingested.

Health Disparities

Substance use disorders span across a variety of races, cultures, and socioeconomic standing. This is because addictive substances act upon the brain's reward system, which is biologically similar across all people. Therefore, every person experiences a certain amount of risk, with genetics accounting for 40–60% of a person's vulnerability to addiction.[5]

Age Disparities

According to NIDA,[6] the younger a person is when he or she engages in substance use, the more likely he or she is to develop an addictive disorder. A 2014 report by the Substance Abuse and Mental Health Services Administration (SAMSHA)[7] indicates that most illicit substance use starts between 16 and 17 years old, and that 9.4% of individuals between 12 and 17 years old were current users of illicit substances. Individuals between the ages of 18 and 25 represented the highest percentage of current illicit substance users at 22%. Factors that predict earlier age of substance use are unstable or volatile family structure, mental illness, abuse, peers, where the individual resides, availability of substances, and lack of oversight from parents.

Gender Disparities

Although men have higher lifetime rates of substance use than women, substance use in women is more severe, persistent, and difficult to treat. Telescoping, or the rapid progress from substance use to substance dependence, is a term used to describe the progression of addiction for women compared to men. This disparity is due to physiological differences in managing stress, societal pressures that women face, and barriers to obtaining treatment for substance use such as child care, pregnancy, greater dependence on social welfare system, changes in insurance policies, and family obligations. Women also have a higher tendency to abuse cocaine and psychotherapeutic substances than men due to biological and neurological mechanisms, and have more persistent alcohol use disorders than men.[8] For women, mental health issues usually precede the onset of a substance use disorder, where for men it is typically the opposite. Approximately 90% of women entering treatment for substance use have had a lifetime history of interpersonal trauma, which can complicate treatment outcomes.[9]

Gender and Sexual Minorities

Gender and sexual minorities are at a disproportionate risk for substance use. Individuals who identified as *mostly* heterosexual, bisexual, and lesbian/gay were more likely to have reported illicit substance use in the past year than individuals who identified as completely heterosexual.[10] Females identifying as bisexual were also more likely to use substances than other sexual orientations. Sexual minorities who experienced discrimination, bullying, and harassment based on their sexual orientation, race, and/or gender were four times more likely to have used substances than individuals identifying as lesbian, bisexual, or gay who did not experience discrimination.[11]

Racial, Ethnic and Socioeconomic Disparities

Addiction affects people similarly across race, ethnicity, and socioeconomic status (SES), but risks for developing an addictive disorder are far greater among individuals in lower SES areas than those in middle and higher SES.[12] One longitudinal study with over 20,000 participants found that Hispanics reported higher initial rates of substance use compared to other racial and ethnic groups, where Caucasian individuals had higher rates of change in substance use (SU) over time and higher levels of use from adolescence into their 30s. Rates of SU were similar across racial and ethnic groups once individuals reached 30 with the exception of African Americans, who had higher rates of cannabis use into their 30s than other racial and ethnic groups.[13] Compared to individuals identifying as white, Hispanic and African Americans were also significantly less likely to receive treatment for substance use unless treatment was provided through the criminal justice system.[14]

Healthy People 2020

Healthy People 2020 set 21 objectives aimed at prevention, screening, and treatment of substance abuse, with the overarching goals to 1) increase the proportion of adolescents who disapprove of and never use substances, 2) reduce the proportion of adults who binge drink or excessively drink alcohol, 3) increase the number of admissions to substance abuse treatment centers or follow-up care and evaluation for substance abuse, 4) reduce steroid use, tobacco use, and the nonmedical use of prescription substances, 5) decrease the rate of alcohol-impaired driving, and 6) reduce substance- and alcohol-induced deaths.

According to Healthy People 2020, adolescent substance abuse has decreased from 18.4% to 17.4% since baseline data collection in 2008 and needs to decrease at the rate of 4.6% in order to meet the of goal 16.6% by 2020. Adult binge drinking, on the other hand, has not changed since 2008 and needs to decrease at the rate of 10% in order to meet the goal of 24.2% by 2020. In adults, there has been a decrease in tobacco use but not much change in teens. Therefore, approaches geared toward lowering the rates of teen smoking need to be adjusted so that Healthy People goals can be met by the year 2020.[15]

Common Substances of Abuse

Alcohol

Alcohol use and our relationship to alcohol can be deceiving, especially in a society that advertises drinking. When we see people drinking in commercials or on billboards, they are attractive, having fun, and often appear to have the kind of life that we all desire. Although drinking alcohol does not typically provide the happy-go-lucky, adventurous lifestyle that television promises us, when used *in moderation and responsibly*, some research has shown that consumption of certain types of alcohol can reduce risk of heart disease *in combination with* other healthy lifestyle behaviors such as regular exercise, maintaining a healthy body weight, and getting regular sleep.[16]

Moderate drinking is defined as consuming *up to one* drink per day for women and *up to two* drinks per day for men.[17] These guidelines may vary depending on individual and environmental factors. Such factors include having a family history of alcohol use disorders, having a smaller body frame, being or trying to become pregnant, having certain medical conditions, and/or being on medication that could interact with alcohol such as prescription opioids. While most individuals use alcohol responsibly, some individuals abuse alcohol and increase their risk for chronic physical and psychological health conditions, social problems, and sometimes death.[18]

In 2014, 17 million people over the age of 12 had an alcohol use disorder (AUD), with the highest use occurring between the ages of 18 and 25. Racially, Hispanics and Native Americans/Alaska Natives represent the highest rates of AUD between 12 and 17 years old. Among individuals 18 and over, Native Americans and Alaska Natives represent the highest 12-month prevalence of AUD, making up approximately 23% of individuals admitted into treatment for alcohol in 2014, and 18% of individuals admitted into treatment for alcohol and another illicit substance. Chronic use of alcohol can result in cancers of the mouth, esophagus, larynx, pharynx, liver, and breast, liver disease, cirrhosis, and Korsakoff's Syndrome (which is a disorder involving amnesia, blackouts, motivation issues, and memory deficits). Individuals with AUD show smaller overall brain mass than moderate drinkers, which indicates that chronic use of alcohol degenerates the brain.

Alcohol consumption can be a slippery slope because people usually place their own definition on what moderate drinking is. For example, while some people think that a 40-ounce bottle of malt liquor is "one beer," it is actually 5.71 beers, since seven ounces of malt liquor is considered "one drink" according to the National Institute on Alcohol Abuse and Alcoholism (NIAAA).[19]

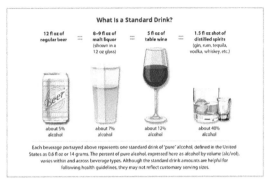

Another slippery factor when consuming alcohol is that while drinking, judgment and decision-making capabilities become impaired, and it can be difficult for people to stop drinking after a certain point. As one continues drinking, and judgment is impaired, the body becomes more and more dehydrated. The body gives a signal to drink water, but the booze-soaked brain perceives this signal as wanting more alcohol. This process can lead to drinking a lot

FIGURE 11.1   Equivalents of one standard drink

of alcohol in a short period of time, posing serious short-term effects on physical health including alcohol poisoning, coma, and death. NIAAA offers drinking guidelines that pose low risk for developing AUD. For women, low-risk drinking is defined as no more than three standard drinks on *any single day* and no more than seven standard drinks *per week*. For men, low-risk drinking is defined as no more than four standard drinks on any single day and no more than 14 standard drinks per week. NIAAA is *not* suggesting that men should consume four drinks every day or 14 drinks on one day during the week. However, if they do, they will be at risk for developing AUD particularly if they have preexisting risk factors, such as family history of substance abuse.[20]

Binge Drinking and College Students

Even if one wants to drink moderately, many factors can contribute to abusing alcohol to a point where an individual develops problematic behaviors around alcohol use. SAMHSA defines *binge drinking* as consuming five or more alcoholic beverages on the same day, and *heavy drinking* as binge drinking for five or more days in the past 30 days. Engaging in binge drinking and heavy drinking increases one's risk for developing AUD.

College students may be thinking this seems like a normal Saturday night. College students are a population in which binge drinking is embedded in the culture and is heavily reinforced by society and the media. In the United States, approximately 20 million students are enrolled in college. Approximately 60% of those college students consume alcohol within a 30-day period and 2/3 of that population engage in binge drinking. That equals approximately eight million people between the ages of 18 and 22 engaging in binge drinking. Additionally, about one in five college binge drinkers meet criteria for AUD or a problematic pattern of alcohol use leading to clinically significant impairment or distress.[21]

There are significant health and socioeconomic concerns for college binge drinkers and their families. One of the most obvious concerns is an increase in academic problems. About 25% of college binge drinkers between the ages of 18 and 22 do poorer on exams, are more absent from classes and fall behind on assignments, and receive overall poorer grades.[22] On campuses that make students share the cost of vandalism, each student may be charged for property damage that occurs when students are drunk and reckless. More severe consequences of regular binge drinking are the increased likelihood of experiencing and perpetrating assault and sexual violence. Approximately 696,000 students are physically assaulted by another student who has been drinking, and 100,000 students are raped when under the influence of alcohol. Sadly, every year almost 2,000 young, bright-minded individuals die from alcohol-related incidents from unintentional injuries, including motor-vehicle accidents and alcohol poisoning. Suicide attempts, unprotected sex, and other high-risk behaviors are also more likely to occur after binge drinking.[23]

Many social, psychological and environmental factors are at play that encourage binge drinking behavior. For many young college students, having freedom from parental supervision paired with greater availability of alcohol and peer pressure creates an environment with fewer immediate and direct consequences of drinking, like getting in trouble with parents. Certain fraternities and sororities promote a culture of wild parties and may also have dangerous and deadly hazing rituals in which individuals are asked to drink lethal amounts of alcohol and often perform some activity while under the influence. Additionally, depression is directly and positively related to binge drinking (i.e., the more depressed a person is, the more he or she drinks). However, females who were depressed AND experienced school stress were less likely to binge drink. Male juniors and seniors also tend to drink more than freshmen and sophomores.[24]

Alcoholism in Older Adulthood

One population that, until recently, has received little attention in addiction research is older adults. Due to projected increases in life expectancy and a larger portion of the population living into old age (21% by 2030),[25] it is expected that there will be more adults with substance use disorders, specifically alcohol abuse and prescription pain medication use. The lack of attention given to this population is due to ageism, lack of awareness, clinician behavior, and comorbid disorders. An underlying assumption in our culture is that treating addiction in older adults is not a worthwhile effort because they were born during a time when alcohol abuse was socially acceptable, or the quality of life of older adults will only be poorer if substances are "taken" from them. This is evidenced by attitudes like "Evening cocktails are the only thing that makes Grandma happy" or "Just let him drink; he won't be around much longer anyway." However, many older adults use substances because they feel lonely, have been injured, or are losing loved ones as they age. They are facing mortality and what their existence has meant up until the present. Additionally, older adults are less likely to drive and have smaller social circles, which make it more difficult to detect substance use disorders. There is also stigma, and many older adults consider substance use a "private matter" that they do not want others to know about or may be too embarrassed to share with their health care provider. Clinicians' behavior also plays a role in not detecting substance use in older adults. They often do not ask about substance use because of assumptions that it is not happening and spend a very short amount of time with their older patients to screen for substance use.[26]

Effects of Alcohol Abuse on the Family

While AUD and alcohol abuse has obvious effects on individuals who endorse these behaviors, it can also tear families apart and contribute to generational trauma for future generations of a family. Families who have a caretaker (or several caretakers) who abuse alcohol throw the family system off balance by not fulfilling their expected roles. For example, caretakers with AUD may have greater missing days of work or hospitalization days and may not be able to fulfill their obligations of paying for housing, food, and school supplies for children, monitoring their children, or getting their children to school. Children of adult alcoholics may have to pick up more responsibilities such as taking on a job, caretaking for younger siblings, or caretaking for parents. This decreases the amount of time children can spend on their own academic work and limits the amount of time they can spend just being a kid.

It is also often the case that if one spouse is an alcoholic, the other spouse takes on the responsibility of two adults in the household. Spouses of alcoholics may spend a lot of time covering up for their significant other or making excuses for their behaviors around drinking. This will often tear the partnership apart and cause either hostile fights or distancing which can also cause an instable structure for children growing up in these households. It also models maladaptive behavioral patterns around addressing problems and may cause dysfunction in the relationships of the children when they become adults.

Opioids

Opioids are central nervous system (CNS) depressants derived from opium poppies. The body has naturally occurring pain relievers that are activated when the body goes through intensive pain or physical trauma. When opioids are ingested, they mimic the body's naturally occurring endorphins and produce the same euphoric and pain-relieving effects. Individuals with chronic pain conditions or recovering from surgery are sometimes prescribed opioid medication (i.e., oxycodone, hydrocodone, Dilaudid) in order to gain increased functioning in daily life or to comfortably get through an intense healing process.

Opioid addiction has quickly become an epidemic in the United States and is becoming increasingly more prevalent in younger populations. In 2014, 435,000 people 12 and older were current heroin users, representing about 2% of the U.S. population. In 2002–2013, heroin dependence doubled from 100,000 to 200,000 people, and there was an astonishing 286% increase in heroin overdose related deaths. Overdose death rates have increased by 26% between 2013 and 2014 alone.[27] People can ingest heroin in many ways. Intravenous heroine use (i.e., via a needle) is the most dangerous and addictive method of ingestion. Injecting heroin can lead to blood-borne viruses such as HIV and Hepatitis C and result in bacterial infections like abscesses. Some individuals smoke or snort heroin, which also increases an individual's likelihood to contract lung diseases such as pneumonia, infection of the heart valves and arteries, and liver disease. Heroin that contains additives may also cause clogging of the blood vessels in the heart, lungs, kidneys, liver, and brain.

Prescription Pain Medications in America

Prescription pain medication prevalence has skyrocketed and is an even larger epidemic than heroin use in the U.S. Approximately 4.3 million people in 2015 were non-medical users of pain relievers. Addiction to pain relievers has increased by 150% since 1999, and prescriptions for pain medication have also increased fourfold since 2002. It is no surprise that with the increased accessibility of prescription pain medication there is a significant increase in pain-medication-overdose deaths. Most individuals using prescription pain medication for non-medical purposes received them from a close relative, friends, or their physician. In fact, 4% of doctors in the United States, many of whom are not pain specialists, are prescribing more than 60% of the pain medication[28].

A documentary on Netflix, "The Oxycontin Express," describes the influence of pill mills, or medical offices that indiscriminately write prescription opioids for individuals who do not have sufficient evidence of a chronic or acute pain condition. Although this significantly contributes to opioid addiction in the U.S., many state public health agencies have been cracking down on these practices. Another factor that contributes to increases in opioid addiction is non-pain specialist doctors prescribing high-dose opioid medication. Physicians who are not trained specifically in pain management can give individuals a strong pain reliever without tapering them off slowly as they complete their course of treatment. In this case, the person will go through withdrawal symptoms and may be compelled to find another (often illegal) method of obtaining opioids.

Withdrawal symptoms from opioids are probably one of the most severe of all substance classes. Symptoms of opioid withdrawal include negative mood, vomiting, diarrhea, insomnia, aching bones and muscles, sweating, fever, and yawning, all at once. Many people describe this experience as having the worst flu and multiplying it by 100. These symptoms can last between two and three weeks, and the only thing that relieves the symptoms is using opioids again or waiting out the symptoms, which can be very difficult to do if the person has other obligations such as school, a job, or a family to care for. The constant struggle between wanting to be free of this substance's grasp and wanting to avoid withdrawal at all costs makes opioid addiction one of the most difficult from which to recover.[29]

Psychologically, many people who use opioids for non-medical purposes or not as prescribed often report wanting to "feel better." Individuals who abuse opioids often have had childhood trauma, witnessed or were a victim to violence, or had chaotic family environments. When individuals are dealt a tough deck of cards early in life, they are more prone to mental and physical health conditions that follow them through adulthood. These individuals may view opioids as a temporary escape from painful emotions and memories.

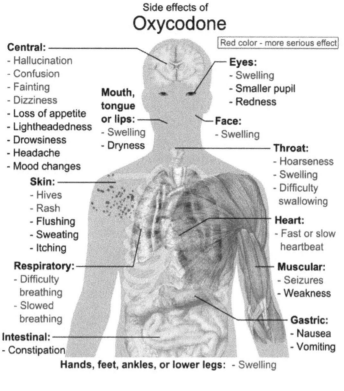

Side effects of
Oxycodone

Red color - more serious effect

Central:
- Hallucination
- Confusion
- Fainting
- Dizziness
- Loss of appetite
- Lightheadedness
- Drowsiness
- Headache
- Mood changes

Mouth, tongue or lips:
- Swelling
- Dryness

Skin:
- Hives
- Rash
- Flushing
- Sweating
- Itching

Respiratory:
- Difficulty breathing
- Slowed breathing

Intestinal:
- Constipation

Eyes:
- Swelling
- Smaller pupil
- Redness

Face:
- Swelling

Throat:
- Hoarseness
- Swelling
- Difficulty swallowing

Heart:
- Fast or slow heartbeat

Muscular:
- Seizures
- Weakness

Gastric:
- Nausea
- Vomiting

Hands, feet, ankles, or lower legs: - Swelling

FIGURE 11.2   Side effects of Oxycodone

Mixing Substances

Some people use opioids in combination with other CNS depressants (i.e. alcohol, anxiolytics) causing a synergistic effect which increases the effect of the substance more than if only one of the substances was taken alone. This can slow the CNS down to a dangerous rate and often results in substance overdose. Jim Morrison, Heath Ledger, Elvis Presley, and Kurt Cobain (who ingested a CNS cocktail before committing suicide) died from this combination. Alternatively, another lethal and highly addictive cocktail of substances is the mixing of opioids and a CNS stimulant, such as cocaine. Some individuals dissolve both of these substances into a single injection (known as a speedball) or snort both of these substances at the same time (crisscross). This mixture confuses the CNS because one substance slows it down while the other speeds it up. This rapid change in physiological functioning can cause heart failure and instant death, much like Chris Farley and John Belushi's death after injecting speedballs.

Opioid Treatment

Although some people quit opioids cold turkey, the most common treatment for opioid addiction is through Medication Assisted Treatment (MAT) programs. Full opioid agonists like methadone or partial agonists like buprenorphine block (or partially block) opioid receptors in the brain, which eventually extinguishes withdrawal symptoms. Not having withdrawal symptoms leads to a decrease in cravings or the need to take illicit opioids. Additionally, opioid blockers stop the effects of any other opioids that are ingested while on MAT so that individuals seeking treatment will not get high from taking their opioid of choice, which reduces the likelihood that people will continue using or paying for opioids if they are not experiencing the "feel-good" effects. The cessation of withdrawal, the decrease in cravings, and lack of behavioral reinforcement can help individuals change their substance abuse behavior and begin to make positive changes in their lives. Since methadone and buprenorphine are opioid-based, however, there is the potential to abuse and become addicted to these substances. With careful monitoring from health care providers and behavioral health care specialists, as well as willingness of individuals with opioid addiction to work hard on their recovery, MAT can be a very successful treatment for stopping opioid use for good.

Naloxone (Narcan)

According to the CDC, over 42,000 people die annually from opioid overdose. In turn, one important way that people can prevent accidental overdose and death from opioids is with rapidly delivered antagonist therapy, which blocks the effects of opioids. This medication has been available since the 1960s and is declared by the World Health Organization to be a crucial medication for emergency and health delivery systems. It is often used in

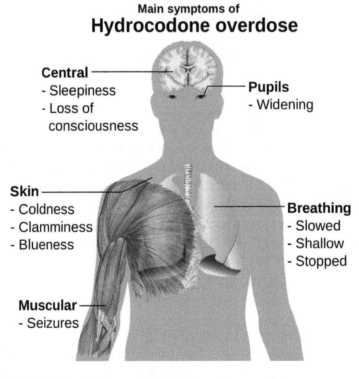

FIGURE 11.3   Main symptoms of Hydrocodone overdose

emergency settings. With the surge of opioid use throughout the U.S., this method is not only routinely used in emergency departments and among emergency transportation personal (emergency medical technicians or ambulance personnel), but now family members and other individuals who live with people who use heavy amounts of opioids and heroin are also often encouraged to have Naloxone on hand in case of emergency. It is now, for instance, available at easy-to-obtain locations, including Walgreens, and active "take home naloxone" campaigns have been initiated by health organizations such as the WHO.[30] Naloxone is delivered orally (via pill) or delivered into the body intravenously or via injection into muscle. When delivered via injection or intravenously, the medication can halt the effects of opioids in less than five minutes; however, it comes with very difficult side effects, including agitation, nausea, and increased heart rate. It often requires multiple injections to sustain effects.

Effects of Opioid Use on Individual, Family and Community Well-being

As with any addiction, opioid abuse can also challenge an individual's social functioning and well-being. As mentioned before, when an individual experiences withdrawal symptoms, there is no way to hide it. As family, friends, and colleagues begin to notice that an individual regularly has "the flu," they begin to wonder what is going on. With addiction comes shame and guilt, isolation from family members, and severe mental health concerns. Even when people with opioid abuse enter into maintenance treatment (i.e., methadone, suboxone), they may experience stigma. Individuals in methadone maintenance treatment report being shunned by recovery communities, as abstinence-based programs (i.e., Narcotics Anonymous) believe that using methadone in treatment is not practicing true abstinence. As discussed, however, people with opioid addiction cannot quit "cold turkey" like with other substances; it has to be a slow, tapering process while building relapse prevention skills and coping skills to manage life stressors without using opioids. It is important for individuals tapering off opioids to have social support and high quality care to successfully manage their addiction. Since opioid use disorder is so prevalent and community clinics often lack the resources needed to support individuals seeking treatment, lowering the rates of opioid use has been challenging. More preventative care, policy changes, and oversight around prescribing opioids must be implemented in order to effectively address this issue.

Substance-Exposed Newborns

Probably the most vulnerable victims of addiction are newborns. Mothers who use substances during their pregnancy subject their newborn babies to withdrawal symptoms as one of their first experiences of being alive in the world. Infant withdrawal, more commonly known as Neonatal Abstinence Syndrome (NAS), occurs when mothers use substances up to a week before giving birth. The substance passes through the placenta, which makes the baby addicted to whatever substance was being used. Once the baby is born, he or she is no longer receiving the substance through the mother and begins to have withdrawal symptoms about one to seven days after birth. NAS can be caused from use of opioids, alcohol, benzodiazepines, barbiturates, and some antidepressant medications.

Symptoms of NAS depend of the substance that was used, the frequency, duration and amount that was used, genetic factors of how the substance breaks down in the body, and if the baby was born full term or prematurely. Symptoms of NAS include excessive crying, motor agitation, sweating, respiratory, digestive, and cardiovascular difficulties, irritability, and seizures, just to name a few. Other complications that can occur in addition to NAS are low birth weight and premature birth, birth defects, smaller head circumference, and developmental and behavioral problems later in life. Again, treatment differs depending on individual factors, but they typically include receiving extra fluid through IV if the baby is dehydrated from vomiting and diarrhea, as well as receiving medication such as methadone or phenobarbital to reduce withdrawal and calm the infant down. Higher calorie diets may also be a part of the treatment for infants with NAS if they are having problems with feeding. Lastly and most importantly, providing infants with extra snuggles during these difficult months will help them to feel loved and supported through their withdrawal and recovery period.

There are many barriers to women receiving the care that they need while pregnant. For one, many women who are economically disadvantaged may not have proper access to prenatal and neonatal care, and the community facilities that are available may have long waitlists for admission and poor treatment implementation. These factors decrease the chances of seeking and adhering to treatment. Second, pregnant women who are addicted to illicit substances likely have partners who are also using illicit substances. They may receive little support from their partner or they may even be discouraged from receiving treatment and care due to the fear of being arrested for possession and use of illegal substances. There is also a real fear of Child Protective Services taking the baby away from the mother if someone finds out she is using while pregnant. This is especially true if other children are residing in the home. Lastly, although one would hope that a pregnant mother on substances would share this information with her health care provider, pregnant mothers often experience stigma and judgment by health care providers, making them less likely to ask for help during this vulnerable time.[31, 32]

Cannabis

In 2014, cannabis was reported as the number one illicit substance used in the United States. It was estimated that 22.2 million people 12 and older are current users of cannabis, with the highest use in people aged 18 to 25. Although rates of cannabis use remained consistent for 18 to 26 year olds, there was an increase in cannabis use in individuals aged 26 and older. In 2013, the average age individuals tried cannabis for the first time was 18 years old, and for 70% of individuals, cannabis was the first illicit substance they tried.[33]

Short-term effects of cannabis after intoxication can differ depending on the strength of chemicals in the cannabis plant. On average, most individuals will experience euphoria, lapses in memory, distortions in time perception, psychomotor and cognitive impairments, elevated appetite, and changes in motivation and energy level. Long-term effects of highly concentrated cannabis include memory and cognitive impairment, diminished executive functioning and IQ, and anxiety.[34]

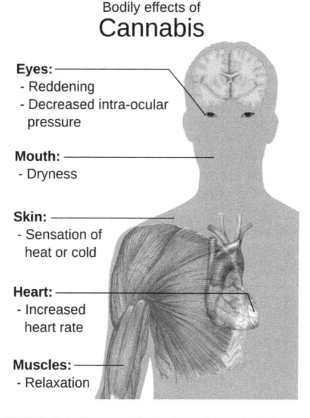

Bodily effects of
Cannabis

Eyes:
- Reddening
- Decreased intra-ocular pressure

Mouth:
- Dryness

Skin:
- Sensation of heat or cold

Heart:
- Increased heart rate

Muscles:
- Relaxation

FIGURE 11.4   **Common effects of cannabis on the body**

Legalization of Cannabis in the United States

Today, there is a great divide in the United States regarding cannabis and its place in our society. Although still considered a felony under federal jurisdiction, laws regarding cannabis vary by state. Alaska, Oregon, Colorado, Washington, California, Nevada, Massachusetts, and Maine are the only states in the U.S. that have legalized cannabis for recreational and medicinal use, while an additional 19 states plus Washington, D.C. have legalized cannabis for medical use and decriminalized possession of cannabis without a medical card. In other states such as Alabama or Wisconsin, possession of cannabis will result in a felony.[35]

The legalization of cannabis has the potential to bring billions of untaxed dollars floating around the black market into the hands of American consumers. In 2014 Colorado made 700 million dollars in cannabis sales, and it is estimated that in 2016, it will be a billion-dollar retail market just for that state alone. Oregon legalized cannabis in July of 2015 with 11 million dollars in legal sales during the first week with a 25% tax rate to go toward public health services. The legalization of cannabis also creates jobs and decreases incarcerated populations. Similar to alcohol laws, restrictions on age and when and where to use cannabis will be set in place. In Oregon, law enforcement is developing a cannabis

Breathalyzer to detect if an individual is intoxicated while driving. Cannabis use is also illegal to individuals under the age of 21.[36]

Cannabis Addiction: "Not Your Father's Weed"

Although many people give an eye roll at the idea of cannabis being an addictive substance, its increasing tetrahydrocannabinol (THC) levels has increased the risk for physiological and psychological dependence. An article entitled "Not Your Father's Weed" describes the increasing dosage of THC in cannabis and the implications it is having on human health and functioning. In 1974, the average amount of THC found in cannabis was >1%, and 3–4% in the 1990s. Today, the average amount of THC found in cannabis is 13%, with the highest concentrations at 37%. Other concentrated forms of THC like Dabs contain upwards of 70–90% THC. High-concentration THC can place individuals at risk for heightened CNS activity such as increased heart rate and blood pressure, feelings of anxiety and panic, and home or automobile accidents. In the last two years, emergency room visits have increased by 19% due to cannabis use. It is no surprise that with rising THC levels, there is a greater incidence of cannabis addiction. Withdrawal from cannabis is not life threatening as with alcohol, cocaine, or opioids. An individual will feel extremely uncomfortable, irritable, and anxious.[37]

Medical Cannabis

With today's technology, scientists are able to modify cannabis plants to control concentrations of state-altering chemicals to produce certain effects. Some studies have provided evidence to suggest that modified cannabis can assist with symptoms related to cancer,[38] neurodegenerative disorders,[39] schizophrenia,[40] and chronic pain,[41,42] while one review showed that there was not enough clinical evidence to suggest its medicinal efficacy due to sample size and lack of randomized-control trials.[43] More research is needed to understand how best to use cannabis for pain or medical management.

Cannabis Use in College Students

Not surprisingly, daily use of cannabis is at the highest that it is has been since 1980 in college students and has tripled since 1994.[44] Although cannabis may seem "harmless" compared to other substances of abuse, the impact of using cannabis regularly on college success is not so harmless. The more frequently college-aged individuals use cannabis, the more they report academic difficulties (e.g., impairments in memory and motivation, poor grades), psychiatric impairment (e.g., depression, anxiety, panic attacks, paranoia), and cannabis-related problems (e.g., legal, financial, and occupational problems). College students who are more likely to use cannabis are those who have at least $100 in spending money a month, smoke cigarettes, use alcohol or other illicit substances, and are sensation seekers.[45] Although some research suggests that cannabis-focused interventions could be useful in reducing cannabis-related problems in college students,[46] college students simply are not very interested in receiving treatment to reduce cannabis use. In one study, the 14% of students who were interested in receiving treatment were more likely to have several and severe cannabis-related problems, family problems, and problems with executive functioning.[47]

Tobacco

Tobacco is the number one most preventable cause of death in the U.S. Approximately 480,000 people die from tobacco-related issues each year.[48] That is more deaths in one year than deaths from HIV, illegal-substance use, alcohol use, motor vehicle accidents, and firearm-related incidents combined. More than 10 times the amount of people in the U.S. have died from smoking than have died from war in all U.S. history. It was estimated in 2015 that 4% of eighth graders, 7.9% of tenth graders, and 13% of twelfth graders were current users of tobacco. Although the prevalence of tobacco use is still alarming, the good news is that these numbers have decreased compared to prior years.[49]

Several kinds of tobacco products can be purchased in the U.S. at 18 years and older. Combustible tobacco refers to tobacco one can light up and smoke such as cigarettes, cigars, and hookah. Although some people believe that smoking hookah is healthier than smoking cigarettes, it actually poses the same health-related risks as cigarettes and may even result in exposing the smoker to more toxins.[50] Cigarettes have over 7,000 chemicals when burned, and 69 of those are known carcinogens.[51] Smokeless tobacco products, like snuff, chew, or dissolvable tobacco are less lethal than combustible tobacco but far from safe. Smokeless tobacco is placed in the mouth, usually between the teeth and gums, and nicotine is absorbed through oral tissue. The use of smokeless tobacco causes oral cancers and periodontal disease. E-cigarettes, or vapor cigarettes, are another form of tobacco that is gaining popularity, especially among people who are trying to quit smoking combustible cigarettes. An alluring aspect of the e-cigarette is that an individual does not have to burn tobacco to inhale the nicotine, which appears to decrease the amount of toxins that are administered to the body when compared to traditional cigarettes.[52] However, not enough data exists to conclude that the e-cigarette is a safer alternative to combustible cigarettes.

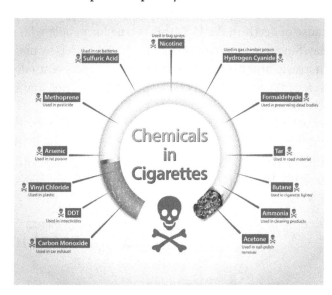

FIGURE 11.5   A selection of the chemicals and carcinogens in cigarettes

Effects of Tobacco on the Body

Although some people may consider tobacco a depressant for its seemingly relaxing effects, nicotine, the addictive substance in tobacco, mimics a neurotransmitter called acetylcholine. The nicotine binds to acetylcholine's receptor site, causing the body's adrenal system to be activated. The boost in CNS activity increases heart rate and blood pressure, and often gives individuals feelings of motivation and focus. Nicotine also causes a release of dopamine, which is the "reward" hormone and is why people have so much difficulty quitting smoking. In chronic smokers, the receptor sites become desensitized and using tobacco no longer activates the body as well as it did during first use.

Tobacco use is associated with a plethora of chronic diseases and cancer of every single organ in the body. Tobacco use is very closely linked to lung cancer but also causes cancers such as oral cancers and bladder cancers. Anywhere the toxins travel, such as through the bladder in urine, will be exposed to the carcinogens. An individual who smokes tobacco is also two to four times more likely to develop coronary heart disease, which is the leading cause of death in the U.S. This is true for people who smoke fewer than five cigarettes a day. Smoking tobacco damages the blood vessels by making them thick and narrow, which increases heart rate, blood pressure, and can eventually cause clotting. Stroke is also two to four times more likely to occur from smoking, and results from blood clots flowing up to the brain.[53]

Tobacco and Lung Cancer

The correlation between smoking tobacco and lung cancer is obvious. Annually, lung cancer care and loss-in-productivity costs totaled an estimated 46.2 billion dollars in the United

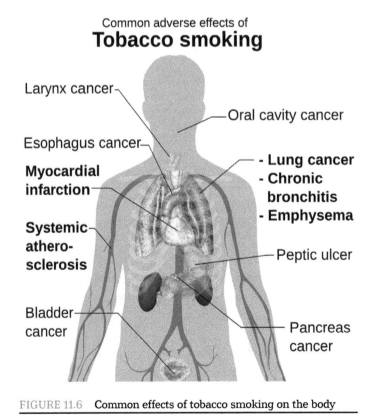

FIGURE 11.6   Common effects of tobacco smoking on the body

States.[54] Smoking increases the risk for developing lung cancer by 25 times, and smoking tobacco causes nine of every 10 incidences of lung cancer. Rates of lung cancer have decreased by 28% for men while increasing by 98% for women over the last 37 years, which is due to a generational shift. Smoking was once considered a "man's habit," but more young women have recently picked up the habit. African American males and females who smoke are the most vulnerable populations for developing lung cancer.[55]

While fewer people over the age of 65 smoke compared to younger folks, more than 65% of people diagnosed with lung cancer are over the age of 65.[56] Individuals who may have smoked in their youth but quit later in life are still at risk for this silent and chronic killer. One of the main reasons why lung cancer is so deadly is because of its late detection and diagnosis. Screening tools used to detect lung cancer are not sensitive enough to determining early stages of cancer, so most lung cancers are detected after they have significantly progressed. Sadly, only 10% of people diagnosed with lung cancer will live past five years. The U.S. task force on prevention recommends that Low-Dosed Computer Tomography be used as the standard screening tool in individuals who smoke 30 packs a year and are current smokers or have quit smoking within 15 years because it is more sensitive to small cellular changes attributed to cancer. Screens are recommended every year until an individual has ceased tobacco use for at least 15 years.[57] Additionally, smoking is related to 80% of individuals who develop Chronic Obstructive Pulmonary Disease, which accounts for the third-leading cause of death in the United States. If no one smoked, cancer rates would be reduced by 33%. Smoking also negatively impacts people around the smoker, as 41,000 non-smokers die each year due to second-hand smoke exposure.[58]

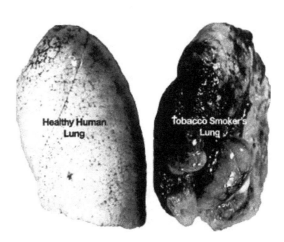

FIGURE 11.7 Healthy lungs vs. lungs of a smoker

Tobacco Use Among Adolescents

Adolescents are more likely to smoke at an earlier age if their parents, friends, and siblings smoke, if they have poor relationships with their parents, and if the teen lacks supervision. Childhood stressors such as abuse and violence in the household increases a teen's risk of smoking by age 14, with continued use into adulthood. Exposure to cigarette advertisements or promotional tobacco items, as well as ease of obtaining tobacco from parents or siblings, predicts earlier onset of smoking in teens. Additionally, Hispanic teens are more likely to smoke or drink than African-American teens, and low socioeconomic status predicts earlier onset of smoking as a teenager.[59,60] Smoking tobacco is also strongly associated with drinking alcohol in social contexts,[61] making adolescence a vulnerable time. On the bright side, as cigarettes get more expensive, it increases the likelihood that adolescents quit smoking.

Substance Abuse: How It Affects the Family's Health and Well-Being

Family members react in many different ways when loved ones develop an addiction. Many families try to intervene and give support when family members are struggling with addiction. Unfortunately, addiction is very difficult to overcome, and relapse is common. The continuous cycle of relapse can become tiring and heartbreaking for family members who are trying to support and help loved ones. Some families may have a difficult time confronting the addiction and may cope in maladaptive and unhelpful ways (e.g., getting very angry). Some family members might compensate for that individual's behavior change by cleaning up after him or her, working more hours due to the person's lack of contribution, or blaming themselves for the addicted family member's behavior. They might decrease their interaction with other family members and friends due to feelings of isolation, shame, or embarrassment. It is also common for family members to feel denial toward the individual(s) in their family who are struggling with addiction and go on functioning as if there is no problem at all. For others, the stress of addiction may eventually become too great, leading to a decision to terminate contact with their loved one.[62]

Children whose parents use substances not only have more challenges growing up but also have challenges in their own adult lives. Parents who are substance users may neglect to meet the very basic needs of their children.[63] Their children may also be put in dangerous situations if their parents allow them around other substance users. Children may face the challenge of unstable housing if parents are unable to keep a steady income or if parents are incarcerated due to substance use. Children may have to move to other relative's homes or may have to be in foster care if no one is available to care for them in place of their parents. Grandparents who take over primary parenting roles are becoming an increasing reality, especially as the number of opioid-related deaths increase in the U.S. When children of parents with addiction grow up, those children have a greater risk to develop addictive or psychological disorders. Even if children do not become substance users themselves, they may not have had a model for healthy relationship functioning, which may impact relationships in their adulthood with their own partners and children.[64] Children who have had unstable relationships with their parents tend to have insecure attachment styles if they have not had a relationship with another stable adult figure in their lifetime.[65] They are at greater risk for developing depression, anxiety, PTSD, or Borderline Personality Disorder.[66,67] Since addiction very clearly impacts everyone in the family, Family Systems Therapy combined with substance abuse treatment can be a particularly effective treatment for addiction. Family therapy allows every person in the family to voice his or her feelings and concerns, reassess roles in the family, obtain information about the disease, problem solve the consequence of the addictive behaviors, and be part of the plan to move forward in recovery.

Community-Level Interventions: Drug-Free Community Programs

Community-level interventions for substance abuse typically involve a coordinated set of preventive interventions throughout the community. A particularly effective approach to preventing and intervening in substance abuse includes community coalitions. Community coalitions are comprised of organizations that work together to provide outreach, education, prevention, service delivery, capacity building, empowerment, community action, community policing and systems change.[68] Created through the Drug Free Communities Act of 1997, the Office of National Drug Control Policy and the Substance Abuse and Mental Health Services Administration fund *Drug-Free Community Programs* (DFCs). DFCs aim to reduce substance use and increase collaboration among community agencies and leaders to address substance-related problems. Drug-free community programs use the proven effective, "Seven Strategies for Change" model which includes 1) providing information, 2) enhancing skills, 3) providing support, 4) enhancing access and reducing barriers, 5) changing consequences, 6) changing physical design, and 7) modifying and changing policies. Each of these strategies is facilitated by different agencies. For instance, modifying and changing policies likely requires efforts at the local government level to alter laws. Changing physical design might include adding lights to parks or surveillance to neighborhoods known for trafficking. Enhancing access and reducing barriers includes providing transportation to treatment or childcare during treatment sessions. Community coalitions have been very successful at decreasing substance use at the middle and high school levels, which results in a broad range of benefits in both families and communities. Other programs, such as Community Oriented Policing Services (COPS) are similar in that they facilitate partnerships between community health agencies and law enforcement. These programs facilitate police and community collaboration, which allows both parties to address underlying issues, change negative patterns of behavior, and make sure resources are allocated to those who need them. Specific initiatives can be found at https://cops.usdoj.gov.

Conclusion

Substance use and abuse results in a wide range of implications for individuals, families, and communities. Although this chapter reviewed only a handful of substances, the impact of substance use and abuse on individuals, families, and communities displays similar patterns across substances. While most people do not plan to use and abuse substances, it is important to remember that people start using substances for good reasons, such as a way to cope with their struggles. There is no one way to treat or prevent substance abuse, and community leaders and agencies must work together to create environments that promote healthy living and productive lives for all living in America.

Case Study

Elliott is a 19-year-old, first-generation female of Puerto Rican decent who was born and raised in a low socioeconomic status neighborhood on the east coast. She is the third of five siblings and was primarily raised by her older sister, who is now away at college. Her mother and father work for several hours a day at minimum wage jobs and do not see their children very often, except for late in the evenings. Elliott has taken the burden of caring for her younger siblings who are 12 and 14 years old because her older brother was incarcerated due to substance trafficking about six months ago. Elliott had a very close relationship with her older brother and felt devastated when her brother was taken to prison. It also placed a greater hardship on her family because her older brother helped pay for household expenses. Although Elliott's older sister tries her best to help out from far away, Elliott's parents have to compensate for the finances that were provided by her older brother, and Elliott had to take fewer classes at her community college so that she could help watch over her younger siblings and care for the house.

Elliott has been experiencing severe mood swings since her brother went to prison. She experiences explosive anger to a point where she will drive recklessly and also punch the walls of her bedroom until her knuckles bleed. When she is not angry, she experiences severe depression. She will not get up from bed except for when she has to walk her younger siblings home from school and sometimes misses class because she has little energy. She often cries alone in her room thinking about what life would have been like if her brother did not get incarcerated. She often has suicidal ideation because of her anger, depression, and greater responsibility to the family. She sometimes wishes that she could have a "normal life" and that her parents would be around more often to care for her siblings so that she could move away like her sister to pursue her education.

Within the last three months she has been drinking heavily by herself in her room. She consumes two 40-ounce bottles of malt liquor everyday before she has to pick up her brothers from school, and when she can, she will consume up to five shots of whiskey a night. Elliott is able to get alcohol from the liquor store that her brother's best friend works at. She has been able to hide this from her parents because they return home from work at 9 p.m., and she often makes the excuse that she is tired from studying. Within the last month her drinking has noticeably increased. Because of this, she has gone to school with hangovers and has not been turning in her coursework. She has also been missing more classes and even dropped out of one class. Lately her parents have been noticing Elliott's behavior and the smell of alcohol coming from Elliott's room. They also once found empty bottles of alcohol hidden in her closet. Elliott's parents are worried about her, but they are fearful to approach her because of her anger outbursts and do not want to make her upset. They are also unsure of how to approach this situation because in their culture, it is shameful for a young woman to have a drinking problem. They feel it reflects badly on their parenting, and they already feel embarrassed that their son was incarcerated for substance trafficking. They pray about Elliott everyday and consult with their pastor about options to help her. Their pastor suggested that she should enter a support group through AA while signing up for intensive treatment. There is usually a long waitlist for the community-based clinic due to the high need for addiction services in their area.

Notes

1 Hallucinogens and dissociative drugs. (2015). NIDA. Retrieved January 11, 2017, from https://www.drugabuse.gov/publications/research-reports/hallucinogens-dissociative-drugs

2 Behavioral health trends in the United States: Results from the 2014 National Survey on Drug Use and Health (HHS Publication No. SMA 15–4927, NSDUH Series H-50). (2015). Center for Behavioral Health Statistics and Quality. Retrieved from http://www.samhsa.gov/data/

3 Hallucinogens and dissociative drugs. (2015). NIDA. Retrieved January 11, 2017, from https://www.drugabuse.gov/publications/research-reports/hallucinogens-dissociative-drugs

4 *Diagnostic and statistical manual of mental disorders, 5th ed. (DSM-5)* (2013). Washington, DC: American Psychiatric Association.

5 Ducci, F., & Goldman, D. (2012). The genetic basis of addictive disorders. *The Psychiatric Clinics of North America, 35*(2), 495–519. http://doi.org/10.1016/j.psc.2012.03.010

6 Hallucinogens and dissociative drugs. (2015). NIDA. Retrieved January 11, 2017, from https://www.drugabuse.gov/publications/research-reports/hallucinogens-dissociative-drugs

7 Behavioral health trends in the United States: Results from the 2014 National Survey on Drug Use and Health (HHS Publication No. SMA 15–4927, NSDUH Series H-50). (2015). Center for Behavioral Health Statistics and Quality. Retrieved from http://www.samhsa.gov/ data/

8 Merikangas, K. R., & McClair, V. L. (2012). Epidemiology of substance use disorders. *Human Genetics, 131*(6), 779–789. http://doi.org/10.1007/s00439-012-1168-0

9 Lev-Ran, S., Le Strat, Y., Imtiaz, S., Rehm, J., & Le Foll, B. (2013). Gender differences in prevalence of substance use disorders among individuals with lifetime exposure to substances: Results from a large representative sample. *The American Journal on Addictions, 22*(1), 7–13. doi:10.1111/j.1521-0391.2013.00321.x

10 Corliss, H. L., Rosario, M., Wypij, D., Wylie, S. A., Frazier, A. L., & Austin, S. B. (2010). Sexual orientation and drug use in a longitudinal cohort study of U.S. adolescents. *Addictive Behaviors, 35*(5), 517–521.doi:http://dx.doi.org/10.1016/j.addbeh.2009.12.019

11 McCabe, S. E., Bostwick, W. B., Hughes, T. L., West, B. T., & Boyd, C. J. (2010). The relationship between discrimination and substance use disorders among lesbian, gay, and bisexual adults in the United States. *American Journal of Public Health, 100*(10), 1946–1952. doi:10.2105/AJPH.2009.163147

12 Redonnet, B., Chollet, A., Fombonne, E., Bowes, L., & Melchior, M. (2012). Tobacco, alcohol, cannabis and other illegal drug use among young adults: The socioeconomic context. *Drug and Alcohol Dependence, 121*(3), 231–239. doi:http://dx.doi.org/10.1016/j.drugalcdep.2011.09.002

13 Chen, P., & Jacobson, K. C. (2012). Developmental trajectories of substance use from early adolescence to young adulthood: Gender and racial/ethnic differences. *Journal of Adolescent Health, 50*(2), 154–163. doi:http://dx.doi.org/10.1016/j.jadohealth.2011.05.013

14 Hatzenbuehler, M. L., Keyes, K. M., Narrow, W. E., Grant, B. F., & Hasin, D. S. (2008). Racial/ethnic disparities in service utilization for individuals with co-occurring mental health and substance use disorders in the general population. *Journal of Clinical Psychiatry, 69*(7), 1112–1121.

15 Healthy People 2020 [Internet]. (n.d.). U.S. Department of Health and Human Services, Office of Disease Prevention and Health Promotion [cited 11/21/2016]. Available from: https://www.healthypeople.gov/2020.

16 Alcohol: Balancing risks and benefits. (2015). Harvard School of Public Health. Retrieved on 11/21/2016 from https://www.hsph.harvard.edu/nutritionsource/alcohol-full-story/

17 College drinking. (2015). NIAAA. Retrieved on 9/22/2015 from http://pubs.niaaa.nih.gov/publications/CollegeFactSheet/CollegeFactSheet.pdf

18 College drinking. (2015). NIAAA. Retrieved on 9/22/2015 from http://pubs.niaaa.nih.gov/publications/CollegeFactSheet/CollegeFactSheet.pdf

19 College drinking. (2015). NIAAA. Retrieved on 9/22/2015 from http://pubs.niaaa.nih.gov/publications/CollegeFactSheet/CollegeFactSheet.pdf

20 College drinking. (2015). NIAAA. Retrieved on 9/22/2015 from http://pubs.niaaa.nih.gov/publications/CollegeFactSheet/CollegeFactSheet.pdf

21 Behavioral health trends in the United States: Results from the 2014 National Survey on Drug Use and Health (HHS Publication No. SMA 15–4927, NSDUH Series H-50). (2015). Center for Behavioral Health Statistics and Quality. Retrieved from http://www.samhsa.gov/ data/

22 College drinking. (2015). NIAAA. Retrieved on 9/22/2015 from http://pubs.niaaa.nih.gov/publications/CollegeFactSheet/CollegeFactSheet.pdf

23 College drinking. (2015). NIAAA. Retrieved on 9/22/2015 from http://pubs.niaaa.nih.gov/publications/CollegeFactSheet/CollegeFactSheet.pdf

24 Pedersen, D. E. (2013). Gender differences in college binge drinking: Examining the role of depression and school stress. *The Social Science Journal, 50*(4), 521–529.

25 Ortman, J. M., Velkoff, V. A., & Hogan, H. (2014). *An aging nation: the older population in the United States.* Washington, DC: U.S. Census Bureau, 25–1140.

26 *Center for substance abuse treatment: Substance abuse among older adults.* (Treatment Improvement Protocol (TIP) Series, No. 26.) (1998). Rockville, MD: Substance Abuse and Mental Health Services Administration (US). Available from: https://www.ncbi.nlm.nih.gov/books/NBK64419/

27 Jones, C. M., Logan, J., Gladden, M., Bohm, M. K. (2015). Vital signs: Demographic and substance use trends among heroin users—United States, 2002–2013. *Morbidity and Mortality Weekly Report, 64*(26), 719–725.

28 Rudd, R. A., Seth, P., David, F., Scholl, L. (2016). Increases in drug and opioid-involved overdose deaths—United States, 2010–2015. *Morbity and Mortality Weekly Report 2016, 65*:1445–1452. DOI: http://dx.doi.org/10.15585/mmwr.mm655051e1.

29 Foster, D., Tanner, C., & van Zeller, M. (Producers). (2009). The oxycontin express [Documentary]. New York: Vangaurd.

30 Naloxone: A take-home antidote to drug overdose that saves lives. (2014, November). World Health Organization. Retrieved January 11, 2018, from http://www.who.int/features/2014/naloxone/en/

31 Cohen, L. R., & Hien, D. A. (2006). Treatment outcomes for women with substance abuse and PTSD who have experienced complex trauma. *Psychiatric Services, 57*(1), 100–106. doi:10.1176/appi.ps.57.1.100

32 Greenfield, S. F., Back, S. E., Lawson, K., & Brady, K. T. (2010). Substance abuse in women. *The Psychiatric Clinics of North America, 33*(2), 339–355. doi:10.1016/j.psc.2010.01.004

33 Hedden, S. L., Kennet, J., Lipari, R., Medley, G., Tice, P. (2015). Behavioral health trends in the United States: Results from the 2014 national survey on drug use and health. *SAMHSA*, 1–64.

34 Hallucinogens and dissociative drugs. (2015). NIDA. Retrieved January 11, 2017, from https://www.drugabuse.gov/publications/research-reports/hallucinogens-dissociative-drugs

35 State marijuana laws. (2016). Governing.com. Retrieved on 11/21/2016 from http://www.governing.com/gov-data/state-marijuana-laws-map-medical-recreational.html

36 Hellerman, C. (2013). Is super weed super bad? CNN. Retrieved on 11/21/2016 from http://www.cnn.com/2013/08/09/health/weed-potency-levels/

37 Hellerman, C. (2013). Is super weed super bad? CNN. Retrieved on 11/21/2016 from http://www.cnn.com/2013/08/09/health/weed-potency-levels/

38 Ramer, R., Merkord, J., Rohde, H., & Hinz, B. (2010). Cannabidiol inhibits cancer cell invasion via upregulation of tissue inhibitor of matrix metalloproteinases-1. *Biochemical Pharmacology, 79*(7), 955–966. doi:http://dx.doi.org/10.1016/j.bcp.2009.11.007

39 Iuvone, T., Esposito, G., De Filippis, D., Scuderi, C., & Steardo, L. (2009). Cannabidiol: A promising drug for neurodegenerative disorders? *CNS Neuroscience & Therapeutics, 15*(1), 65–75. doi:10.1111/j.1755-5949.2008.00065.x

40 Leweke, F. M., Piomelli, D., Pahlisch, F., Muhl, D., Gerth, C. W., Hoyer, C., Koethe, D. (2012). Cannabidiol enhances anandamide signaling and alleviates psychotic symptoms of schizophrenia. *Translational Psychiatry, 2*, e94. doi:10.1038/tp.2012.15

41 Lynch, M. E., & Campbell, F. (2011). Cannabinoids for treatment of chronic non-cancer pain: A systematic review of randomized trials. *British Journal of Clinical Pharmacology, 72*(5), 735–744. doi:10.1111/j.1365-2125.2011.03970.x

42 Martín-Sánchez, E., Furukawa, T. A., Taylor, J., & Martin, J. L. R. (2009). Systematic review and meta-analysis of cannabis treatment for chronic pain. *Pain Medicine, 10*(8), 1353–1368. doi:10.1111/j.1526-4637.2009.00703.x

43 Belendiuk, K. A., Baldini, L. L., & Bonn-Miller, M. O. (2015). Narrative review of the safety and efficacy of marijuana for the treatment of commonly state-approved medical and psychiatric disorders. *Addiction Science & Clinical Practice, 10*(1), 1–10. doi:10.1186/s13722-015-0032-7

44 Hallucinogens and dissociative drugs. (2015). NIDA. Retrieved January 11, 2017, from https://www.drugabuse.gov/publications/research-reports/hallucinogens-dissociative-drugs

45 Buckner, J. D., Ecker, A. H., Cohen, A. S. (2010). Mental health problems and interest in marijuana treatment among marijuana-using college students. *Addictive Behaviors, 35*(9), 826–833.

46 Lee, C. M., Kilmer, J. R., Neighbors, C., Atkins, D. C., Zheng, C., Walker, D. D., Larimer, M. E. (2013). Indicated prevention for college student marijuana use: A randomized controlled trial. *Journal of Consulting and Clinical Psychology, 81*(4), 702–709.

47 Suerken, C. K., Reboussin, B. A., Sutfin, E. L., Wagoner, K. G., Spangler, J., & Wolfson, M. (2014). Prevalence of marijuana use at college entry and risk factors for initiation during freshman year. *Addictive Behaviors, 39*(1), 302–307.

48 Fast Facts. (2016, December 20). CDC. Retrieved January 11, 2017, from https://www.cdc.gov/tobacco/data_statistics/fact_sheets/fast_facts/

49 Fast Facts. (2016, December 20). CDC. Retrieved January 11, 2017, from https://www.cdc.gov/tobacco/data_statistics/fact_sheets/fast_facts/

50 Fast Facts. (2016, December 20). CDC. Retrieved January 11, 2017, from https://www.cdc.gov/tobacco/data_statistics/fact_sheets/fast_facts/

51 Health risks of secondhand smoke. (n.d.). Cancer.org. Retrieved January 16, 2017, from http://www.cancer.org/cancer/cancercauses/tobaccocancer/secondhand-smoke

52 Hallucinogens and dissociative drugs. (2015). NIDA. Retrieved January 11, 2017, from https://www.drugabuse.gov/publications/research-reports/hallucinogens-dissociative-drugs

53 Health risks of secondhand smoke. (n.d.). Cancer.org. Retrieved January 16, 2017, from http://www.cancer.org/cancer/cancercauses/tobaccocancer/secondhand-smoke

54 *Trends in tobacco use* (Rep. No. 1). (2011, July). American Lung Association. Retrieved January 11, 2017, from http://www.lung.org/assets/documents/research/tobacco-trend-report.pdf

55 *Trends in tobacco use* (Rep. No. 1). (2011, July). American Lung Association. Retrieved January 11, 2017, from http://www.lung.org/assets/documents/research/tobacco-trend-report.pdf

56 De la Cruz, C. S., Tanoue, L. T., & Matthay, R. A. (2011). Lung cancer: Epidemiology, etiology, andpPrevention. *Clinics in Chest Medicine, 32*(4), 10.1016/j.ccm.2011.09.001. http://doi.org/10.1016/j.ccm.2011.09.001

57 Moyer V. A. (2014). On behalf of the U.S. Preventive Services Task Force. Screening for lung cancer: U.S. Preventive Services Task Force recommendation statement. *Annals of Internal Medicine,160*, 330–338. doi:10.7326/M13-2771

58 Hallucinogens and dissociative drugs. (2015). NIDA. Retrieved January 11, 2017, from https://www.drugabuse.gov/publications/research-reports/hallucinogens-dissociative-drugs

59 Selya, A. S., Dierker, L. C., Rose, J. S., Hedeker, D., & Mermelstein, R. J. (2012). Risk factors for adolescent smoking: Parental smoking and the mediating role of nicotine dependence. *Drug and Alcohol Dependence, 124*(3), 311–318.

60 Tyas, S. L., & Pederson, L. L. (1998). Psychosocial factors related to adolescent smoking: a critical review of the literature. *Tobacco Control, 7*(4), 409–420.

61 Bobo, J. K., & Husten, C. (2000). Sociocultural influences on smoking and drinking. *Alcohol Research and Health, 24*(4), 225–232.

62 Behavioral health trends in the United States: Results from the 2014 National Survey on Drug Use and Health (HHS Publication No. SMA 15–4927, NSDUH Series H-50). (2015). Center for Behavioral Health Statistics and Quality. Retrieved from http://www.samhsa.gov/ data/

63 Barnard, M., & McKeganey, N. (2004). The impact of parental problem drug use on children: What is the problem and what can be done to help? *Addiction, 99*(5), 552–559.

64 Behavioral health trends in the United States: Results from the 2014 National Survey on Drug Use and Health (HHS Publication No. SMA 15–4927, NSDUH Series H-50). (2015). Center for Behavioral Health Statistics and Quality. Retrieved from http://www.samhsa.gov/ data/

65 Lander, L., Howsare, J., & Byrne, M. (2013). The impact of substance use disorders on families and children: From theory to practice. *Social Work in Public Health, 28*(0), 194–205. http://doi.org/10.1080/19371918.2013.75900

66 Anda, R. F., Whitfield, C. L., Felitti, V. J., Chapman, D., Edwards, V. J., Dube, S. R., & Williamson, D. F. (2002). Adverse childhood experiences, alcoholic parents, and later risk of alcoholism and depression. *Psychiatric Services, 53*(8), 1001–1009.

67 Repetti, R. L., Taylor, S. E., & Seeman, T. E. (2002). Risky families: Family social environments and the mental and physical health of offspring. *Psychological Bulletin, 128*(2), 330.

68 Prevention of substance use and mental illness. (2016). Substance Abuse and Mental Health Administration. Retrieved on 11/21/2016 from http://www.samhsa.gov/prevention

Figure Sources

1 Figure 11.1: Source: https://www.niaaa.nih.gov/alcohol-health/overview-alcohol-consumption/what-standard-drink.

2 Figure 11.2: Source: https://commons.wikimedia.org/wiki/File:Side_effects_of_Oxycodone.png.

3 Figure 11.3: Source: https://commons.wikimedia.org/wiki/File:Main_symptoms_of_Hydrocodone_overdose.png.

4 Figure 11.4: Source: https://upload.wikimedia.org/wikipedia/commons/thumb/e/ef/Bodily_effects_of_cannabis.svg/2000px-Bodily_effects_of_cannabis.svg.png.

5 Figure 11.5: Copyright © 2014 Depositphotos/harshmunjal.

6 Figure 11.6: Source: https://upload.wikimedia.org/wikipedia/commons/thumb/c/c5/Adverse_effects_of_tobacco_smoking.svg/2000px-Adverse_effects_of_tobacco_smoking.svg.png.

7 Figure 11.7: Source: https://upload.wikimedia.org/wikipedia/commons/c/c6/Healthy_lung-smokers_lung.jpg.

CHAPTER TWELVE

Sexual and Reproductive Health

Coauthors:
Lindsay Hylek, B.A., Sue K. Adams, Ph.D., Sarah W. Feldstein Ewing, Ph.D.

@PPFA

Introduction

A debate is ongoing both nationally and internationally as to whether or not sexual and reproductive health, and health care in general, is a right or a privilege. On the one hand, if sexual and reproductive health are considered fundamental human rights, the government has a responsibility to provide access to care, regardless of whether or not individuals can afford it. On the other hand, if sexual and reproductive health are considered a privilege, then only those who can afford it will be granted high quality care. Although sexual and reproductive health affects males, much of the burden of the social and political debate fight falls squarely on the shoulders of women. Along with defining sexual and reproductive health as they relate to human development, this chapter will help deconstruct this societal discord.

What Is Sexual and Reproductive Health?
Defining Sexual Health
The WHO defines sexual health as a "state of physical, mental, and social well-being in relation to sexuality. It requires a positive and respectful approach to sexuality and sexual relationships, as well as the possibility of having pleasurable and safe sexual experiences, free of coercion, discrimination, and violence."[1] Here, sexuality refers to "a core dimension of being human which includes gender, sexual identity, sexual orientation, eroticism, emotional attachment/love, and reproduction. It is experienced or expressed in thoughts, fantasies, desires, beliefs, attitudes, values,

activities, practices, roles, relationships. Sexuality is the result of the interplay of biological, psychological, socio-economic, cultural, ethical, and religious/spiritual factors."[2] A number of challenges preclude individuals from practicing a healthy sexual life. Key issues include concerns related to body integrity, sexual safety, eroticism, gender, sexual orientation, and emotional attachment. Sexual health care involves promoting sexual health at the societal level, educating individuals about sexuality, and providing assessments and treatments for abovementioned problems through counseling services and other types of care.[3]

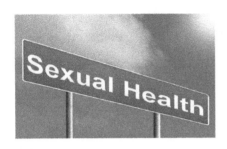

FIGURE 12.1

Defining Reproductive Health

Reproductive health is an important component of sexual health and often discussed in its own right. According to the WHO, reproductive health "addresses the reproductive processes, functions, and system at all stages of life...[and] implies that people are able to have a responsible, satisfying, and safe sex life, that they have the capacity to reproduce, and the freedom to decide if, when, and how often to do so. Implicit in this are the right of men and women to be informed of and to have access to safe, effective, affordable, and acceptable methods of fertility regulation of their choice, and the right of access to appropriate health care services that will enable women to go safely through pregnancy and childbirth and provide couples with the best chance of having a healthy infant."[4] There is a lot of overlap between sexual health and reproductive health concerns. For example, some categorize sexually transmitted infections or STIs as a sexual health issue, while others view it as a reproductive health issue. In this chapter, key reproductive health issues will include concerns related to contraception, abortion, adolescent pregnancy, pregnancy-related services, maternal mortality, pregnancy aftercare for both mother and child, and sterility/infertility.[5]

Human Rights in Sexual and Reproductive Health

The WHO asserts that human beings possess certain sexual and reproductive health rights surrounding body integrity, sexual safety, eroticism, gender, sexual orientation, emotional attachment, and reproduction. Certain issues result from conditions on individual, relational, or societal levels that may require identification, prevention, and treatment before people can lead truly healthy lives. The WHO, in collaboration with the Pan American Health Organization (PAHO) and the World Association for Sexology, released a list of challenges and problems that need to be addressed in order to advance sexual and reproductive health.[6] The following describes these areas of concern:

- Body integrity and sexual safety. Human beings have the right to freedom from sexual coercion and violence, body mutilations, the contraction and transmission of STIs, sexual consequences of physical or mental disabilities, and impacts on sexual life of medical conditions or treatments.

- *Sexual coercion and sexual violence* takes on different forms. The Center for Disease Control and Prevention (CDC) divides sexual violence into the following: completed or attempted forced penetration of a victim, completed or attempted alcohol/drug-facilitated penetration of a victim, completed or attempted forced acts in which a victim is made to penetrate a penetrator or someone else, non-physically forced penetration, which occurs after a person is pressured verbally or through intimidation or misuse of authority to consent or acquiesce, unwanted sexual contact, and non-contact unwanted sexual experiences.[7] In 2000, the National Institute of Justice and CDC's Injury Center sponsored the National Violence Against Women Survey, which revealed that about 1.9 million women and 3.2 million men are physically assaulted annually in the United States.[8] Certain individual, relationship, community, and societal factors are associated with a greater likelihood of becoming a perpetrator of sexual violence. A number of physical, psychological, and social consequences for victims of sexual violence will be described in detail later in this chapter.[9]

con-sent 🔊 [*kuhn*-sent]

verb

1. To permit, approve, or agree; comply or yield: *He consented to the proposal. We asked her permission and she consented.*

2. When applied to sexual contact, it means that at the time of the act, there are actual words or physical conduct indicating freely given agreement.

FIGURE 12.2

- Body mutilations namely refer to female genital mutilation (FGM).[10] FGM primarily refers to procedures that remove external female genitalia for non-medical reasons. Over three million girls between infancy and adolescence within certain regions of Africa, the Middle East, and Asia are at risk annually. FMG is said to be performed due to sociocultural factors, including views surrounding appropriate sexual behavior. FGM is often thought to ensure premarital virginity and marital fidelity, making women more suitable for marriage according to the communities where it is performed. FGM has no health benefits and makes women susceptible to a number of immediate and long-term health complications.[11]

- *STIs* are the result of bacteria, viruses, and/or parasites transmitted through sexual contact, including vaginal, anal, and oral sex.[12] According to Healthy People 2020, an estimated 19 million new cases of STIs are diagnosed in the United States annually.[13] The four most common curable STIs are syphilis, gonorrhea, chlamydia, and trichomoniasis. The four most common incurable STIs include hepatitis B, herpes simplex virus (HSV), human immunodeficiency virus (HIV), and human papillomavirus (HPV). It is possible to contract an STI without experiencing symptoms, but the most common symptoms include vaginal discharge, urethral discharge or burning, genital ulcers, and abdominal pain. Although incurable, viral infection symptoms can be reduced through treatment. In some cases, STIs lead to other negative reproductive health consequences, such as infertility, which will be described in detail later in this chapter.[14]

- Eroticism. Human beings have the right to know about sexual response and pleasure; recognize the value of sexual pleasure in a safe and responsible manner; and practice consensual, non-exploitative, honest, and mutually pleasurable relationships.
- Gender. Human beings have the right to gender equality, nondiscrimination based on gender, and respect for gender differences.
- Sexual orientation. Human beings have the right to nondiscrimination based on sexual orientation and the expression of sexual orientation.
- Emotional attachment. Human beings have the right to freedom from exploitative, coercive, violent, or manipulative relationships; information on family options; skills that enhance personal relationships like decision-making, communication, assertiveness, and negotiation; expression of love; and divorce.
- Reproduction. Human beings have the right to make informed decisions about reproduction regardless of age, sex, and marital status; access reproductive health care; safe motherhood; and infertility prevention and care.[15]

Health Disparities in Sexual and Reproductive Health

Some people have a higher susceptibility to sexual and reproductive health issues. For example, take sexual violence. More females are victims of sexual violence than men. A national representative survey conducted by the CDC showed that 11.8% of adolescent girls experienced sexual violence as opposed to 4.5% of adolescent boys. In addition, 18.3% of adult women experience sexual violence as opposed to 1.2% of men. There are also racial and ethnic disparities in sexual violence. Among adolescents, the CDC estimates that 13.5% of multiracial teens, 12.5% of American Indian/Alaska Native teens, 10.5% of Native Hawaiian/Pacific Islander teens, 8.6% of black teens, 8.2% of Hispanic teens, and 7.4% of white teens were coerced into sexual intercourse between grades 9–12. Among adult women, 35.5% of multiracial women, 26.9% of American Indian/Alaska Native women, 22% of black women, 18.8% of white women, and 14.6% of Hispanic women are estimated to suffer from an attempted or completed rape.[16]

STI contraction and transmission is another sexual health concern that plagues some groups more than others. With regards to racial and ethnic health disparities, black and Hispanic women experience higher rates of sexually transmitted infections than other group of Americans. Specifically, black and Hispanic women contract STIs at higher rates than white women, accounting for 80% of reported female HIV/AIDS diagnoses even though they represent only 25% of the female population.[17] Black men and women account for 44% of new HIV/AIDS infections, 47% of new gonorrhea cases, 31% of new chlamydia cases, and 38% of new syphilis cases even though they represent only 12% of the United States population.[18] Hispanic men and women are three times more likely to contract HIV, twice as likely to contract gonorrhea, and twice as likely to contract chlamydia as white men and women. Black and Hispanic women also experience higher rates of reproductive cancers as a result of high STI prevalence; Hispanic women are more likely to be diagnosed with cervical cancer than women of any other racial background,[19] and black women are twice as likely to die from cervical cancer as white women.[20]

In addressing global health disparities, the United Nations Population Fund (UNFP) identified three key reproductive health indicators: adolescent birth rates, contraceptive prevalence, and unmet need for family planning. Adolescent birth rate, the number of births per 1,000 15- to 19-year-old girls, is suggestive of the opportunities available to girls as well as vulnerabilities they face during adolescence. For example, girls often have greater access to primary education in countries where adolescent birth rates are low. When girls are knowledgeable about their right to exercise reproductive health, they feel more empowered to decide if and when they want to become pregnant. Contraceptive prevalence rate, the percentage of 15- to 49-year-old partnered women who are using contraception, hints at how many sexually active women who do not want to become pregnant are taking precautionary measures. The unmet need for family planning, contrarily, refers to the proportion of partnered women of reproductive age who do not want to become pregnant, but are *not* using contraception. These two indictors are reflective of contraception availability as well as social norms surrounding the decision to actively choose various forms of contraception. Taken together, they help organizations like the UNFP get a sense of the percentage of women getting their needs met with regards to family planning and, therefore, call attention to inequalities surrounding access to reproductive health services.[21]

Health Disparities Within the United States

Within the United States, certain populations have limited access to reproductive health services. Namely, black and Hispanic populations often experience higher adolescent birth rates, lower prevalence of contraception use, and higher rates of an unmet need for family planning. As such, black and Hispanic women experience higher instances of unintended pregnancies, low-income Hispanic women are twice as likely as low-income white women to have an unintended pregnancy, and low-income black women are three times as likely as low-income white women to have an unintended pregnancy.[22] Consequently, black and Hispanic women also have higher rates of abortion. Black women are three times as likely as white women to have an abortion, and about four in 10 unintended pregnancies among Hispanic women end in abortion.[23]

Causes of Racial and Ethnic Disparities

It is difficult to pinpoint why and how these reproductive health inequalities manifested. The Guttmacher Institute is a research and policy organization dedicated to advancing sexual and reproductive health nationally and internationally. According to its former board chair, "The root causes are manifold: a long history of discrimination; lack of access to high-quality, affordable health care; too few educational and professional opportunities; unequal access to safe, clean neighborhoods; and, for some African Americans, a lingering mistrust of the medical community."[24] One particular obstacle for black and Hispanic populations within the United States is lack of health insurance. More Hispanic Americans, about 31%, are uninsured than any other racial or ethnic group,[25] followed by black Americans at 15.9% and white Americans at 9.8%. As a result, black and Hispanic women are often forced to postpone care because they are unable to pay for it.[26]

Healthy People 2020: Goals for Sexual and Reproductive Health

Part of the Health People 2020 agenda is to improve sexual and reproductive health services because enhancing care will help eliminate health disparities. Sexual and reproductive health services, such as STI testing and treatment, often become an entry point into the medical system. As a result, individuals seeking services related to pregnancy prevention or prenatal care may also receive screenings for intimate partner violence, referrals to substance-abuse treatment, and counseling on nutrition and physical activity, which cut costs in the long term. For example, publicly funded family planning services prevent an estimated 1.94 million unintended pregnancies, including 400,000 teen pregnancies, per year. The government saves about four dollars in Medicaid pregnancy-related care expenses for every dollar spent on contraception-related care.[27] Moreover, aside from saving money, promoting sexual and reproductive health services is likely to advance overall health for the country as a whole, the primary goal of the Healthy People 2020 initiative.

In 2014, the Healthy People 2020 initiative released a progress report with regard to sexual and reproductive health indicators. For instance, from 2006 to 2010, 78.6% of sexually active females between 15 and 44 received reproductive health services within the past year.[28] By 2020, Healthy People hopes to increase that number by about 10% by 2020. While there was no statistically significant change between the 2006–2010 data and the 2011–2013 data, Healthy People remains optimistic about reaching the goal of 86.5% by 2020.[29]

Healthy People 2020 aims to address sexual and reproductive health disparities for the LGBT population by conducting more research to understand how environmental factors impact quality of health care, implementing trainings on culturally competent care, increase anti-bullying policy efforts in schools, providing social services against suicide and homelessness, and improving STI prevention and treatment. Through these efforts, Healthy People 2020 hopes to reduce the transmission and progression of STIs, enhance mental and physical well-being, decrease health care costs, and increase longevity.[30]

Sexual and Reproductive Health Across Development

Adolescents

A major reproductive health issue that adolescents face is teenage pregnancy. In 2014, about 250,000 girls age 15–19 gave birth to a child, a birth rate of about 24 per 1,000 teenagers. Teen birth rates vary by race and ethnicity in the United States with American Indian/Alaska Native teens at 12%, black teens at 11%, Asian/Pacific Islander teens at 11%, Hispanic teens at 9%, and white teens at 7%.[31] Other risk factors for teen pregnancy include being raised by a single mother, having parents with low levels of education, and growing up in poverty. About 82% of pregnancies that occur among women under 20 years old are unintended.[32] As a result, teen pregnancy has a number of social and economic costs due to increased health care, foster care, and incarceration rates among children as well as lower school attainment and income among teen parents. For instance, about 90% of women who do not have children during their teenage years graduate from high school, where only 50% of women who have children during their teenage years obtain a high school diploma by age 22.

The CDC, along with a number of other organizations, has made efforts toward reducing teen pregnancy rates in the United States. The implementation of evidence-based teen pregnancy prevention programs, such as sexuality education programs, youth development programs, and abstinence-education programs have all shown to help reduce instances of teen pregnancy. As a result of such progress in preventative care, teenage birth rates fell 11% for girls age 15–16 and 7% for girls age 18–19 from 2013 to 2014. Currently, the birth rates amongst teenage girls in the United States is at an historic low.[33]

Births per 1,000 Females Aged 15–19 Years, by Race and Hispanic Ethnicity, 2007-2015

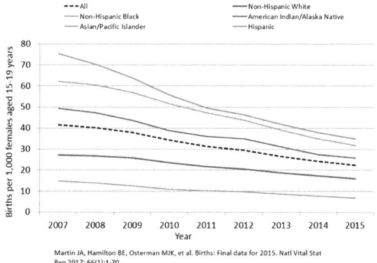

Martin JA, Hamilton BE, Osterman MJK, et al. Births: Final data for 2015. Natl Vital Stat Rep 2017; 66(1):1-70

FIGURE 12.3   Births per every 1,000 Females Aged 15–19 Years, by Race and Hispanic Ethnicity: CDC, 2007–2015

Adults

An important component of sexual health throughout the lifespan is establishing and maintaining healthy relationships with sexual partners. Emotional attachment becomes particularly significant during adulthood when people start entering into more committed relationships. It is considered normative behavior for Americans to get married and have children in their 20s and 30s. However, according to the CDC, fewer individuals are actually getting married and entering into other types of partnerships instead. In 2000, 8.2 out of 1,000 people got married, and 4.0 out of 1,000 people got divorced, while in 2014, 6.9 out of 1,000 people got married and 3.2 got divorced.[34]

Regardless of whether or not individuals choose to enter into a marriage, they have the right to consensual partnerships founded on mutual respect and admiration. However, not all relationships are built on a secure attachment style. Securely attached relationships are based on honesty, openness, and equality. In these relationships, partners feel connected and reciprocate support but allow one another to comfort themselves independently. Insecure attachment styles include anxious preoccupation, dismissive avoidant, and fearful avoidant attachment. People with anxious preoccupation attachment seek a sense of safety from their partners and can become clingy, demanding, or possessive. People with dismissive avoidant attachment distance themselves from their partners to maintain a sense of independence as a protective mechanism. People with fearful avoidant attachment are ambivalent and vacillate between fears of getting too close or too distant.

These attachment styles influence sexual health because they play a role in how individuals relate to one another sexually. Couples with an anxious preoccupation attachment may seek out sexual activity too frequently where couples with a dismissive avoidant attachment may avoid it all together. Fearful avoidant attachment often leads to dramatic relationships with highs and lows that may manifest themselves in sexual and physical abuse. Fortunately, maladaptive attachment styles can be addressed through sex therapy and other forms of care so that individuals can sustain satisfying, loving adult relationships.[35]

Infertility

A reproductive-health concern for many adults is infertility. Currently, 20% of women are waiting to have their first child after age 25, and about 33% of couples over 35 struggle with infertility (only 6% of partnered women and 7.5% of partnered men between 15 and 44 years old are infertile).[36] Infertility affects women and men. Individuals are deemed infertile once the woman is unable to get pregnant after a year of unprotected sex. Some people are more susceptible to infertility than others. For women, conditions such as polycystic ovarian syndrome, functional hypothalamic amenorrhea, diminished ovarian reserve, premature ovarian insufficiency, and menopause all cause anovulation or the absence of an ovulation cycle. Menopause is an age-appropriate decline in ovarian function and typically occurs between 45 and 55 years of age. Not only does aging decrease a woman's chances of getting pregnant, but it also increases the risk of miscarriage as well as genetic abnormalities for the child. For men, risk factors for infertility include varicoceles, diabetes, cystic fibrosis, trauma, infection, testicular failure, chemotherapy or radiation treatment, testosterone supplementation, anabolic steroid use, and exposure to environmental toxins. Both women and men run the risk of becoming infertile from unhealthy habits like heavy alcohol use, smoking, and illicit drug use.

Some options for a couple deemed infertile include medicine, surgery, intra-uterine insemination, or assisted reproductive technology.[37] Without health insurance coverage, the costs of these procedures can be in excess of $28,000.[38] Moreover, the procedures do not always work for everyone. Infertility can be difficult to cope with, and many partners begin couple's therapy in order to navigate this challenge, as well as decide if other avenues of family planning (e.g., adoption) will be pursued.

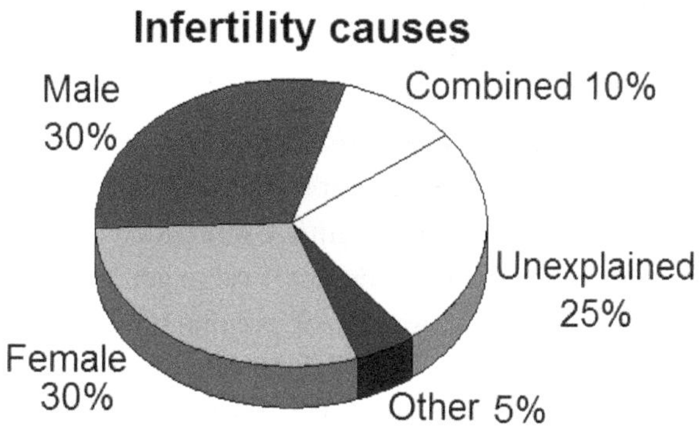

Infertility causes

Male 30%
Combined 10%
Unexplained 25%
Female 30%
Other 5%

FIGURE 12.4   Infertility is often caused by multiple factors and sometimes a cause cannot be determined

Older Adults

Society often misconstrues older adulthood as a period of asexuality. However, the belief that people can have sex up only to a certain age can be considered an act of ageism. In reality, studies show that many couples maintain a healthy sex life well into old age. According to one study, a significant amount of men and women over the age of 60 reported having sex at least once a month. For those couples that have sex less frequently, their abstinence may not be due to lack of desire. A host of physical ailments may impede both elderly males and females from engaging in sexual activity. For example, men may suffer from erectile dysfunction or delayed ejaculation where women may experience arousal disorder, female orgasmic disorder, or genitopelvic pain. Some of these issues may stem from emotional issues, such as no longer feeling sexually desirable, which is amplified by society's negative attitude toward sexuality during this period of development. As such, the treatment of various sexual dysfunctions may include reassurance from partners, sex education, sex counseling, and/or prescribed medications.[39]

Unfortunately, older adults do not always receive adequate care when it comes to sexual health. Younger populations are often targets of sexual health care reform efforts, leaving older populations by the wayside. According to the United Nation's Convention on the Elimination of all Forms of Discrimination Against Women, "Post-menopausal, post-reproductive, and other age-related and gender-specific physical and mental health conditions and diseases tend to be overlooked by research, academic studies, public policy, and service provision."[40] This pattern is becoming particularly problematic as the average lifespan continues to increase. In other words, the number of older men and women with unaddressed sexual health issues will rise as the population continues to grow.[41] Concerted action is necessary to educate the public about the needs of older adults when it comes to sexual health. Hopefully, dispelling ignorance will eliminate ongoing discrimination against this group, empower individuals to advocate for themselves, and prompt policymakers and health care providers to prioritize treatment for older adults facing sexual health issues.[42]

Family Functioning and Couples

Not only does sexual and reproductive health affect intimate partnerships, but it also has a bearing on family functioning. Unintended pregnancies can either result from a mistimed pregnancy (the woman did not want to get pregnant until later) or an unwanted pregnancy (the woman did not want to be pregnant at all). Forty-two percent of unintended pregnancies end in abortion. When the mother chooses to keep the child, mothers may choose to put the child up for adoption or try to raise him or her themselves (58% of the unintended pregnancies).[43] Children that are not initially adopted or deemed unsafe under the care of their biological parents may enter into the foster care system. Foster care can be traumatic for children who are forced to move in between families. These children may develop abandonment issues later on in life, which may manifest in one of the aforementioned insecure attachment styles (anxious preoccupation, dismissive avoidant, and fearful avoidant). Even children who are adopted into loving homes may experience difficulties later on in life. Adopted children may acquire feelings of insecurity due to the belief that their biological parents did not love them enough to keep them. Both fostered children and adoptees are more likely to be diagnosed with oppositional defiant disorder, attention-deficit/hyperactivity disorder (ADHD), conduct disorder, major depressive disorder, and separation anxiety disorder.[44]

There are negative consequences in cases where mothers decide to keep the child of an unintended pregnancy as well. Over 40% of children born from unintended pregnancies come into the world with unmarried parents. Moreover, marriages that result from unintended pregnancy usually end in divorce. If the father is present and resentful that he has to help raise the child, then he may take it out on the mother and the child, which could result in domestic violence. If the father is absent, then mothers may be forced to raise the child themselves without adequate resources, which has negative impacts. For instance, children raised by single parents are more likely to drop out of school and less likely to attend or graduate college.[45] Indeed, the poor mental, physical, and emotional health of children of unintended pregnancies is yet another reason to improve sexual health education in hopes of preventing unintended pregnancies from happening in the future and enhancing family functioning nationwide.

Lesbian, Gay, Bisexual, and Transgender Health

The lesbian, gay, bisexual, and transgender (LGBT) community is diverse and includes people from all races, ethnicities, ages, socioeconomic statuses, and geographic locations.[46] Thus, the LGBT community is important to consider when addressing health disparities in the United States. It is particularly vital to focus on eliminating discrimination against this group in order to improve their sexual and reproductive care. For example, LGBT individuals may suffer from family disownment and hate crimes because they are not readily accepted. At the most extreme, people in the LGBT community may face legal discrimination with regards to access to health care as well as employment, housing, marriage, adoption, and retirement benefits. The stigmatization against LGBT individuals has been linked with high rates of substance abuse, suicide, and psychiatric disorders as a result.

Impacts of Sexual and Reproductive Health on Wellbeing

Sexual and reproductive health issues have major biological, psychological, and social consequences. In this chapter, four major sexual and reproductive health issues will be discussed in detail with regards to their biological, psychological, and social impacts: sexual violence, contraception, the contraction and transmission of STIs, and abortion.

Sexual Violence

Victims of sexual violence suffer from immediate and chronic biological consequences. These include bruising; broken or dislocated bones; trouble walking; genital injuries; STIs; cervical cancer; gastrointestinal disorders; gynecological complications, such as bleeding, infection, chronic pelvic pain, pelvic inflammatory disease, and urinary tract infections; migraines; and chronic pain. Increased stress levels after the event can lead to fatigue, shortness of breath, muscle tension, involuntary shaking, changes in eating and sleeping patterns, sexual dysfunction, and infertility.[47] Sexual assault may also lead to an unintended pregnancy that results in abortion, which has its own biological consequences.[48]

Initially, after an episode of sexual violence, men and women may experience shock, fear, denial, confusion, anxiety, shame, guilt, withdrawal, and distrust. Oftentimes, men and women start experiencing post-traumatic stress disorder (PTSD) symptoms such as emotional detachment, sleep disturbances, and flashbacks after instances of rape and other forms of sexual violence, which lead to a PTSD diagnosis later on in life.[49] Indeed, research conducted in the United States, New Zealand, and France indicates that women are 50% to 95% likely to develop PTSD after being raped. Furthermore, studies show that 33% of women with a history of sexual abuse and 15% of women with a history of physical abuse show signs of psychiatric disorders where only 6% of women without a history of physical abuse experience psychiatric symptoms.[50]

Other long-term psychological consequences include low self-esteem, loss of interest in sexual activities, self-harm, suicidality, depression, generalized anxiety, and sleep disorders.[51] As victims struggle to deal with such a traumatic event, they may start to engage in destructive coping mechanisms in order to self sooth. These health-risk behaviors include engaging in risky sexual behavior such as unprotected sex, early sexual initiation, having multiple sexual partners, and trading sex for money or other items; using harmful substances, such as smoking cigarettes, drinking alcohol, and taking drugs; disordered eating, such as fasting, vomiting, and overeating; committing crimes; and avoiding healthy behaviors, such as wearing a seatbelt. Researchers believe that these behaviors are not only consequences of sexual violence but also increase one's vulnerability to future victimization.

As a result of the biological and psychological consequences of sexual violence, victims' worldview and outlook on life may be negatively impacted. The experience of losing control frequently causes individuals to become reluctant to trust others and withdraw from social situations.[52] This behavior may impact individuals' social life. Such repercussions include strained relationships with family, friends, and intimate partners; less frequent contact and emotional support from friends and family; and decreased likelihood of marriage.[53]

Contraction and Transmission of STIs

Contracting STIs can have a number of biological ramifications. As mentioned previously, there are four common bacterial STIs: syphilis, gonorrhea, chlamydia, and trichinosis. Common symptoms of these STIs are vaginal discharge, urethral discharge or burning, genital ulcers, and abdominal pain. Bacterial STIs are curable and can be eliminated with relatively simple antibiotic regimens.[54] If left untreated, these STIs can have more severe long-term consequences. For example, chlamydia and gonorrhea can increase the risk of chronic pelvic pain and cause infertility.[55] However, the four common viral STIs, hepatitis B, herpes, HIV, and HPV, are incurable. Treatment options for these types of STIs include antiviral medications to manage the disease.[56] Unfortunately, because these STIs do not have a true cure, individuals must manage additional health problems along with the symptoms of the disease. These health problems may include difficulties for both mother and child during pregnancy, infections in other parts of the body, organ damage, cervical cancer, and death.[57]

According to the CDC, 15–25 year olds contract 50% of newly diagnosed STIs every year even though they account for only 27% of the sexually active population. The most commonly transmitted STI on college campuses is HPV, followed by chlamydia, and genital herpes. Adolescents and young adults are particularly at risk due to insufficient screening methods, concerns regarding health care providers' adherence to confidentiality measures, biological susceptibility among young women, lack of insurance and transportation to access prevention services, and multiple sexual partners. Youth may suffer also from long-term consequences. For example, undiagnosed STIs like chlamydia cause 24,000 women to become infertile per year.[58] Also, two types of HPV (types 16 and 18) cause 70% of cervical cancers in females, 95% of anal cancers, and 70% of oropharyngeal (tonsils, tongue and palate) cancers. Since HPV can be transmitted by all forms of sexual activity including vaginal, anal and oral sex, all areas of the body used for sexual purposes can be affected by HPV.[59]

Contracting an STI affects people in different ways, but many experience anger, shame, and depression after the diagnosis. People may blame themselves for not practicing safer sex, which lowers self-esteem. Depression is particularly common when individuals contract more severe STIs, such as herpes or HIV, which are incurable. Not only do studies show that STIs lead to major depressive disorder, but depressive symptoms also proceed STI acquisition. Researchers postulate that people who are depressed may lack self-confidence and engage in riskier sexual behaviors as a result.

Typically, individuals do not become depressed after contracting an incurable STI due to symptom management. Instead, people get depressed because of how the STI diagnosis may impact their relationships. Infected individuals may become torn between the moral responsibility of disclosing their diagnosis to sexual partners and keeping it a secret in fear of rejection. Consequently, men and women with STIs may avoid intimacy all together.[60] The stigma surrounding STIs is pervasive in American society, and many believe that it is a negative reflection of someone's character. It becomes easy for individuals to feel embarrassed after noticing symptoms, and they may avoid getting tested and treated because they are so ashamed. However, much of the stigma surrounding STIs is based on misinformation and ignorance, not scientific fact. For example, HIV was originally associated with gay men during a period of heightened homophobia in the United States. Part of the reason that it became such an epidemic was that heterosexual Americans did not think that they were susceptible to this disease. As a result, more people ended up acquiring HIV, fewer people knew how to prevent it, and preventative care was limited due to lack of government funding. As such, some argue that the stigmatization of STIs is more detrimental than the diseases themselves.[61]

Abortion

Roughly 25% of pregnancies end in abortion. Between 2010 and 2014, about 56 million abortions occurred around the world annually, or, in other words, 35 abortions per 1,000 women between age 15 and 44 years old.[62] Depending on whether or not the abortion is

FIGURE 1. Number, rate,* and ratio† of abortions performed by year — selected reporting areas,§ United States, 2005–2014

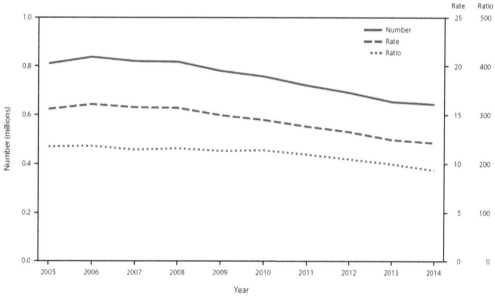

* Number of abortions per 1,000 women aged 15-44 years.

† Number of abortions per 1,000 live births.

§ Data are for 48 reporting areas; excludes California, Louisiana, Maryland, and New Hampshire.

FIGURE 12.5   **Number, rate,* and ratio† of abortions performed by year in United States: CDC, 2005–2014**

induced in a safe manner, women can experience a number of biological complications from the procedure. These include heavy bleeding, infection, uterine perforation, injury to the genital tract and internal organs, and death.

Unintended pregnancies that end in abortion can be very emotionally taxing, and women may experience psychological problems in the weeks and months after the procedure. For example, women may be haunted by thoughts of whether or not the abortion was the right decision. Some may develop what has been referred to as post-abortion syndrome, which is thought to be a form of PTSD. However, most women do not face such severe mental health consequences after the procedure. In fact, studies show that psychological distress actually decreases after abortions. Thus, pro-choice advocates argue that abortion should remain a viable option for women.

Stigma surrounds abortions both nationally and internationally based on moral, religious, and ethical beliefs against the procedure. This stigmatization creates barriers to accessing this reproductive health care option. Oftentimes, countries may have restrictive laws that ultimately lead to unsafe abortion procedures if women feel as though they have no other choice.[63] Specifically, in the United States, debate surrounds whether or not abortions should be available without restrictions, the extent to which government funds should pay for abortions, and whether or not parents should have to consent to the procedure. Women who ultimately decide to have an abortion, as well as health care professionals who carry out the procedure, may face hostility and violence from the community at large.[64]

Despite the controversy, a woman's right to access safe, legal abortion is protected by the U.S. Supreme Court decision of Roe v. Wade (1973). In this case, two female law school graduates filed a lawsuit against the Dallas County District Attorney Henry Wade on behalf of a pregnant woman named Norma McCorvey—"Jane Roe"—who asserted that it was unconstitutional for states to ban abortions. At the time, Texas law criminalized all abortions except those preventing the death of the mother. Roe reported that she did not have the funds to travel out of state for the abortion and believed she had a right to medical care within her state of residence. Ultimately, after much debate, the Supreme Court decided that states could not prevent pregnancy termination in the first trimester but could modulate abortions in later trimesters if they so choose.[65]

Reproductive Health Advocacy Efforts
Planned Parenthood
A number of efforts have been made to address sexual and reproductive health concerns nationally and internationally. The oldest non-profit organization dedicated to this cause is Planned Parenthood, which was founded in 1916 to educate women about birth control options. According to its mission statement, "Planned Parenthood believes in the fundamental right of each individual, throughout the world, to manage his or her fertility, regardless of the individual's income, marital status, race, ethnicity, sexual orientation, age, national origin, or residence."[66] Specifically, Planned Parenthood is dedicated to providing extensive sexual and reproductive health care including pregnancy services, birth control,

emergency contraception, abortions, STI testing and treatment, body image counseling, education around healthy relationships and sexuality, and more. Due to various ethical and religious qualms around the nature of the Planned Parenthood mission, it has a long history of fighting for its own survival. In 2016, Planned Parenthood launched an "100 Years Strong" campaign, essentially articulating to the world that it is here to stay despite whatever resistance is encountered in the coming years.

Guttmacher Institute

Founded in 1968, the Guttmacher Institute is approaching its 50th anniversary. It is a non-profit policy research institute committed to expanding nonpartisan social science research efforts and policy analysis to inform policymakers on decisions surrounding sexual and reproductive health issues. Its findings are accessible to the public so as to educate readers on the facts. Specifically, the institute publishes two peer-reviewed journals, *Perspectives on Sexual and Reproductive Health* and *International Perspectives on Sexual and Reproductive Health* as well as the public policy journal *Guttmacher Policy Review*.[67] An example of one of organization's findings is that there was a decline in abortion from 2011–2014 in the United States, which was believed to be driven by increased access to contraception and, thus, fewer unintended pregnancies.[68]

Center for Reproductive Rights

More recently, the Center for Reproductive Rights was founded in 1992 with the goal of advocating for women's autonomy surrounding reproduction. Akin to Planned Parenthood and similar agencies, the Center believes that reproductive freedom is a fundamental human right. The activist tool of choice is the law. The Center is comprised of attorneys who specialize in both U.S. constitutional and international human rights law in order to fight for reproductive rights. Their work has expanded access to reproductive health care from birth control to obstetric services in over 50 countries.[69]

Conclusion

While organizations like the WHO affirm that all human beings should have access to sexual and reproductive health care, it is clear that significant inequities exist in the U.S. which limit access to reproductive health care for certain groups of people. These inequities impact the rates of STIs, access to treatments for sexual diseases and reproductive services, and the long-term consequences of STIs on a person's health. The political and social debate over the role of access to reproductive health care is far from resolved, and many uncertainties remain in how political decisions will impact the rights of women and men to access various services such as birth control, reproductive technologies, and abortions. Certain organizations like Planned Parenthood have filled an important role in underserved communities to provide health care to women and men no matter what. However, these services are not guaranteed. Returning back to the introduction of this chapter, we ask you, the reader, to consider if reproductive and sexual health care should be a privilege or a right?

Caroline was a junior in college when she found out that she had contracted HIV. Four months prior, she had broken up with her long-term boyfriend and started sleeping with multiple partners. She learned about STIs in health class in high school, but none of her friends had one (at least that she knew about), so she did not think they were that common. Caroline *did* know people that got pregnant unintentionally and had to get an abortion, so she made sure to get an IUD while she was with her now ex-boyfriend. When Caroline began having sex with other people, she started off wearing condoms just to be safe, but over time she became less concerned about it in the moment. If her sexual partner forgot to bring a condom, she would reassure him that she was on birth control, so neither of them had anything to worry about.

About six weeks after Caroline had sex with someone on New Year's Eve, she started feeling really sick. She thought she might have the flu because she had a fever, but then she noticed a rash.[70] She went to the health center to see if she was having some sort of allergic reaction. The health practitioner asked her some questions about her sexual activity and told her she might have an STI. The health practitioner took urine and blood samples to test her for STIs. One week later, Caroline received a call from the health center asking her to come back in so they could discuss her results. She had tested positive for HIV. Caroline was in shock and asked how that was even possible; she thought that HIV was only transmitted through anal sex. The health practitioner explained that HIV is usually transmitted through sexual behaviors and syringes. Specifically, contact with body fluids like blood, semen, pre-seminal fluid, rectal fluids, vaginal fluids, and breast milk can spread HIV from one person to another. The health practitioner told Caroline that it was possible that she slept with someone who was HIV-positive, and the virus entered her body through the mucus membranes that line the vagina and cervix.[71]

She went on to explain the three stages of HIV: acute HIV infection, chronic HIV infection, and AIDS. During the first stage, individuals may experience flu-like symptoms when the virus multiples and spreads throughout the body, attacking the immune system's infection-fighting CD4 cells. During the second stage, the virus continues to multiply but much less rapidly. Individuals with chronic HIV infection may not experience any HIV-related symptoms. During the third stage, which usually takes about 10 years to reach, people are diagnosed with AIDS after the virus has damaged the immune system to the point where the body cannot fight off new infections. Specifically, HIV-positive individuals are diagnosed with AIDS after their CD4 count is less than 200 cells/mm, they have at least one opportunistic infection, or both.[72] The health practitioner reassured Caroline that significant advancements had been made in HIV treatment over the years and that certain medications prevent HIV from developing into AIDS.[73]

Caroline immediately burst into tears and slowly entered into a deep depression. She eventually started seeing a counselor, as recommended by the health practitioner, who helped her cope with her new diagnosis. Years into her new identity as woman who is HIV-positive, she settled into an HIV regimen that worked for her and felt empowered to continue to pursue her dreams of becoming a doctor. Now, she works at a non-profit that advocates for STI education, prevention, and treatment in adolescents and young adults. Specifically, she treats individuals who test positive for HIV in hopes of helping them maintain life satisfaction despite contracting the disease, much like she did.

Notes

1 Sexual health. (2017). World Health Organization. Retrieved from http://www.who.int/topics/sexual_health/en/.

2 *Promotion of Sexual Health: Recommendation for Action.* (2000, May). Pan American Health Organization. Retrieved from http://www1.paho.org/hq/dmdocuments/2008/PromotionSexualHealth.pdf.

3 Sexual health issues. (2017). World Health Organization. Retrieved from http://www.who.int/reproductivehealth/topics/sexual_health/issues/en/.

4 Reproductive health. (2017). World Health Organization. Retrieved from http://www.who.int/topics/reproductive_health/en/.

5 Fact sheets: reproductive health. (2017). World Health Organization. Retrieved from http://www.who.int/topics/reproductive_health/factsheets/en/.

6 *Promotion of Sexual Health: Recommendation for Action.* (2000, May). Pan American Health Organization. Retrieved from http://www1.paho.org/hq/dmdocuments/2008/PromotionSexualHealth.pdf.

7 Sexual violence: Definitions. (2014). Centers for Disease Control and Prevention. Retrieved from https://www.cdc.gov/violenceprevention/sexualviolence/definitions.html.

8 *Findings From the National Violence Against Women Survey.* (2000). National Institute of Justice. Retrieved from https://www.ncjrs.gov/pdffiles1/nij/183781.pdf.

9 Sexual violence: Risk and protective factors. (2016). Centers for Disease Control and Prevention. Retrieved from https://www.cdc.gov/violenceprevention/sexualviolence/riskprotectivefactors.html.

10 Sexual health issues. (2017). World Health Organization. Retrieved from http://www.who.int/reproductivehealth/topics/sexual_health/issues/en/.

11 Fact sheets: Female genital mutilation. (2016). World Health Organization. Retrieved from http://www.who.int/mediacentre/factsheets/fs241/en/

12 Fact sheets: sexually transmitted infections (STIs). (2016). World Health Organization. Retrieved from http://www.who.int/mediacentre/factsheets/fs110/en/

13 Reproductive and Sexual Health. (2017). Healthy People 2020. Retrieved from https://www.healthypeople.gov/2020/leading-health-indicators/2020-lhi-topics/Reproductive-and-Sexual-Health

14 Fact sheets: sexually transmitted infections (STIs). (2016). World Health Organization. Retrieved from http://www.who.int/mediacentre/factsheets/fs110/en/.

15 Sexual health issues. (2017). World Health Organization. Retrieved from http://www.who.int/reproductivehealth/topics/sexual_health/issues/en/

16 Facts at a glance: Sexual violence. (2012). Centers for Disease Control and Prevention. Retrieved from https://www.cdc.gov/violenceprevention/pdf/sv-datasheet-a.pdf.

17 Addressing disparities in reproductive and sexual health care in the U.S. (2016). Center for Reproductive Rights. Retrieved from https://www.reproductiverights.org/node/861.

18 Addressing sexual and reproductive health disparities among African Americans. (2015). Planned Parenthood. Retrieved from https://www.plannedparenthood.org/files/3614/2773/6927/AA_Disparities.pdf.

19 Addressing sexual and reproductive health disparities among Latinos. (2015). Planned Parenthood. Retrieved from https://www.plannedparenthood.org/files/2814/2773/6927/Latino_Disparities.pdf.

20 Addressing sexual and reproductive health disparities among African Americans. (2015). Planned Parenthood. Retrieved from https://www.plannedparenthood.org/files/3614/2773/6927/AA_Disparities.pdf.

21 Universal access to reproductive health: Progress and challenges. (2016). United Nations Population Fund. Retrieved January 24, 2017, from https://www.unfpa.org/sites/default/files/pub-pdf/UNFA_Reproductive_Paper_20160120_online.pdf

22 Addressing disparities in reproductive and sexual health care in the U.S. (2016). Center for Reproductive Rights. Retrieved from https://www.reproductiverights.org/node/861.

23 Addressing sexual and reproductive health disparities among Latinos. (2015). Planned Parenthood. Retrieved from https://www.plannedparenthood.org/files/2814/2773/6927/Latino_Disparities.pdf.

24 Black history month: Addressing health disparities. (2010). Guttmacher Institute. Retrieved from https://www.guttmacher.org/article/2010/02/black-history-month-addressing-health-disparities.

25 Addressing sexual and reproductive health disparities among Latinos. (2015). Planned Parenthood. Retrieved from https://www.plannedparenthood.org/files/2814/2773/6927/Latino_Disparities.pdf.

26 Addressing sexual and reproductive health disparities among African Americans. (2015). Planned Parenthood. Retrieved from https://www.plannedparenthood.org/files/3614/2773/6927/AA_Disparities.pdf.

27 Reproductive and sexual health. (2017). Healthy People 2020. Retrieved from https://www.healthypeople.gov/2020/leading-health-indicators/2020-lhi-topics/Reproductive-and-Sexual-Health.

28 Reproductive and sexual health. (2014). Healthy People 2020. Retrieved January 25, 2017, from https://www.healthypeople.gov/2020/leading-health-indicators/2020-lhi-topics/Reproductive-and-Sexual-Health/data

29 Leading health indicators: Reproductive and sexual health. (2014, May). Healthy People 2020 Retrieved January 25, 2017, from https://www.healthypeople.gov/sites/default/files/HP2020_LHI_Repro_Sex_Hlth.pdf

30 Lesbian, gay, bisexual, and transgender health. (2017). Healthy People 2020. Retrieved from https://www.healthypeople.gov/2020/topics-objectives/topic/lesbian-gay-bisexual-and-transgender-health.

31 About teen pregnancy. (2016). Centers for Disease Control and Prevention. Retrieved from https://www.cdc.gov/teenpregnancy/about/index.htm.

32 Haider, S., Stoffel, C., Donenberg, G., & Geller, S. (2013). Reproductive health disparities: A focus on family planning and prevention among minority women and adolescents. *Global Advances in Health and Medicine, 2*(5). Retrieved from https://www.ncbi.nlm.nih.gov/pmc/articles/PMC3833575/.

33 About teen pregnancy. (2016). Centers for Disease Control and Prevention. Retrieved from https://www.cdc.gov/teenpregnancy/about/index.htm.

34 National marriage and divorce rate trends. (2015). Centers for Disease Control and Prevention. Retrieved from https://www.cdc.gov/nchs/nvss/marriage_divorce_tables.htm.

35 Firestone, L. (2013). How your relationship style impacts your relationship. *Psychology Today*. Retrieved from https://www.psychologytoday.com/blog/compassion-matters/201307/how-your-attachment-style-impacts-your-relationship.

36 Infertility in America 2015. (2015). Reproductive Medicine Associates of New Jersey. Retrieved January 24, 2017, from http://www.rmanj.com/wp-content/uploads/2015/04/RMANJ_Infertility-In-America-SurveyReport-_04152015.pdf

37 Infertility FAQs. (2016). Centers for Disease Control and Prevention. Retrieved from https://www.cdc.gov/reproductivehealth/infertility/index.htm.

38 Cost of fertility treatment for women and men: National average, ranges—and our prices. (2016). Advanced Fertility Center of Chicago. Retrieved from http://www.advancedfertility.com/fertility-treatment-costs.htm.

39 Dominguez, L. J. & Barbagallo, M. (2016). Ageing and sexuality. *European Geriatric Medicine*, *7*(6). Retrieved from http://www.sciencedirect.com/science/article/pii/S1878764916300675.

40 General recommendation No. 27 on older women and protection of their human rights. (2010, October). United Nations Convention on the Elimination of All Forms of Discrimination against Women. Retrieved January 25, 2017, from http://www2.ohchr.org/english/bodies/cedaw/docs/CEDAW-C-2010–47-GC1.pdf

41 Aboderin, I. (2014). Sexual and reproductive health and rights of older men and women: Addressing a policy blind spot. *Reproductive Health Matters*. Retrieved from http://www.rhm-elsevier.com/article/S0968-8080(14)44814-6/pdf.

42 Weg, R. B., ed. (1983). *Sexuality in the later years: Roles and behavior*. New York: Academic Press. Retrieved from https://books.google.com/books?hl=en&lr=&id=Tn6LBQAAQBAJ&oi=fnd&pg=PP1&dq=elderly+sexuality&ots=CUu7TZYrbR&sig=rDc1UdPI9OkWlKCzcrf-1MMAjo4#v=onepage&q=elderly%20sexuality&f=false.

43 *Unintended pregnancy in the United States*. (2016). Guttmacher Institute. Retrieved from https://www.guttmacher.org/fact-sheet/unintended-pregnancy-united-states.

44 Kaplan, A. (2009). Adoption and mental illness. *Psychiatric Times*. Retrieved from http://www.psychiatrictimes.com/articles/adoption-and-mental-illness.

45 Brown, S. & Eisenberg, L., eds. (1995). *The best intentions: Unintended pregnancy and the well-being of children and families*. Washington, DC: National Academies Press. https://www.ncbi.nlm.nih.gov/books/NBK232137/.

46 Lesbian, gay, bisexual, and transgender health. (2014). Centers for Disease Control and Prevention. Retrieved from https://www.cdc.gov/lgbthealth/.

47 Effects of sexual assault and rape. (2015). Joyful Heart Foundation. Retrieved from http://www.joyfulheartfoundation.org/learn/sexual-assault-rape/effects-sexual-assault-and-rape.

48 Health consequences of sexual assault. (2006). Stop Violence Against Women. Retrieved from http://www.stopvaw.org/health_consequences_of_sexual_assault.

49 Sexual violence: Consequences. (2016). Centers for Disease Control and Prevention. Retrieved from https://www.cdc.gov/violenceprevention/sexualviolence/consequences.html.

50 Health consequences of sexual assault. (2006). Stop Violence Against Women. Retrieved from http://www.stopvaw.org/health_consequences_of_sexual_assault.

51 Effects of sexual violence. (2016). RAINN. Retrieved from https://www.rainn.org/effects-sexual-violence.

52 Effects of sexual assault and rape. (2015). Joyful Heart Foundation. Retrieved from http://www.joyfulheartfoundation.org/learn/sexual-assault-rape/effects-sexual-assault-and-rape.

53 Sexual violence: Consequences. (2016). Centers for Disease Control and Prevention. Retrieved from https://www.cdc.gov/violenceprevention/sexualviolence/consequences.html.

54 Fact sheets: sexually transmitted infections (STIs). (2016). World Health Organization. Retrieved from http://www.who.int/mediacentre/factsheets/fs110/en/

55 Sexually transmitted infections. (2017). Office on Women's Health, U.S. Department of Health and Human Services. Retrieved from https://www.womenshealth.gov/publications/our-publications/fact-sheet/sexually-transmitted-infections.html

56 Fact sheets: sexually transmitted infections (STIs). (2016). World Health Organization. Retrieved from http://www.who.int/mediacentre/factsheets/fs110/en/

57 Sexually transmitted infections. (2015). Office on Women's Health, U.S. Department of Health and Human Services. Retrieved from https://www.womenshealth.gov/publications/our-publications/fact-sheet/sexually-transmitted-infections.html.

58 Sexually transmitted infections among young Americans. (2013). Centers for Disease Control and Prevention. Retrieved from https://www.cdc.gov/std/products/youth-sti-infographic.pdf.

59 HPV and cancer. (2015). National Cancer Institute. Retrieved from https://www.cancer.gov/about-cancer/causes-prevention/risk/infectious-agents/hpv-fact-sheet.

60 Davis, M. (2013). Sexual health news: Sexually transmitted diseases. *Sexual Health*. Retrieved from https://www.sexualhealth.com/sexually-transmitted-diseases-may-affect-mental-health_n_1483/.

61 Corinna, H. (2011). Unpacking a bag full of STI stigma. *Rewire News*. Retrieved from https://rewire.news/article/2011/04/25/unpacking-full-stigma/.

62 Induced abortion worldwide. (2016, August 03). Guttmacher Institute. Retrieved January 25, 2017, from https://www.guttmacher.org/fact-sheet/induced-abortion-worldwide

63 Fact sheet: Preventing unsafe abortion. (2016). World Health Organization. Retrieved from http://www.who.int/mediacentre/factsheets/fs388/en/.

64 Brown, S. & Eisenberg, L., eds. (1995). *The best intentions: Unintended pregnancy and the well-being of children and families.* Washington, DC: National Academies Press. https://www.ncbi.nlm.nih.gov/books/NBK232137/.

65 McBride, A. (2006). Roe vs. Wade (1973). *PBS*. Retrieved from http://www.pbs.org/wnet/supreme-court/rights/landmark_roe.html.

66 Mission. (2014, May 21). Planned Parenthood. Retrieved January 25, 2017, from https://www.plannedparenthood.org/about-us/who-we-are/mission

67 *About Us*. (2017). Guttmacher Institute. Retrieved from https://www.guttmacher.org/about.

68 Wind, R. (2017). Contraception and fewer unintended pregnancies likely drove 2011–2014 abortion decline. *Guttmacher Institute*. Retrieved from https://www.guttmacher.org/news-release/2017/contraception-and-fewer-unintended-pregnancies-likely-drove-2011-2014-abortion.

69 About us. (2017). Center for Reproductive Rights. Retrieved from https://www.reproductiverights.org/about-us.

70 Fact sheets: HIV overview. (2017). AIDS Info. Retrieved from https://aidsinfo.nih.gov/education-materials/fact-sheets/19/46/the-stages-of-hiv-infection.

71 HIV transmission. (2016). Centers for Disease Control and Prevention. Retrieved from https://www.cdc.gov/hiv/basics/transmission.html.

72 Fact sheets: HIV overview. (2017). AIDS Info. Retrieved from https://aidsinfo.nih.gov/education-materials/fact-sheets/19/46/the-stages-of-hiv-infection.

73 Overview of HIV treatments. (2015). HIV.gov. Retrieved from https://www.aids.gov/hiv-aids-basics/just-diagnosed-with-hiv-aids/treatment-options/overview-of-hiv-treatments/.

Figure Sources

1 Figure 12.1: Copyright © Nick Youngson (CC BY-SA 3.0) at http://www.picserver.org/s/sexual-health.html.

2 Figure 12.2: Source: https://media.defense.gov/2012/Nov/07/2000098754/-1/-1/0/121107-F-JZ007-965.JPG.

3 Figure 12.3: Source: https://www.cdc.gov/teenpregnancy/about/index.htm.

4 Figure 12.4: Source: https://upload.wikimedia.org/wikipedia/commons/7/79/Infertility_causes.png.

5 Figure 12.5: Source: https://www.cdc.gov/mmwr/preview/mmwrhtml/ss6410a1.htm.

CPSIA information can be obtained
at www.ICGtesting.com
Printed in the USA
LVHW020714060121
675689LV00002B/13